Lippincott's
QUICK REFERENCE
BOOK FOR NURSES

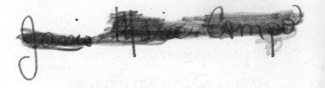

Lippincott's

QUICK REFERENCE

AUTHOR PANEL

BETH L. CAMERON, R.N., M.A.

Associate in Nursing

MARCIA MARY GATCHELL, B.S.

Instructor in Nutrition

ELIZABETH S. GILL, R.N., M.A.

Director of Nursing and Professor of Nursing

LOUISA M. KENT, R.N., M.A.

Associate in Nursing

HELEN F. PETTIT, R.N., M.A.

Professor of Nursing

DOROTHY E. REILLY, R.N., M.S.

Associate Professor of Nursing

*Department of Nursing, Faculty of Medicine,
Columbia University; Presbyterian Hospital
School of Nursing, New York*

AND

LOUISE J. SCHLICHTING, R.N., M.A.

Instructor, School of Nursing

*Orange Memorial Hospital unit of
The Hospital Center at Orange
Orange, New Jersey*

J. B. LIPPINCOTT COMPANY

BOOK for NURSES

EIGHTH EDITION

Prepared under the direction of
ELEANOR LEE, R.N., A.B.

HELEN YOUNG, R.N.

> *Late Director of Nursing*
> *The Presbyterian Hospital in the City of New York*

ELEANOR LEE, R.N., A.B.

> *Professor Emeritus and formerly Professor of*
> *Nursing and Associate Dean (Nursing), Faculty*
> *of Medicine, Columbia University; and Director of*
> *Nursing of The Presbyterian Hospital in the City*
> *of New York*

PHILADELPHIA · TORONTO

Preface to the Eighth Edition

Once again a thorough revision of this book, with its wealth of new material, has necessitated a complete re-setting of its pages. New type has been used advantageously to facilitate immediate assimilation of information on the part of the reader.

A new section, *Nursing of Children,* has been added. It follows *Maternity Nursing,* thus providing the continuity of care which is the philosophical basis of current maternal-child health concepts. Included in this new section are principles of growth and development of the child from infancy through school age. Special nursing needs and considerations are emphasized in the pediatric medical-surgical content.

Also new in this edition is a special index of emergency conditions, located in the end papers for instant availability.

Every section has been expanded and brought up-to-date. New procedures, treatments and approaches to nursing care have been incorporated in the *Nursing Technics* and *Medical and Surgical* sections. Important new additions to the latter include tables of laboratory tests and new clinical entities. *Normal and Therapeutic Diets* (formerly titled *Diet Therapy*) has been reorganized for easier reference, and the material dealing with infant diets has been completely revised.

The *Pharmacology* section is more comprehensive than ever. Many new approved drugs have been added, and those divisions covering steroids and anti-infectives have been enlarged. This entire section has been rearranged to permit revision of it at frequent intervals.

This book continues its tradition of presenting a maximum of pertinent and current nursing information in a volume of minimum bulk, and of maintaining a high degree of convenience in locating facts despite its ever-growing content.

The authors wish to express their thanks to the fol-

PREFACE TO THE EIGHTH EDITION

lowing members of the staff of the Faculty of Medicine of Columbia University for their invaluable assistance in the preparation of this edition: Janet Alley, Jane Andrews, Dr. Daniel W. Benninghoff, Hester A. Brown, Carolyn Dawson, Dolores Farrell, Glenda L. Fregia, Dr. John G. Gorman, Dr. Calderon Howe, Catherine Lang, Edith Luik, Dr. John T. McCarthy, Jane McConville, Eunice K. Macdonald, E. Marion Mike, Priscilla C. Parke, Dr. Thomas V. Santulli and Dr. Henry O. Wheeler. Thanks are due also to Dr. Joseph F. Lutz, of the Hospital Center at Orange, New Jersey, for his help and advice.

Contents

CONTENTS

Section I
Nursing Technics

Many important factors in the nursing care of the patient are considered by the nurse as she carries out specific technics. Details of the less tangible factors, essential to the patient's comfort and well-being, of necessity must be reduced to a minimum in any quick reference text.

Although particular equipment and procedures are suggested in the following pages, it is important to adapt them to meet the needs of particular patients. Having "a way of doing things" contributes to the development of skill, but this must be flexible enough to meet varying requirements in individual situations.

It must be borne in mind that the efficacy of any procedure is enhanced if the patient understands what is to be done and is able to co-operate in carrying it out. Simple, clear explanations offered by the nurse in obtaining this co-operation are well rewarded by the patient's reaction to her as well as to the treatment.

Since nursing care is given in a wide variety of situations, the amount that is recorded is left to a large extent to the discretion of the nurse. It is assumed that when the care of the patient is shared by several people this aspect of his care will receive particularly careful consideration.

ARTIFICIAL RESPIRATION

Mouth-to-Mouth (Mouth-to-Nose) Method of Artificial Respiration

If there is foreign matter visible in the mouth, wipe it out quickly with your fingers or a cloth wrapped around your fingers.

Tilt the head back so that the chin is pointing upward (Fig. 1, Part 1). Pull or push the jaw into a jutting-out position (Fig. 1, Parts 2 & 3).

ARTIFICIAL RESPIRATION
MOUTH-TO-MOUTH (MOUTH-TO-NOSE) METHOD

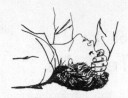

(1) If there is foreign matter visible in the mouth, wipe it out quickly with your fingers or a cloth wrapped around your fingers.

Tilt the head back so the chin is pointing upward.

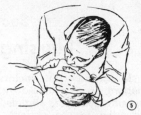

(2) ⬆ Pull or push ⬇ the jaw into a jutting-out position.

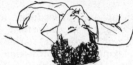

(3)

(4) Open your mouth wide and place it tightly over victim's mouth. At same time pinch victim's nostrils shut.

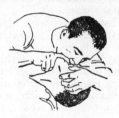

(5) Or close the nostrils with your cheek.

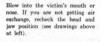

(6) Or close the victim's mouth and place your mouth over the nose.

Blow into the victim's mouth or nose. If you are not getting air exchange, recheck the head and jaw position (see drawings above at left).

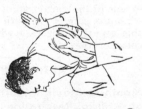

(7) If you still do not get air exchange, quickly turn the victim on his side and administer several sharp blows between the shoulder blades in the hope of dislodging foreign matter.

Resume breathing procedure.

The illustrations on pp. 2 to 11 are from the American National Red Cross.

FIGURE 1

These maneuvers should relieve obstruction of the airway by moving the base of the tongue away from the back of the throat.

Open your mouth wide and place it tightly over the victim's mouth. At the same time pinch the victim's nostrils shut (Fig. 1, Part 4) or close the nostrils with your cheek (Fig. 1, Part 5). Or close the victim's mouth and place your mouth over the nose (Fig. 1, Part 6). Blow into the victim's mouth or nose. (Air may be blown through the victim's teeth, even though they may be clenched.)

The first blowing efforts should determine whether or not obstruction exists.

Remove your mouth, turn your head to the side, and listen for the return rush of air that indicates air exchange. Repeat the blowing effort.

For an adult, blow vigorously at the rate of about 12 breaths per minute. For a child, take relatively shallow breaths appropriate for the child's size, at the rate of about 20 per minute.

If you are not getting air exchange, recheck the head and jaw position (Fig. 1, Parts 6 & 7). If you still do not get air exchange, quickly turn the victim on his side and administer several sharp blows between the shoulder blades in the hope of dislodging foreign matter (Fig. 1, Part 7).

Again sweep your fingers through the victim's mouth and remove foreign matter.

Those who do not wish to come in contact with the person may hold a cloth over the victim's mouth or nose and breathe through it. The cloth does not greatly affect the exchange of air.

Mouth-to-Mouth Technic for Infants and Small Children

If foreign matter is visible in the mouth, clean it out quickly as described previously.

Place the child on his back and use the fingers of both hands to lift the lower jaw from beneath and behind, so that it juts out.

Place your mouth over the child's mouth AND nose, making a relatively leakproof seal, and breathe into the child, using shallow puffs of air. The breathing rate should be about 20 per minute.

If you meet resistance in your blowing efforts, recheck the position of the jaw. If the air passages are still blocked, the child should be suspended momentarily by the ankles or inverted over one arm and given two or three sharp pats between the shoulder blades, in the hope of dislodging obstructing matter.

Manual Methods of Artificial Respiration

Rescuers who cannot, or will not, use mouth-to-mouth or mouth-to-nose technics, should use a manual method. The rescuer should not be limited to the use of a single manual method for all cases, since the nature of the injury in any given case may prevent the use of one method, while favoring another.

It has already been pointed out that the base of the tongue tends to press against and block the air passage when a person is unconscious and not breathing. *This action of the tongue can occur whether the victim is in a face-down or face-up position.*

The Chest Pressure-Arm Lift (Silvester) Method

If there is foreign matter visible in the mouth, wipe it out quickly with your fingers or a cloth wrapped around your fingers.

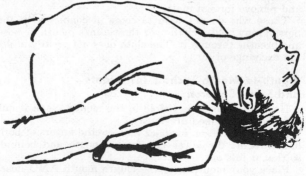

FIGURE 2

Place the victim in a face-up position and put something under his shoulders to raise them and allow the head to drop backward (Fig. 2).

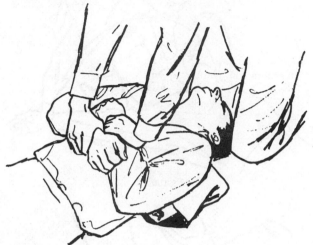

FIGURE 3

Kneel at the victim's head, grasp his arms at the wrists, cross them, and press them over the lower chest (Fig. 3). This should cause air to flow out.

Immediately release this pressure and pull the arms outward and upward over his head and backward as far as possible (Fig. 4). This should cause air to rush in.

Repeat this cycle about 12 times per minute, checking the mouth frequently for obstructions.

When the victim is in a face-up position, there is always danger of aspiration of vomitus, blood, or blood clots. This hazard can be reduced by keeping the head extended and turned to one side. If possible, the head should be a little lower than the trunk. If a second rescuer is available, have him hold the victim's head so that the jaw is jutting out (Fig. 5). The helper should

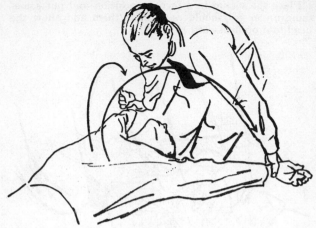

FIGURE 4

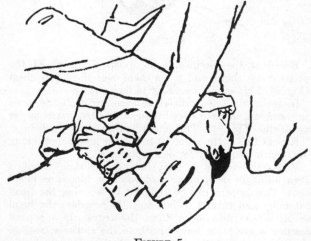

FIGURE 5

be alert to detect the presence of any stomach contents in the mouth and keep the mouth as clean as possible at all times.

The Back Pressure-Arm Lift (Holger-Nielsen) Method

If there is foreign matter visible in the mouth, wipe it out quickly with your fingers or a cloth wrapped around your fingers.

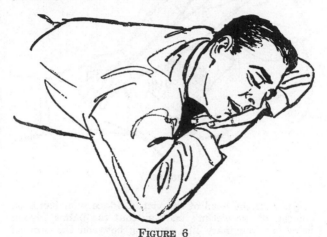

FIGURE 6

Place the victim face-down, bend his elbows and place his hands one upon the other, turn his head slightly to one side and extend it as far as possible, making sure that the chin is jutting out (Fig. 6).

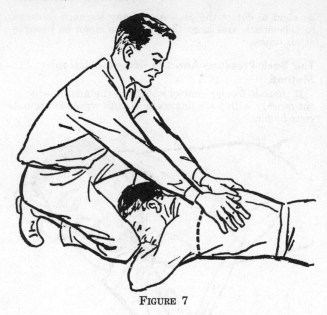

FIGURE 7

Kneel at the head of the victim. Place your hands on the flat of the victim's back so that the palms lie just below an imaginary line running between the armpits (Fig. 7).

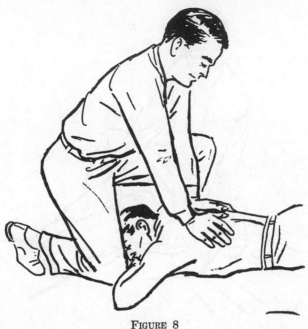

FIGURE 8

Rock forward until the arms are approximately vertical and allow the weight of the upper part of your body to exert steady, even pressure downward upon the hands (Fig. 8).

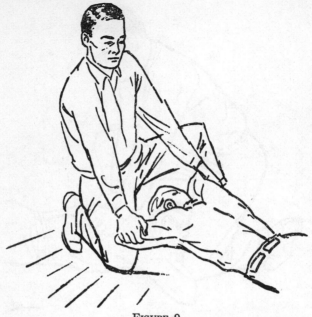

FIGURE 9

Immediately draw his arms upward and toward you, applying enough lift to feel resistance and tension at his shoulders (Fig. 9). Then lower the arms to the ground. Repeat this cycle about 12 times per minute, checking the mouth frequently for obstruction.

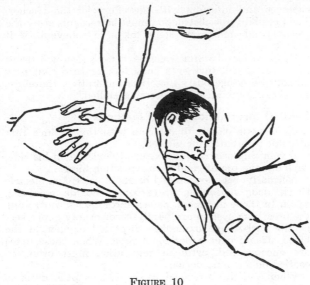

FIGURE 10

If a second rescuer is available, have him hold the victim's head so that the jaw continues to jut out (Fig. 10). The helper should be alert to detect any stomach contents in the mouth and should keep the mouth as clean as possible at all times.

Artificial Respiration for Water Cases

Individuals who die as a result of a water accident usually die from the lack of air, and not because of water in the lungs or the stomach.

A drowning victim may be either active or passive. Unless unconscious, the drowning victim usually struggles to remain on the surface or to regain the surface, in order to secure air. These efforts are energy-consuming and may result in the victim swallowing varying quantities of water. This water, along with food remaining in the stomach, could, if regurgitated, obstruct the air

11

passages and interfere with the efforts of the rescuer. The possibility of obstruction must be recognized by the rescuer and immediate steps taken to relieve it if it occurs.

Evaporation of water from the victim's skin will result in lowering still further a body temperature that may already be dangerously low. It is imperative, therefore, to keep the victim from becoming chilled.

Related Information for All Methods

Time your efforts to coincide with the victim's first attempt to breathe for himself.

If vomiting occurs, quickly turn the victim on his side, wipe out the mouth, and then reposition him.

Normally, recovery should be rapid, except in electric shock, drug poisoning, or carbon monoxide poisoning cases. In these instances, nerves and muscles controlling the breathing system are paralyzed or deeply depressed, or the carbon monoxide has displaced oxygen in the blood stream over a period of time. When these cases are encountered, artificial respiration must often be carried on for long periods.

When a victim is revived, he should be kept as quiet as possible until he is breathing regularly. He should be kept covered and otherwise treated for shock until suitable transportation is available, if he must be moved.

Artificial respiration should be continued until the victim begins to breathe for himself, or until a physician pronounces the victim dead, or until the person appears to be dead beyond any doubt.

A doctor's care is necessary during the recovery period, as respiratory and other disturbances may develop as an aftermath.

BANDAGES

PRINCIPLES OF APPLYING BANDAGES

Position of Patient

Comfortable for the patient, convenient for the nurse.

Position of Part to Be Bandaged

As it is to remain after the bandage is applied, usually in a position of function, well supported, elevated if necessary.

Position of Nurse

Directly in front of patient, or facing part to be bandaged.

Important Points

Skin surfaces should be separated. Pad with absorbent cotton or separate with sterile dressing.

Place outer surface of initial extremity of the bandage against part to be bandaged.

Anchor bandage by at least two circular turns around part at its smallest diameter.

Bandage to the right.

Exert even pressure.

Avoid useless turns.

When possible, leave fingers and toes exposed for observation of circulatory changes.

Signs of undue pressure are:

Pallor	Tingling
Coldness	Numbness
Blueness	Swelling

If this condition is not relieved, damage to the part may occur.

After applying bandage, secure terminal extremity by pinning with safety pins, tying or strapping with adhesive.

It is best not to pin or tie in the following places:

Over injured part or inflamed surface

Over bony prominence

Inner surface of limb

Where patient may lie on it

Where it may cause discomfort

NURSING TECHNICS

Remove bandages by gathering folds in a loose mass, passing mass from one hand to the other, as the bandage is unwound. Cut with bandage scissors if the bandage is soiled, in an emergency or to avoid pain.

Materials Used

Gauze, muslin, crinoline, flannel, Canton flannel, plaster of Paris, rubber, rubber and wool, rubber and silk.

(*See also* Local Application of Drugs.)

Size

Variations in width and length of the roller bandage:

	WIDTH	LENGTH
Finger	¾-1 in.	1-3 yds.
Hand	1½-2½ in.	3 yds.
Arm	2 -2½ in.	6 yds.
Head	2 -2½ in.	6 yds.
Eye	2 in.	3 yds.
Foot	1½-3 in.	3 yds.
Leg	2½-3 in.	9 yds.
Body	3 -6 in.	10 yds.

ROLLER BANDAGES

The following 5 types of turns are used in applying a roller bandage: circular, spiral, spiral reverse, figure-of-8, recurrent.

Circular

Several turns around a part, each turn exactly covering the preceding one.

Examples: Wrist, neck, forehead

Spiral

Anchor with a circular turn.

Carry bandage slightly upward and around the part, each turn paralleling the preceding one, which it overlaps from one half to one third.

Examples: arm, fingers, trunk

Spiral Reverse

Anchor with 2 circular turns.

Make 1 spiral turn.

Place thumb of left hand on the upper edge of the last turn and hold firmly to prevent loosening bandage where reverse is to be made.

Unwind the roll which is in the right hand about 6 in.

Pronate the right hand so bandage is directed downward instead of upward (reverse).

Carry the roll around the limb firmly.

Continue these turns, making sure that the reverses are uniform and in line, and that each turn is evenly spaced.

USES

To retain dressings or splints.

To apply pressure and afford support. Suitable for a tapering part, such as a forearm or leg.

Figure-of-8

This consists of oblique turns that alternately ascend and descend after encircling the part. Each turn crosses the preceding one in front, overlapping it one half or two thirds, making a figure-of-8.

USES

To retain dressings in place

To apply pressure and afford support

To immobilize joints

It may be used in combination with the spiral reverse.

Recurrent

Fix or anchor the bandage by circular turns.

Reverse and pass backward and forward over the part covered, applying the first turn over the center and each succeeding turn alternating on each side.

Complete the bandage by applying 2 or 3 circular turns over the first or fixation turns.

USES. To hold dressing on the head, the extremities or an amputation stump.

USES OF ROLLER BANDAGES

The following examples of bandaging include one or more of the basic turns.

NURSING TECHNICS

Hand

GAUNTLET. *Bandage 8 yds. × 1 in.*

1. Anchor the bandage by 2 circular turns around the wrist.

2. Carry the bandage over the back of the hand and around the base of the thumb (if left hand) or little finger (if right hand).

3. Continue up thumb or finger in spiral turns.

4. Cover the tip with recurrent turns.

5. Descend with spiral turns.

6. Carry bandage over the back of the hand and encircle the wrist.

7. Repeat the above for each finger in turn.

8. Anchor the bandage by 2 circular turns around the wrist. Secure.

NOTE: This technic may be modified to include only the affected finger or fingers.

MITTEN. *Bandage 8 yds. × 2 in.*

1. Separate the fingers with compresses or pieces of muslin.

2. If the thumb is to be bandaged, do so now, using a spiral or spica of the thumb.

3. Anchor the bandage by 2 circular turns around the wrist.

4. Cover the hand by recurrent turns over the tips of the fingers (fan shape).

5. Secure recurrent turns by figure-of-8 turns around the hand.

6. Anchor the bandage by 2 circular turns about the wrist. Secure.

Leg

SPIRAL REVERSE. *Bandage 8 yds. × 2½ or 3 in.*

1. Anchor the bandage obliquely across the right ankle joint; carry the bandage diagonally down over the dorsum of the foot to ball of great toe on the right foot—base of little toe on left foot—under the foot and around the base of the small toe.

2. Make a circular turn and then 1 or 2 spirals until the instep is reached, when *reverses* are used up to the point of the instep.

3. Carry the next turn up around the ankle (low

16

down), then over the instep and around the foot, up the outside of the foot and around the angle (*figure-of-8 turn*), covering one half of the previous turn.

4. Carry the bandage up the leg with spiral and, as needed, *spiral reverse turns* until the upper edge of the last turn reaches the lower border of the patella (with leg extended).

5. Pass the next turn directly over the patella, a succeeding turn over the lower half of the patella and another turn over the upper half of the patella.

6. Carry the bandage up the thigh with spiral reverse turns. Complete bandage with 2 circular turns. Secure.

NOTE: This bandage is difficult to retain in place if the leg is dependent or in use. For ambulatory patients the figure-of-8 is preferred.

FIGURE-OF-8. *Bandage 8 yds. × 2½ or 3 in.*

1. The bandage is similar to the spiral reverse of the lower extremity until, on ascending the calf, reverses are needed.

2. Incline the bandage rapidly upward by spiral or oblique turns. Make a turn around the leg and return in downward direction in front of the leg across the first turn just outside the crest of the tibia.

3. Successive turns similar to the *figure-of-8* are made overlapping one half of each previous turn as the bandage ascends the leg. It will be noted that there is a gap posteriorly between the 2 loops of the 8 and that the lower edge of the upper loop does not lie flat.

4. Complete the bandage by 2 circular turns. Secure.

SPIRAL. *Elastic Bandage 2 to 3 in. Wide*

1. Anchor bandage by 2 circular turns around the instep.

2. Make a single figure-of-8 around the ankle.

NOTE: Ascertain whether or not the physician wants the heel to be covered. If so, make initial figure-of-8 turn over the heel and continue turns, alternating above and below initial turn (overlapping each by ½ to ⅓) until heel is covered.

3. Carry bandage by spiral turns, maintaining slight *even* pressure, up to the knee.

4. Anchor with 2 circular turns. Secure.

NURSING TECHNICS

SUBSTITUTES FOR BANDAGING

Patches

Eye and small dressings on the scalp frequently are secured with plastic tape or adhesive instead of roller bandage, thus replacing the monocle or similar elaborate bandages.

EYE

1. Cut plastic tape or adhesive in lengths slightly longer than the dressing.

2. Apply strips over the dressing overlapping each by one half to one third until the dressing is sealed.

NOTE: Slight pressure should be used to keep the eye closed.

SCALP. Follow steps above or

1. Cut a circular piece of adhesive slightly larger than the dressing to be covered.

2. Make a slit along the radius at one point.

3. Cover the dressing overlapping the cut edges of the adhesive (slit) to make patch fit.

Stockinette

Tubular bandage of varying weights of material and in varying widths is available for securing many dressings. It is supplied by the roll, and directions for its use are prepared by the manufacturer. It is useful particularly in covering the head (caps may be made from it quite easily), for extensive coverage of an extremity, particularly if the patient is apt to scratch the area, and for simple bandaging of a finger.

Nonstick—follow manufacturer's directions

Pressure—follow manufacturer's directions

BATHS

GENERAL

Equipment

Patient's face towel, bath towel, washcloth

Patient's gown

Necessary bed linen (if bed is to be made after the bath)

18

Bath tub

Alcohol 25 per cent or commercial skin lotions; mineral oils as indicated

Powder

Orangewood stick, scissors, nail brush s.o.s.

Bath blanket ⎱
Dish with soap ⎰ should be in patient's unit

Procedure

1. Secure privacy for the patient.
2. Replace top bed covers by a bath blanket.
3. Remove the patient's gown.
4. Bathing the patient:

Face. Use firm motion down sides of face and in crevices. Wash from the inner angle of the eye to the outer. Do not neglect the ears.

Shoulders, Chest and Arms. Give special attention to the axillae. Powder.

Abdomen. Cleanse the umbilicus. Powder.

Back. Protect the bed with a towel.

Give light massage, using appropriate solution.

Legs and Feet. Soak the feet in the tub. Cut the nails. Powder.

Genitalia. Cleanse gently and thoroughly.

5. Put on the nightgown. Draw up the bed covers or make the bed. See that the patient is comfortable.
6. Replace equipment within the unit. Make provision for wet or damp articles to dry.
7. Wash and rinse the tub thoroughly. Sterilize s.o.s. (*See* Equipment, Cleaning and Sterilization.)

ALKALINE BATH*

Purpose

To relieve itching associated with certain skin conditions (urticaria, eczema, jaundice, etc.).

Composition of Bath

Sodium bicarbonate and carbonate of soda are the

---

* If there is residual ointment on the skin, great care should be taken in assisting the patient in and out of the tub in order to avoid an accident.

NURSING TECHNICS

two substances commonly used for the alkaline bath. The proportions of each per gallon of water are:

8 oz. of bicarbonate of soda (or 2 oz. per quart for local application)

2 oz. of carbonate of soda (or ½ oz. per quart for local application)

Temperature
92° to 98° F.

Duration
10 to 20 minutes

Procedure
Add measured amount of soda to half-filled tub and assist patient to bathe. Be certain that all skin areas are moistened thoroughly with the solution.

BRAN BATH

Purpose
To relieve skin irritations of various kinds.

Procedure
1. Place 2 cups of bran in a loose muslin bag.
2. Run hot water on the bag and squeeze it into the tub half filled with water.
3. Follow the procedure as outlined for Oatmeal Bath observing precautions regarding chilling, cleanliness, etc.

OATMEAL BATH

Purpose
To soothe and to allay itching in various skin diseases

Composition of the Bath
3 cups of cooked oatmeal in cheesecloth bag
1 cup of sodium bicarbonate
NOTE: Commercial preparations are available.

Temperature
90° to 100° F.

Duration

10 to 15 minutes

Procedure

1. Fill the tub halfway (approximately 30 gallons).
2. Soak the oatmeal bag in the tub until the water becomes milky.
3. While the patient is in the bath, pat his skin gently with the oatmeal bag.
4. When he is removed from the tub again rub the bag gently over his skin.
5. Allow the oatmeal solution to dry on the surface of the body. (Do not rub it off with a towel.)

Important Points

1. Avoid allowing the patient to become chilled.
2. Maintain strict cleanliness in handling the patient in order to avoid infection.

POTASSIUM PERMANGANATE BATH

Procedure

1. Dissolve the prescribed amount of potassium permanganate crystals in a small amount of very hot water. Amount should be measured carefully. All crystals *must* be dissolved.
2. Add the dissolved crystals to the tub of water. (1 level tbsp., 15 Gm., of these crystals, when added to an average size bathtub of 40 to 50 gallons, will make a 1:10,000 solution.)

To Clean the Bathtub After Use

Scrub as usual with soap, and flush with large quantities of hot water. After a potassium permanganate bath, which leaves a stain, fill the tub with clean water containing 30 Gm. of oxalic acid crystals. Allow to stand 30 minutes, drain and flush with hot water.

STARCH BATH

Procedure

1. Mix 2 cups (1 lb.) of cornstarch or laundry starch with 1 qt. of hot water. Remove lumps.

2. Add starch to tub of water and stir well.

3. Permit starch water to dry on patient's skin by patting him dry.

SITZ BATH

Definition

A bath given to apply heat to the pelvic region.

Equipment

IN BATHROOM
   Large tub
   Bath towel
   Safety pin—large
   Straight chair
   Footstool or box, s.o.s.
ADDITIONAL EQUIPMENT
   Bath towel }
   Bath blanket } from patient's unit
   Clothes for the patient
   Wheelchair

Procedure

1. See that the bathroom is warm.

2. Draw half a tub of water at about 110° F.

3. Assist the patient into the tub. See that the water covers the pelvic region.

4. Be sure that the patient is warm enough. Use the bath blankets and towels, s.o.s.

5. If the doctor wishes the patient's feet out of the water elevate them on the stool or box.

6. Add hot water to bring the temperature of the tub to between 115° to 118° F. in accordance with the patient's tolerance.

7. The patient should stay in the tub, with the temperature of the water maintained, for about 20 minutes.

8. Dress the patient warmly. Help her back to bed.

9. Record time and duration of the treatment and its effect on the patient's symptoms.

SPONGE BATH

Purpose

To relieve restlessness and general discomfort associated with fever and to reduce body temperature temporarily.

Equipment

TRAY
  2 towels—tray covers
  3 bath towels
  1 protecting sheet—2 *additional rubbers* for tepid sponge
  3 face cloths
  1 half sheet—when bath blanket is not used over patient
  1 face basin with ordered solution
  Small bowl for ice, s.o.s.

ADDITIONAL EQUIPMENT
  Hot-water bag with cover
  Ice bag with cover
  Bath blanket—in patient's unit

Procedure

1. Prepare solution in face basin according to order.
    ALCOHOL SPONGE. Alcohol 50% and ice, at a temperature of 65° to 75° F.
    COOL SPONGE. Water 85° to 95° F.; ice, s.o.s.
    TEPID SPONGE. Water 95° to 100° F.
2. Fill and cover ice bag and hot-water bag.
3. Arrange equipment at bedside. Uncover tray.
4. See that the surroundings are as conducive to sleep as possible.
5. Fan down top covers with the bath blanket.
6. Remove patient's gown.
7. Place a bath towel (with rubber, s.o.s.) under patient's arms.
8. Place a bath towel and protecting rubber under both legs.
9. When patient is not covered with the bath blanket during the treatment place a half sheet over the groin and fanfold the bath blanket to the bottom of the bed.

10. With a washcloth apply solution and follow with friction in this order:

One side of chest and arms—4 minutes.

Thigh and leg on same side—4 minutes.

Other side of chest and other arm—4 minutes.

Other thigh and leg—4 minutes.

Back—4 minutes.

NOTE: Alternate washcloths so that the applied solution is as cool as possible.

11. Observe patient throughout treatment. Discontinue immediately if any adverse signs are noted.

12. Remove protecting towels, replace bath blanket, remove half sheet.

13. Keep skin surfaces separated—replace top covers.

14. See that the patient is comfortable. Offer him some warm fluids as indicated.

15. Replace gown.

16. Remove bath blanket, hot-water bag and icecap as indicated. (Care for these in the usual manner.)

17. Hang washcloths and towels to dry if procedure is likely to be repeated—otherwise discard in laundry.

18. Reset tray, s.o.s.

19. Take patient's temperature 1 hour after treatment —if patient is awake.

20. Record time; patient's reaction during and after treatment; patient's temperature after 1 hour—if taken.

If the child's condition permits, the use of the bath tub may be the most effective method to reduce his fever.

Procedure

1. Place the child in a bath tub of tepid water (temperature approximately 100° and gradually reduce temperature of water to approximately 80° or the tolerance of the patient.

2. After 20 minutes remove the child from the tub and dry, creating friction with the towel to stimulate the flow of blood to the cooled skin surface and cause vasodilation.

3. Replace the gown and cover lightly allowing for air circulation.

4. Check the temperature 30 minutes following the treatment.

BEDMAKING

GENERAL

Equipment

Spread, 3 sheets, 2 pillowcases, 2 blankets

Rubber sheet or other water-repellent sheeting or mattress cover

Procedure

1. Turn the mattress.

2. Spread the first sheet over the mattress and, at the foot, place the hem at the edge of the mattress next to the springs. Turn the remainder of the sheet under the mattress at the head of the bed. Miter the upper corner and tuck the sheet in along the side of the bed.

3. Put the water-repellent material in place.

4. Spread the draw sheet crosswise over the mattress. Turn the upper salvage edge under 2 in. and tuck this sheet in along the side.

5. Go to the other side of the bed and fold back draw sheet and bed protection. Miter upper corner of lower sheet. Tuck it in tightly and smoothly.

6. Straighten protecting sheet and secure if possible.

7. Spread the draw sheet out, draw it tight and tuck it well in under the mattress. Pull first at the center, then at the foot and then at the head.

8. Spread the top sheet (right side down) over the bed, turn the upper hem over on itself and place it at the upper edge of the mattress. Gather the sheet at the foot and tuck it under the mattress.

9. Spread the blankets on separately, bringing the upper edges 9 in. from the edge of the mattress. Gather them together at the foot and tuck them under the mattress. Miter both corners loosely and tuck them in.

10. Stretch the spread out evenly to the top of the mattress, tuck it in at the foot, miter the corners and leave the sides hanging.

11. Shake the pillows, put them well into the corners of the cases, fold any surplus out of the way and flatten the pillows. Place them one on top of the other with the open ends away from the door of the ward or room.

NURSING TECHNICS

NOTE: To arrange top covers, if bed is to be opened, turn the spread under the blankets at the head of the bed and fold the top sheet over it. Fan the covers down once.

STRIPPING A BED

Procedure

1. Pull the over-the-bed table out far enough to walk around the foot of the bed.
2. Put the bedside table and chair behind the bed.
3. Remove both pillows at one time to the patient's chair. Take off pillow cases if they are not to be used again and discard in the hamper.
4. Loosen the bedding all around the bed. Put the left hand under the mattress, and draw out the sheets with the right hand.
5. If the spread is to be used again, fold it neatly and hang it on the back of the chair.
6. Take off the top blanket by slipping the left hand under the blanket and picking it up in the center with the right hand and placing it over the back of the chair. Remove the second blanket and top sheet in the same way.
7. Discard the draw sheet in the hamper, hang the protecting sheet over the head of the bed and put the bottom sheet in the hamper.
8. Turn the mattress from top to bottom.

TURNING A MATTRESS WITH PATIENT IN BED

Method I

Equipment

3 pillows, small pillow, bandage

Procedure

1. Explain to the patient what you are going to do.
2. Lower the Gatch and substitute one small pillow for the large pillows.
3. Remove the spread and the upper blanket. Fold the

sides of the upper sheet and the remaining blanket back over the patient; turn the bottom part of this fold under the legs.

4. Loosen the lower sheets and bring the upper edge of the under sheet over the pillow around the patient's head and its corners down with the sides. This will prevent the pillow from falling out when the patient is lifted.

5. Roll the sides of the lower sheets as tightly as possible until the rolls touch the patient on each side. Tie the bottom of the rolls around the patient's ankles.

6. Have an assistant and lift the patient to the edge of the mattress.

7. Move the mattress until one half of the springs show, cover the springs with the 3 pillows.

8. Lift the patient on to the pillows and have the assistant turn the mattress head to foot.

9. Reverse the procedure. Lift the patient on to the mattress, remove the pillows, push the mattress in place and lift the patient to the middle of the bed.

10. Arrange the bed and make the patient comfortable.

METHOD II

1. Have 4 assistants.

2. Arrange the patient as above.

3. Have 2 persons on each side of the bed. Lift the patient a few inches from the mattress. The fifth person pulls the mattress out at the foot of the bed, turns it and slips it in place again.

4. The patient is lowered to the center of the mattress, the bedclothes arranged, and the patient made comfortable.

CHANGING A MATTRESS WITH PATIENT IN BED

Equipment
Mattress, small pillow

Procedure
1. *See* Turning a Mattress *steps 1 to 6.* Move the mattress until one half of the springs are exposed.

NURSING TECHNICS

2. Place the fresh mattress on the exposed springs. Curve the mattress up so the patient can be lifted.

3. Lift the patient to the new mattress and slip the used mattress out of the way.

4. Draw the new mattress into place.

5. Move the patient to the middle of the bed and arrange the bed.

FRACTURE BED

Making a Balkan Frame Fracture Bed

1. With a fracture of the upper extremity, no modification of the bed is necessary.

2. With fractures of the lower extremities, the under part of the bed is made as usual.

3. Two sets of bedclothes are used, and they are applied in cross sections. The upper section covers the patient from above the shoulders to the thighs or as far as the ropes and pulleys of the suspended limb will permit. The lower section starts where the upper section leaves off, covers the uninjured leg and reaches across to the opposite side of the bed under the suspended leg and is tucked in under the mattress.

4. Each article is folded in two, hem to hem, and the folded edges of the upper and lower sections are pinned together.

NOTE: Sheets, spreads and blankets can be made especially for these beds. Take measurements of these articles on a bed made as above. From the lower hem of a sheet draw a line up to half the length of the sheet. At this point draw a circle about the diameter of an average thigh. Cut along these lines. Bind the circle and the two straight edges with tape and attach tapes to the straight edges to tie the lower parts together.

OCCUPIED BED

Equipment

Sheet and pillowcase

Procedure

1. Arrange the unit to facilitate making the bed.

2. Remove the spread, fold it and hang it on the back of the chair.

3. Loosen the blanket and the top sheet. Remove one of the blankets.

4. Take out pillows. Place them on a chair.

5. Spread the clean sheet over the remaining blanket.

6. Draw out the blanket and the sheet, separate them, put the sheet on the chair and the blanket over the patient again.

7. Flex the patient's knees, help him to move to the edge of the bed and to turn on his side.

8. Fold the covers up over the patient so that the sheets covering the mattress are exposed.

9. Loosen the draw sheet and fold it closely to the center of the bed and as far under the patient as possible.

10. Tighten the bottom sheet and rearrange the protecting sheet.

11. Use the discarded top sheet as the fresh draw sheet. Fold or gather one half of it and tuck it well under the patient's back. Spread the remainder out smoothly and tuck it under the mattress.

12. Fold back the covers and assist the patient to turn to the opposite side. Fold the covers up over the patient as before.

13. Loosen the draw sheet, draw it from under the patient and remove it by rolling it toward the foot of the bed.

14. Bring the fresh draw sheet through and tuck it in tightly under the mattress.

15. Allow the patient to turn on his back again, replace the pillows and finish the bed.

Important Points

Disturb the patient as little as possible.

Keep the patient warm.

Do not expose the patient.

OPERATIVE BED

Equipment

An open bed or the bedding used to make an open bed.

1 small pillow

NURSING TECHNICS

Pillow cases:
    Waterproof—1 large; 1 small
    Linen—1 small
1 half sheet
1 protecting sheet, 18 × 36 in. (elastic or water-repellent)
Extra half sheet and protecting sheets when needed for further protection of the bed
1 hand towel
2 emesis basins, medium size
2 tongue depressors bandaged together with **gauze** (eliminate for reacted patient)
q.s. mouth wipes
Paper bag
Scotch tape
Fluid slip
Vital signs sheet
NOTE: Shock blocks, stethoscope, sphygmomanometer and intravenous pole to be available in central location in the ward.

Procedure

1. Clear the tops of the over-the-bed table and the bedside stand.

2. Put bedside table and chair behind bed, or to one side, to allow room for stretcher.

3. Strip the bed and turn the mattress.

4. Make the bottom of the bed in the usual manner.

5. Place small protecting sheet at top of mattress.

6. Unfold half sheet until it is in half lengthwise. Place across small protecting sheet with selvage edges toward head of the bed. Tuck the excess sheet at the head of the bed just under the small protecting sheet. Draw the ends of the half sheet tightly under the mattress.

7. When additional protection of the bed is necessary, it should be added where needed.

8. Place top sheet, bed blanket and spread on the bed and finish at the top as for open bed.

9. Turn all covers up even with the foot of the mattress.

10. Fold the upper bedclothes even with the edge of

30

the mattress on the side of the bed near the door. Fold over once, about one third the width of the bed. Fanfold once, bringing folds together close to edge on opposite side of bed.

11. Cover the small pillow with waterproof and then linen case, and place at head of bed.

12. Cover the large pillow with waterproof and then linen case, and place on chair beside the bed.

13. Arrange emesis basins, tongue depressors and wipes in towel on bedside table. Secure paper bag on side of table.

14. Secure fluid slip and vital signs sheet on the over-the-bed table.

15. Check availability of shock blocks, stethoscope, sphygmomanometer and intravenous pole in central location in the ward.

Important Points

Be sure that mattress and pillows are well protected.

See that the unit is free of drafts and is conducive to rest.

Have free space on both sides of the bed for the stretcher and any persons necessary for lifting the patient.

BEDPAN

Equipment

Bedpan with cover, toilet tissue, washcloth and towel, small basin with warm water.

Procedure

1. Secure privacy for the patient.

2. Assist the patient to flex her knees and lift her hips. Arrange the bedpan in place.

3. If possible leave the patient alone after being sure that she has some means of summoning aid.

4. If the patient is able to complete her own toilet see that the toilet tissue and equipment for washing her hands are accessible.

5. When the patient is unable to complete her own toilet, the nurse should cleanse her with toilet tissue

or wash the perineal area and buttocks with warm water and soap, being sure to dry the area thoroughly afterward.

NOTE: Alternative technic. (*See* Perineal Care.)

6. Assist the patient into a comfortable position.

7. Before emptying the bedpan observe the contents, noting amount, color, odor and any abnormal constituents that may be present.

8. Wash and rinse equipment. Sterilize, s.o.s. (*See* Equipment, Cleaning and Sterilization of.)

9. If a record is being kept of the patient's intake and output record the amount of urine voided.

BINDER, ABDOMINAL

To Apply the Scultetus or Many-tailed Binder

The body of the binder is placed under the patient so that the lower edge and the inner tails will come down 3 or 4 in. below the iliac crests. The strips then are brought one by one from either side obliquely over the abdomen so that they cross each other directly in the mid-line. Considerable traction is used so as to give firm support, the patient's comfort being the guide as to the degree of traction used. Pin the last two tails in place. Also pin at the points in the mid-line where the tails cross.

Important Points

The length of the binder should be 1½ times the hip measurement.

The first two tails should reach well over the hip bones and should anchor the binder. The tails should overlap each other from one half to two thirds, depending upon the contour of the abdomen.

The shaft of the safety pin should be at right angles to the pull of the material.

If a tail is too long, turn it back upon itself. Have no wrinkles over the bony prominences of the hips.

Abdominal binders should be inspected frequently and reapplied whenever necessary.

NOTE: The application of an abdominal or scultetus binder for a postoperative patient differs from that for an obstetric patient. In the former case, the pressure is usually made from below upward to give proper support for the abdominal muscles and to avoid strain on the sutures. In the latter case the tails are applied from above downward, as a downward pressure brings the greatest tension over the fundus. In many hospitals the abdominal binder no longer is used in obstetrics, or, if needed for an unusual case, often is discarded after 24 hours.

For Breast Binders, *see* Maternity Nursing.

BLOOD PRESSURE

I. PURPOSE: To measure the pressure of the blood within the arteries

II. EQUIPMENT: sphygmomanometer and stethoscope

III. PROCEDURE

1. See that the patient is in a comfortable position. (Whether the patient is lying down or sitting up, his arm must be well supported.)

2. Wrap the cuff around the upper arm, using circular turns. The cuff must be wrapped evenly and without pressure. The rubber cuff should be placed over the brachial artery. Secure by tucking the end under the last turn.

3. Inflate the cuff until the radial pulse is obliterated. Pump the rubber bulb until the mercury has been raised an additional 20 points.

4. Place the bell of the stethoscope over the large vein in the crease of the elbow or at the place where the brachial artery pulse is felt.

5. Open the valve on the bulb and allow the mercury to descend slowly.

6. Listen carefully for the first definite beat and note the reading on the mercury column (systolic pressure).

7. Continue to let the mercury fall. The beats will vary in volume and sound again becoming sharp and hammerlike, finally fading out entirely. *The last definite beat* is recorded as the diastolic pressure.

8. When the cuff is completely deflated remove it from the patient's arm. (If repeated blood pressure

readings are to be taken the bulb may be detached from the cuff and the cuff left in place.)

9. The readings should be recorded as a fraction. The systolic pressure is represented as the numerator, and the diastolic as the denominator of the fraction. (*See* Blood Pressure *under* Medical and Surgical Nursing.)

CATHETERIZATION

Equipment

TRAY

Sterile covered catheter dish with 2 metal catheters, 2 rubber or plastic catheters (No. 12 or 14 French), thumb forceps, cotton balls, q.s., sterile vegetable lubricant, q.s.

Sterile covered jar with sterile water or normal saline; small cotton balls, q.s.

Emesis basin large—1 unsterile

Emesis basin medium—1 unsterile or paper bag

Dressing towel—unsterile

ADDITIONAL EQUIPMENT: Draping equipment, standing lamp, sterile gloves

Procedure

1. Move the bedside table to the foot of the bed and arrange the equipment.

2. Screen and drape the patient.

3. Adjust the standing lamp.

4. Place the emesis basins conveniently. Uncover the sterile dishes.

5. Put on sterile gloves.

6. Separate the vulva with the thumb and forefinger of the left hand, exposing the meatus.

7. Handling the cotton balls in the cleansing solution with the thumb forceps, cleanse the meatus. Use each cotton ball for one downward stroke only.

8. Keeping the left hand in place, lubricate and insert the catheter into the meatus without allowing it to be contaminated. (This must be done very gently and with the utmost care to avoid trauma.)

9. Insert the catheter until the urine begins to flow and no further.

10. When a sterile specimen is required, receive the urine into a sterile tube or bottle.

11. When the urine stops flowing, withdraw the catheter slightly and wait a moment to see if more urine will flow.

12. Withdraw the catheter, hold it over the basin and allow it to empty.

13. Place the catheter in the emesis basin with discarded sponges.

14. Dry the patient using the cotton balls.

15. Replace emesis basins on the tray.

16. Remove gloves.

17. Draw up the covers, remove the draping sheet, and make the patient comfortable.

18. Note and record:
    Amount of urine
    Whether the urine is clear or cloudy
    Whether there are signs of blood or pus
    Whether these abnormalities appear at the beginning, end or throughout the flow.

MALE

Equipment

As for female catheterization, but use rubber catheters only. Add: Kelly clamp; stylette, s.o.s.

Procedure

1. Assist the patient into a dorsal recumbent position.

2. Fold the top covers down to the patient's mid-thighs; place a shawl or blanket over his chest.

3. Place the emesis basin between patient's thighs.

4. Scrub your hands (unless a clamp is used to hold the catheter).

5. Cleanse the meatus.

6. Holding the penis in an upright position over the pubis, gently introduce the catheter into the meatus. As the catheter is advanced from the urethra to the bladder the penis should be lowered to an angle of about 60°.

7. Continue as described for female catheterization.

NURSING TECHNICS

CHEST DRAINAGE

Chest drainage, with or without suction, is used to drain air and/or fluid from the pleural cavity.

Equipment

2 1-gallon bottles
2 rubber stoppers—one with 3 holes, one with 2 holes, must fit bottles well
2 straight glass tubes—long
3 "L" tubes
Hard rubber tubing, q.s.
Sterile distilled water—1,000 cc.
Sterile compresses
Sink with special suction faucet, Chapman pump connection for regular faucet or suction machine
1 glass connecting tube
Adhesive tape, q.s.
Clamp—to be kept in patient unit

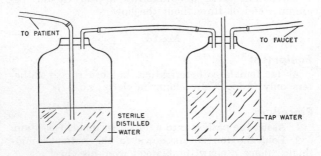

Preparation of Equipment

1. Sterilize the following:
   1 1-gallon bottle
   2-holed rubber stopper
   1 straight glass tube
   1 "L" tube
Rubber tubing—connects bottle and chest catheter

2. Assemble the above equipment as shown in the illustration above (*left*).

3. Put 1,000 cc. sterile distilled water into sterile bottle.

4. Cover the open ends of "L" tube and connecting tube with sterile compresses, secured with elastic bands.

5. Mark the water level on bottle with adhesive tape, and print *1,000 cc.* on the adhesive tape.

6. The second bottle (unsterile), the 3-holed rubber stopper, the 2 "L" tubes and the straight glass tube are assembled as shown in the illustration on page 36.

7. Put 1,000 cc. tap water into the unsterile bottle. Attach hard rubber tubing to suction faucet and to the "L" tube of unsterile bottle. Turn on the suction and watch for gentle and continuous bubbling in the bottle.

8. Tape all tube connections and the stoppers to prevent them from pulling apart. Bottles should be marked *"Do Not Open."*

9. The bottles are placed under the bed so they will not be in the way or knocked over.

Points to Check for Proper Functioning

Fluid (often bloody) and air will be seen draining from patient's catheter into the sterile bottle.

The long glass tube that extends below the water level in the sterile bottle, will show a fluid level that rises and falls with the patient's respirations.

The water in the unsterile bottle should bubble gently and continuously.

Points to Check When Apparatus Is Not Functioning Properly

1. Are all connections tight and taped?

2. Are there any kinks in the tubing? Often a rolled bath towel, a small pillow or a sandbag must be placed at the patient's side to prevent him from lying on the tube.

3. Are the faucets or suction turned on? A sign should be placed over the sink that is being used for suction, to warn everyone *not* to turn off the faucet.

NOTE: Notify the doctor.

NURSING TECHNICS

Warning

The nurse should *never open the bottles* or disconnect the tubing, as this may cause pneumothorax.

The nurse is responsible for seeing that orderlies, nurse aides, etc., do not disturb the bottles or the sink faucet.

If the apparatus accidentally comes apart, the nurse must *immediately* clamp off the tube coming from the patient and call the doctor.

CHEST DRAINAGE WITHOUT SUCTION

The sterile bottle is set up as described and only this is used.

COLD COMPRESSES

Equipment

Small basin with a moderate-sized piece of ice
2 compresses to fit the part

Procedure

1. Pour 8 oz. of water over the ice.
2. Moisten the compresses, wring them dry and place on the ice.
3. Apply the compresses to the affected area with a firm but gentle motion.
4. Change compresses frequently.

COUGH MACHINE
(COF-FLATOR)

Purpose

The Cof-flator is a mechanical method employed to produce a high expiratory flow rate from the lungs to aid in the elimination of bronchopulmonary secretions.

Its use is of great importance in the treatment of patients with ineffective coughs resulting from poliomyelitis, myasthenia gravis, and other neurologic disorders involving paralysis of the muscles of respiration, and in a variety of clinical illnesses and postoperative states in

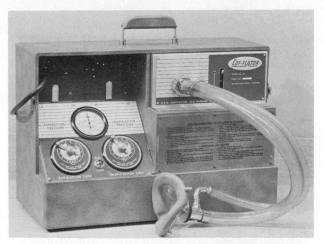

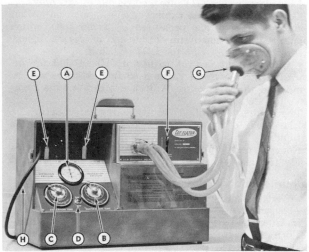

Cof-flator: (A) Pressure gauge. (B) Inspiration time regulator. (C) Expiration time regulator. (D) Motor and valve switch. (E) Positive and negative pressure regulators. (F) Volume control. (G) Tubing and mask. (H) Electric cord and plug. (O.E.M. Cof-flator: a product of Shampaine Industries, Inc., St. Louis, Mo.)

which there is impairment of the physiologic mechanism of coughing. The Cof-flator also may be used for resuscitation and for pressure breathing.

Methods of Operation

In adults, the lungs are gradually inflated with a positive pressure of 20 to 40 mm./Hg over 2 to 2.5 seconds; then the pressure is dropped automatically and quickly to 20 to 40 mm./Hg negative pressure. This negative pressure is maintained for 1.5 to 2.0 seconds after which the next inspiratory cycle follows.

A cough consists of a complete respiratory cycle, inspiration and expiration.

A treatment consists of 30 to 60 coughs given at intervals during one sitting.

Preparation of the Machine

Plug electric cord (H) into electric outlet, AC only.

Cork or block off the tubing or mask, turn on switch (D) and observe the pressures of gauge (A) which should register a maximum of plus and minus 40. Adjust pressure regulators (E) to "LO" position.

Adjust inspiration time regulator (B) so that the *inspirating* interval from vacuum to full pressure will be completed in 2.5 seconds. Adjust *expiration* time regulator for 1.5 seconds.

The volume control (F) may be regulated according to the needs of the treatment and the comfort of the patient.

Remove cork, turn off switch and the machine is ready for use.

Administration of the Treatment

Orient the patient to the machine and to his role in the treatment. His co-operation is *very* important.

Instruct the patient to inhale and exhale normally.

Turn the switch (D) on, and during the machine's inspiratory phase place the mask gently but snugly against the patient's face. Time this to meet the patient's inspiratory phase. Starting pressures should be 20 mm./Hg plus and minus, and gradually be increased to the desired pressure.

If the patient has a tracheostomy, cork the tracheostomy and proceed as otherwise directed. Remove cork p.r.n. for suctioning.

One treatment usually consists of 5 coughs, repeated 6 to 12 times with 1 minute normal breathing periods in-between to avoid hyperventilation. At any one sitting, 30-60 coughs are given and may be repeated at 3-hour intervals or more or less, depending on the individual needs of the patient.

If bronchospasm is present, the inhalation of a bronchodilator aerosol (e.g., 2.25 racemic epinephrine) may be ordered prior to the treatment.

The patient may complain of pain over the sides or front of the thorax; these probably originate in the chest musculature and usually disappear in 1 to 2 days.

After-Care of the Equipment

Remove the mask and tubing, cleanse with soap and lukewarm water. Replace.

Soak the mask and tubing in Zephiran Chloride 1:1,000 aqueous solution for 20 minutes.

CRUTCH-WALKING

Important Considerations

Crutch-walking for fractures or other disabilities of the lower extremity requires good posture and balance, strong finger flexors and triceps and strong abdominal and quadriceps muscles. Exercises to strengthen these muscles should be given to the patient in preparation for using crutches.

Strong triceps and quadriceps are particularly important, for weak elbows and knees make crutch-walking both difficult and dangerous.

Procedure

1. Measure crutches in the erect position, 1 to 2 in. below armpit. (There is no need to pad armpit rests, for the body weight is taken on hands and arms and *not on rests*.)

NOTE: Crutch paralysis may result from crutches that are too long, or wrong posture allowing the body to sag on the rests. Insist on good posture.

2. Place crutches in forward position, carrying weak leg ahead at the same time. Keep weak leg and foot parallel with the strong leg, checking its tendency to slant outward. Let weak leg hang down in normal manner.

3. Let body weight fall forward on hands and arms as sound leg steps through, simulating a normal gait, even though no weight is borne on weak foot.

4. Now bring crutches forward again with weak leg, and repeat. (Do not step through too far as it will upset balance.)

CULTURES

BLOOD

Equipment

Equipment for skin preparation
Syringe—20 cc.
Needle—18 or 19 x 1½ } Sterilized by dry heat
2 culture flasks with appropriate media and labeled, flasks No. 1 and No. 2

Procedure

1. Prepare the patient as for any venipuncture.

2. When the blood has been obtained, approximately 5 cc., it should be put in each flask.

3. Make the patient comfortable and remove the equipment.

4. Identify the cultures, the patient's name, etc., and place in incubator immediately.

5. Sterilize the syringe and needle.

NOTE: Flasks containing a meat broth media should be heated to liquefy the media and then should be cooled to room temperature before they are used.

BODY FLUID

Equipment

Sterile test tube with a cotton plug

Procedure

1. Remove cotton plug.

42

2. Collect fluid in test tube.
3. Replace cotton plug.

BODY SURFACES

Equipment
Sterile test tube with applicator

Procedure
1. Visualize area to be cultured.
2. Remove applicator from test tube.
3. Gently swab area with applicator (applicator must be saturated with material to be cultured).
4. Replace applicator in tube.
NOTE: Cultures must be sent to the laboratory while they are fresh.

ECZEMA MASK

Purpose
Application of an ointment to face and head.

Equipment
Cottonseed oil or albolene
Cotton balls
Ointment
Tongue depressors
Old muslin
Needle and thread
Arm restraints

Procedure
1. Apply arm restraints.
2. Clean the skin thoroughly with cotton balls dipped in the oil.
3. Mark on the muslin the position of eyes, nose and mouth and cut holes accordingly. (See illustration, p. 44).
4. Tear and cut the muslin as per diagram.
5. Apply the prescribed ointment generously.
6. Apply the mask snugly.
7. Put the openings for the eyes, etc., in place.

8. Cover the top of the head to the nape of the neck (No. 1).

9. Bring tails No. 2 up and cross them at the back of the head.

10. Bring tails No. 3 down and cross them at the back of the head.

11. Bring tails No. 4 straight around the head covering the other tails.

12. Sew these in place so that the mask will fit snugly.

13. Arrange opening for eyes, nose and mouth so the patient will be as comfortable as possible.

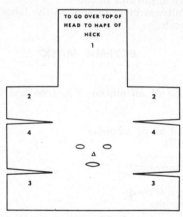

Eczema Mask

ENEMAS*

Equipment

Pitcher containing 250 to 1,000 cc. of soap solution at 105° F.

---

* Commercially prepared sets are available for enemas of many kinds. Directions for their use will be found with the sets.

Funnel
Rectal tube No. 24 French
Rubber tubing 12 in. long
Glass connecting tube
Lubricant
Emesis basin
Treatment sheet and half sheet
Bedpan and toilet paper
Solution bowl with warm water

Procedure

1. Connect the rectal tube, rubber tubing and funnel. Prepare the required solution.

2. Protect the bed with the treatment sheet and the half sheet. Turn the patient on her side in a relaxed and comfortable position.

3. Lubricate the rectal tube, expel the air and insert the tube 3 or 4 in. into the rectum.

4. Hold the funnel a few inches above the rectum and allow the fluid to run in very slowly. Pinch the rectal tube near the rectum and draw it out gently.

5. Cover the patient and allow her to rest quietly for a few minutes. Then place the patient on the bedpan to expel the enema.

6. Proceed as when removing any bedpan.

7. If the patient has been able to complete her own toilet, offer her the small basin in which to wash her hands. If you are going to complete the patient's toilet, use the solution in the basin for this, s.o.s.

8. Make the patient comfortable.

9. Remove equipment from the bedside.

10. Observe the returns before discarding.

11. Wash and rinse equipment. Sterilize, s.o.s. (*See* Equipment, Cleaning and Sterilization of.)

MODIFICATIONS

When a small amount of solution is given to be retained (retention enema), substitute an 18 or 20, French, catheter for the rectal tube, use a small graduate instead of the pitcher and proceed as above. The catheter may be left in the rectum for a few minutes after the treatment if there is any danger of the fluid's being expelled, and a safety pin or a small rubber band may be used as a clamp. Pressure with a towel over the rectum will minimize the possibility of the expulsion of the fluid.

When an oil retention enema has been retained for from 1½ to 2 hours, a soapsuds enema should be administered.

When a cleansing enema is ordered, the procedure is to be repeated until the returns are clear.

SOLUTIONS FOR RECTAL TREATMENTS

Carminative

1. M.G.W.

   Magnesium sulfate ⎱ 60 cc. $\overline{aa}$ Temperature
   Glycerine   ⎰ 105° to 110° F.
   Water

2. Milk   ⎱ 120 cc. $\overline{aa}$ Temperature 105° to
   Molasses ⎰ 110° F.

3. Glycerine   60 cc. ⎱
   Magnesium sulfate   60 cc. ⎰
   Fels bovis   30 cc. ⎰ Temperature
   Turpentine   15 cc. ⎰ 105° to 110° F.
   Hot water or
     soapsuds   240 cc. ⎰

Evacuating

Ivory, castile or any mild unperfumed soap and water, from 250 to 1,000 cc. as necessary. Temperature from 105° to 110° F.

Retention

OIL: Cottonseed or a similar oil, 120 cc.

STARCH: Dissolve 1 tsp. in small amount of cold water. Add 100 cc. boiling water. Boil 30 seconds. Cool to 100° to 105° F.

NOTE: If medication is ordered: Use 2 tsp. starch. Add medication to starch solution after cooking. Dilute with water until solution can be poured. Total amount should not exceed 100 cc.

Miscellaneous

To stimulate voiding:

Glycerine 120 cc. }
Water 60 cc. } Temperature 105° to 110° F.

EQUIPMENT, CLEANING AND
STERILIZATION OF*

Catheters, Rubber (Except Gastric Tubes)

Rinse with cold water. Wash with warm soapy water. (The handle of a hand brush rotated along the outside of the catheter will help to dislodge material clogging it.) Rinse well. Boil 10 minutes.

Enamelware, Stainless Steel, Glassware

Wash in warm soapy water. (Bon Ami, s.o.s.)
Boil 10 minutes.
NOTE: Syringe to be used for taking unsterile blood specimens may be dried by rinsing with acetone.

Gastric Tubes

Clean as described for other catheters.
Soak in Aqueous Zephiran 1:1,000 for 1 hour.
Rinse with clear water. Dry.

Hot-Water Bag, Icebag, Rubber or Plastic Sheeting

Wash with water and soap; rinse; dry. Inflate bags to prolong usefulness.

Instruments, Sharp and Dull

Wash with cold water, then warm soapy water. Scrub with an abrasive, s.o.s.

Boil 10 minutes. (If the cutting edges of sharp instruments are protected with gauze they will not be dulled by boiling.)

NOTE: Instruments that will be damaged by boiling may be soaked in Zephiran Tr. 1:1,000 for 1 hour.

---

* Autoclaving may be used to sterilize many of these items. Pressure and time recommended for the particular machine should be used.

NURSING TECHNICS

Mattresses, Pillows

Whisk with a damp brush. Air in sun 6 hours.

To remove stains—particularly blood—cover spot with paste of starch and ammonia. Allow to dry. Remove with brush or vacuum cleaner.

Thermometers, Mouth or Rectal

INDIVIDUAL EQUIPMENT. Cleaned p.r.n. (at least once a week) as described for terminal disinfection.

TERMINAL DISINFECTION. Wash with cool soapy water; rinse; soak in Aqueous Zephiran 1:1,000 for 1 hour.

Rinse—store dry.

NOTE: For other disinfectants, *See* Pharmacology.

ESOPHAGEAL BALLOON

NOTE: The following is to supplement, for the nurse, the data accompanying the tube. If discrepancies are evident the data provided by the manufacturer should be followed. In any instance, the procedure should be approved by the patient's physician.

Equipment

1. As for Miller-Abbott Tube

2. Additional: Esophageal varices tube with balloons attached

Mercury manometer or aneroid gauge of the Tycos sphygmomanometer

Rubber tubing, q.s.

"Y" tube (glass) to connect manometer to upper sausage balloon

50-cc. syringe with adaptor

2 clamps or hemostats; pad blades with rubber tubing

Circular sponge rubber pad 2 in. in diameter $\times$ $\frac{1}{2}$ in. cut as for any tube dressing; sponge should fit snugly around the tube.

Procedure

1. The nose and the throat probably will be cocainized.

2. Tube will be lubricated and passed through the

nasopharynx into the stomach to the 50 cm. mark. (Assisting the patient to take sips of water while the tube is being introduced may facilitate its passage.)

3. The stomach contents will be aspirated, and the pressure in the balloon established.

NOTE: The tube leading from the gastric balloon must be securely clamped *immediately and at all times*.

Subsequent Treatment

Practice continuous irrigation and aspiration until the stomach is empty of old blood.

Check the pressure in the esophageal balloon frequently, at least every hour, to see that no leakage has occurred. Constant pressure should be maintained unless otherwise ordered.

Gastric tube may be attached to continuous suction.

Secure the tube at the patient's nose, placing around it the sponge rubber cuff fixed to the tube by adhesive, to protect the skin.

Aspirate through the tube at least every ½ hour to *note the appearance of fresh blood*. Irrigate the tube at this time or as ordered.

Keep an accurate record of:

The amount and character of material aspirated

The amount of irrigating solution used

The amount of return from the irrigation

See that the patient swallows nothing, not even saliva, once the tube is in place.

Special mouth care always is important.

Water progressing to high-protein, high-caloric, low-sodium tube feedings as tolerated probably will be ordered after bleeding has been controlled for 12 or more hours. (*See* Gavage.) Be sure to follow the feeding with a small amount of water to keep tube patent.

NOTE: Following removal of the tube and the instigation of oral feedings, the patient should be encouraged to:

Eat small amounts frequently

Eat slowly, chew food well, swallow small portions.

NURSING TECHNICS

After-Care of Equipment

TUBE
1. Wash carefully with a detergent
2. Rinse and dry
3. Store in original package in a cool place

OTHER EQUIPMENT
Care for as usual

EYES

APPLICATION OF OINTMENTS

Equipment

Ointment in small tubes for ophthalmic use should be used exclusively for one patient
Gauze compresses

Procedure

1. If necessary, cleanse the lids before applying ointment.
2. Gently pull down lower lid with index finger of left hand, instruct the patient to look up. Squeeze sufficient ointment along the inside of the lid and in the conjunctival sac.
3. The lower lid is released, and the patient is instructed to close his eye.

ARTIFICIAL EYE (PROSTHESIS)

Artificial eyes are made of a plastic material in the form of a hollow shell.

Care of Eye Socket

The artificial eye and the socket must be cleansed frequently. Normal saline is a satisfactory solution for this purpose. The condition of the socket must be observed, as roughened edges of the artificial eye may cause irritation and inflammation.

The artificial eye must be replaced by a new one when necessary.

Removal of Artificial Eye

Draw the lower lid down with one finger of the left

hand. Insert the end of a small blunt instrument or the thumb nail of the right hand under the lower edge of the artificial eye, thereby loosening it and allowing it to drop out over the lower lid into the hand.

Insertion of Artificial Eye

With the left hand, raise the upper lid sufficiently to insert the artificial eye under this lid with the right hand. Then the upper lid is released, and the lower lid is drawn down and forward with the left hand to allow the insertion of the lower edge of the artificial eye.

NOTE: As soon as the patient is able to assume the responsibility of caring for the socket and the prosthesis, he should receive the required instructions.

BATHING OF EYES

Equipment

 Clean cotton balls
 Normal saline
 Basin or paper bag for used cotton

Procedure

1. Moisten cotton ball with solution, bathe closed eyelids with moistened cotton ball from inner to outer canthus, avoiding pressure on eyeball.

2. To remove secretions from lashes, place moistened cotton ball against lashes with eye closed and instruct patient to open his eye.

3. Dry lids with unmoistened cotton balls.

COMPRESSES

COLD

Equipment

UNSTERILE: Metal tray
STERILE: Bowl containing small pieces of ice. Smaller bowl of saline inside bowl of ice. Compresses (2 × 2 in. or larger). Kelly clamp and thumb forceps

Procedure

1. With clamp and forceps, the nurse squeezes one compress dry and applies it to the closed eye.

2. Three more compresses, squeezed dry, are placed on top of the first one.

3. The second compress is changed frequently, and the top one removed to the bowl of cold solution. This procedure usually is continued for 10 minutes, as often as ordered.

4. After completion of the treatment, the lids are dried gently.

HOT

Equipment

UNSTERILE: Metal tray 12 × 18 in., electric plate, tube of white petrolatum

STERILE

> Dressing towel
> Metal bowl for solution
> Normal saline
> 1 Kelly clamp
> 1 thumb forceps
> 8 gauze compresses (2 × 2 in.)
> 3 gauze sponges

Procedure

1. The patient must be flat in bed and should be made as comfortable as possible.

2. The basin is half filled with the solution which is brought to the boiling point on the electric plate.

3. The compresses are put into the solution.

4. The heat is regulated as necessary but usually kept at low during the treatment.

5. The nurse washes her hands thoroughly.

6. The eye should be bathed gently to remove any discharge, before beginning the treatment.

7. Petrolatum on a gauze sponge is applied to the closed lids and surrounding skin as a protection against burning.

8. With clamp and forceps, the nurse squeezes one compress dry and applies it to the closed eye.

9. Three more compresses, squeezed dry, are placed one at a time on top of the first one.

10. The second compress is changed frequently, and

the top one removed to the basin of hot solution, thus maintaining a fairly constant temperature.

11. This procedure is continued for 15 or 20 minutes, as ordered, and is given several times a day.

12. After completion of the treatment the lids are dried gently with a gauze sponge.

INSTILLATION OF DROPS

Equipment

Drugs as ordered

Eye drops are usually dispensed in a small bottle with a dropper attached to the screwtop or in a plastic squeeze bottle with a small opening under the protective screwtop which releases only 1 drop of the solution when the bottle is squeezed. These bottles should be used exclusively for one patient.

If the medication is in a bottle with an ordinary top, a sterile medicine dropper is used.

Gauze compress

Procedure

1. The patient should be lying down or seated in a chair with a firm head support.

2. The eye should be bathed, if necessary.

3. Check the label on the bottle of the drug carefully.

4. If a dropper is used, draw up a small amount of the drug into the dropper, as 1 drop is usually sufficient or squeeze bottle to obtain desired amount.

5. Draw down the lower lid gently with the left index finger.

6. Approach the eye from the side with the dropper or bottle in the right hand.

7. The side of this hand should rest gently on the patient's face to lessen the danger of the dropper's touching the eye if the patient moves his head suddenly.

8. Instructing the patient to look up, the nurse expresses the drop of the drug into the cup made by the everted lower lid.

9. She then releases the lid and tells the patient to look down. (Any overflow may be absorbed by the gauze compress.)

NURSING TECHNICS

Passage of the drug through the puncta into the lacrimal duct can be prevented by gentle pressure with the gauze compress on the inner canthus of the eye. This procedure should always be carried out when giving atropine to children.

IRRIGATION

Purpose
Usually for mechanical cleansing

Equipment
STERILE

Towel containing bowl for solution

Bulb syringe with glass tip

Gauze sponges

Solution as ordered (such as physiologic saline solution—usually at body temperature)

UNSTERILE

Metal tray about 8 × 10 in.

Cellucotton in 4-in. square pieces or cotton balls to receive and absorb solution

Emesis basin or paper bag

Procedure

1. The patient should be sitting in a chair with a firm head rest or, preferably, lying down with the head turned slightly to the side of the eye to be irrigated.

2. The eyelids should be bathed to remove any secretions.

3. With her left hand, the nurse holds sufficient cellucotton against the outer angle of the eye and separates the lids gently with the index finger and thumb of that hand.

4. With her right hand, she directs the flow of the solution from the bulb syringe from the inner to the outer angle of the eye, never against the cornea.

5. The irrigation is continued until the eye is cleansed thoroughly.

6. The cellucotton is discarded in the emesis in or paper bag, and the lids are dried with the gau ige.

REMOVAL OF FOREIGN BODIES

FROM THE CONJUNCTIVA

The eye should be inspected carefully. Use a bright light. If the foreign body is found to be on the bulbar conjunctiva, usually it can be removed easily with a cotton swab moistened in water or normal saline. To examine the inner surface of the upper lid, the latter should be everted in the following manner. Instruct the patient to look down. Place a toothpick swab horizontally across the lid about ½ in. from the lid margin. Grasp the lashes with the left hand and gently pull the lid down and forward. Fold the lid back over the swab. Hold in place by pressing the lashes with the left thumb against the eyebrow. Using the right hand, the foreign body may be removed with a swab. To return the lid to normal position, grasp the lashes, gently pull the lid forward and down, instructing the patient to look up.

FROM THE CORNEA

The nurse may attempt to remove a foreign body from the cornea by gentle irrigation with normal saline solution or water. If the foreign body is not removed readily in this manner, the patient should be referred to an ophthalmologist. When the foreign body is imbedded in the cornea the doctor uses a local anesthetic and a sharp instrument called a spud. An antiseptic ointment is instilled into the conjunctival sac, and a firm patch is applied for 24 hours to allow the cornea to heal.

FIXED DRESSING—UNNA'S BOOT

Equipment

Basin—warm water and soap
Wash cloth and towel
Alcohol 95 per cent
Warm gelatin paste
Soft paint brush
Roller bandage—2 in.
Adhesive—to secure final bandage
Ointment or medicated paste, if ordered

NURSING TECHNICS

Procedure

1. Melt and warm the gelatin. (A double boiler may be used.)

2. Cleanse the part with soap and water, then with alcohol.

3. Apply ointment of medicated paste.

4. Bandage the part, using roller bandage.

NOTE: Omit steps 3 and 4 unless specifically ordered.

5. Apply gelatin paste with paint brush.

6. Bandage the part. Secure with adhesive.

NOTE: If a cast is to be made of the jelly bandage:

1. Reapply gelatin paste over bandage—omit adhesive.

2. Apply another layer of bandage.

3. This may be repeated until the cast is from 3 to 6 layers thick.

4. Powder the cast with talcum (after cast is dry)

5. Watch for circulatory disturbances in the parts distal to the bandage. Cut or remove the bandage, s.o.s.

NOTE: Commercially prepared bandages are available which may be applied as any other roller bandage.

GASTROSTOMY FEEDING

Equipment

Tray and tray cover

Containers for feeding—tumblers, pitchers, etc.

Napkin

Glass syringe or syringe barrel

Glass of water

Small sponges or pieces of muslin

Elastic band

(For the feeding recipe, *see under* Tube Feeding *in* Diet Therapy.)

Procedure

1. Prepare the feeding on the tray. (Make it as attractive as possible.)

2. Arrange patient as for any meal with the tray in sight.

3. Place napkin around gastrostomy tube.

4. Open end of gastrostomy tube and, using the

syringe, introduce or pour through the barrel of the syringe a small amount of water to test the patency of the tube.

5. Assist the patient with the feeding:

A. Introduce slowly.

B. If several foods are given, introduce them as the patient would eat them normally. Example: tomato juice first, perhaps eggnog last.

C. Talk to the patient, making the occasion as pleasant as possible.

6. Introduce a small amount of water.

7. Cover end of tube with a sponge or a piece of muslin.

8. Bend tube over and secure with an elastic band.

Application to Pediatrics

EQUIPMENT

Small tray

Asepto syringe

20-cc. syringe for aspiration

Emesis basin for discard

Intravenous bottle and set-up to connect to tubing

1. Usually the gastrostomy tube is aspirated before feeding to evaluate residual. If the patient is a small baby, the gastric fluid should be reinserted if more than 5 cc. This should be done before the feeding is begun and the amount subtracted from the total amount of the feeding.

2. The feeding is then allowed to drip in by gravity, either

A. By Murphy drip setup: Asepto syringe, Murphy drip, adaptor, gastrostomy tube.

B. By I.V. bottle setup: run approximately 200 cc. in 30-60 minutes, or by continuous drip.

3. The feeding should be followed by 5 to 20 cc. of water to clear the gastrostomy tube.

4. The nurse should be in attendance during the feeding because of the possibility of vomiting and aspiration.

GAVAGE

Gavage is the introducing of liquid food or medication into the stomach through a tube.

NURSING TECHNICS

Equipment

2 towels—tray covers

Water repellent bib or towel and rubber

Long catheter No. 10 to No. 20 French—rubber or plastic—in a bowl with ice

Lubricant

Tissues

Emesis basin

Container with fluid to be administered

Funnel, syringe or reservoir and connecting tubing as indicated

NOTE: If the patient is to learn to feed himself or if the treatment is to be continued over a period of time, the feeding should be served as any fluid diet.

Procedure

1. Assist the patient into a sitting position, if possible. (This is not essential.)

2. Protect the patient's clothing with the bib or towel and rubber.

3. Lubricate the catheter and pass it into the patient's stomach through his nose or mouth.

NOTE: This should be done gently, and the patient should be encouraged to take deep breaths and swallow frequently.

4. Note the patient's color carefully. Place open end of catheter under water if there is any question as to whether or not the catheter is in the trachea. Fine bubbles of air rising through the water indicate that the catheter is in the trachea. Reinsert the catheter.

5. Introduce the fluid slowly.

6. Pinch off the catheter and remove it gently but quickly.

NOTE: If the catheter is to be left in place, introduce from 60 to 100 cc. of clear water, cover the end of the catheter with gauze, fold the end of the catheter over and secure it with an elastic band. The catheter should be supported and kept out of the patient's line of vision.

7. Make the patient comfortable.

8. Remove and cleanse all equipment. Sterilize, s.o.s.

9. Record: time of the treatment; amount and nature

of fluid administered; patient's reaction to the treatment.

Modifications in Children

In a young child or an infant who cannot co-operate, a mummy restraint should first be applied.

Measure the distance from the child's nose to his stomach and mark the spot on the catheter.

Lubricate the catheter and follow procedure.

NOTE: Chemicals rather than heat often are used to sterilize the catheter. This is safe and will prolong the life of the catheter.

GOWN TECHNIC

When a Gown Is Worn Once

A supply of clean gowns is kept near the patient's unit. A clean gown is put on before entering the patient's unit. After gown is taken off, it is (1) placed in a laundry hamper, if grossly soiled; (2) placed in a bag in which it may be autoclaved, if contaminated but not grossly soiled.

When the Same Gown Is Worn Repeatedly and by Different Persons

A gown is hung in patient's unit. The inside of the gown is considered clean. The outside of the gown is contaminated. The scrub sink is considered clean.

To Put on the Gown

1. With clean hands, palms toward each other, open the rear of the gown and slip the hands into the sleeves.
2. Button the neck and the wrist bands.
3. Bring the edges of the gown together behind, roll to fit body and tie the belt securely.

To Remove the Gown

1. Untie one loop of the belt and unbutton the wrist bands.
2. Proceed to the scrub stand or scrub sink. If a scrub stand is used (no running water), scrub the hands in soap solution for 1 minute. If a sink is used, turn the

faucets with a brush kept in a disinfecting solution and wash hands for 1 minute with soap and water.

3. Unbutton the neck band, slide the hands inside the sleeves, loosen the belt. Remove the gown and fold it down the middle so that the inside surfaces come together. Hang it on the hook through the armhole with the open edges toward the entrance of the unit.

4. Return to the scrub sink and again wash the hands with soap and water.

HYPOTHERMIA

For the Prolonged Application of Cold
(Therm-o-rite Machine)

Equipment
Therm-o-rite Machine
Cotton blankets
5 gallons of 50% Ethanol without adulterant
110-volt AC outlet

PREPARATION OF EQUIPMENT

1. Fill tank with 50% Ethanol (4 to 5 gallons required). Do not use adulterant as (a) organic adulterant apt to destroy tubing; (b) inorganic adulterant apt to damage pump. Fill tank ¼″ *above* refrigerating pipes.

2. Turn outlet valves *off*.

3. Turn pressure valve *low*.

4. Turn pump *on* only *after* these things have been done. No pressure will occur, but this will circulate the fluid.

5. Turn temperature regulation switch *on* and set thermostat somewhat below temperature desired. *Refer to chart* attached to machine. This chart is only an approximation of the thermostat numbers.

6. When the temperature gets down or up to the desired levels (refrigerating or heating element goes off automatically) connect as many thermal blankets as desired, but first do as follows:

7. Wrap extremity or body with a single thin towel or sheet. Then wrap the thermal blankets about the part with the cloth sides inward, being very careful *not* to

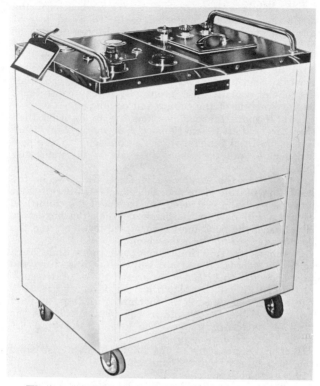

Therm-o-rite machine for hypothermia. (Therm-
o-rite Products Corporation, Buffalo, N. Y.)

bend the blankets in the opposite direction of the rubber
pipes that are enclosed within the blanket. *Do not kink
or bend any of the rubber tubes* either in or outside of
thermal blanket. Then wrap the entire part and surrounding thermal blankets with several layers of woolen
or cotton blankets. This prevents excessive heat absorption of the thermal blankets.

8. Connect blankets to the machine as follows:

NURSING TECHNICS

A. While unit is precooling (or preheating), the applicators may be connected to it. To avoid loss of solution, always hold ends of the lead-tubes as high or higher than the top of the unit, and also higher than the applicators, when connecting or disconnecting them. The coupling nuts *operate freely,* making it unnecessary to twist the lead-tubes. Twisting them may block or impair the flow of coolant. Also, eventually it may cause leaks at the junction of the tubing and couplings.

B. If more thermal blankets are to be used than there are outlets, then connect 2 or more blankets in series: the first blanket's female connector to the second's male, and the second's female to the machine's male.

C. When the headpiece is used, the flow in the hood line of the large top thermal blanket-applicator must be *partially restricted* (by means of the clamp) to ensure a full flow in the blanket. When the headpiece is *not used,* the hood lines are coupled together, and the flow is *pinched off* with the clamp.

9. When all the connections are tight, then turn valves to tubing in use *on.* Only *after* this, turn the pressure valve to *high.* Do not exceed 10 lbs. of pressure.

10. Then it will be seen that the level of the 50% Ethanol in the tank of the machine will drop, as fluid has now displaced the air in the blankets. Refill the tank as necessary to have the level of the fluid $\frac{1}{4}''$ above the refrigerator pipes.

11. The temperature of the fluid will then rise from the heat gained from the blankets.

12. Leave both switches *on.*

13. If the pump should make a lot of noise, due to oil on the pump valves, then turn the pump *on* and *off* a few times. It should go away.

Care While Machine Is in Use

1. Keep 50% Ethanol level above refrigerator pipes. There is a small loss due to evaporation and minute leaks. Check level b.i.d.

2. Keep pressure of fluid at 10 lbs. while machine is in use.

3. Check the temperature of the fluid. Thermostat will

be set, but it may have been accidentally moved or may have to be reset. Check the temperature q. 3 h.

4. Be very careful of the thermal blankets and the tubing. The pump is powerful, and the tubing may break proximal to an obstruction. If it does, a blanket is ruined, and 50% Ethanol will be all over the bed and the patient. Do not bend the thermal blankets against the direction of the enclosed tubing, as this will obstruct the flow of fluid and break the tubing. Be careful not to kink or bend the tube to and from the machine.

5. Try to keep the thermal blankets dry.

6. Keep the thermal blankets wrapped with several woolen or cotton blankets, to prevent excessive temperature loss or gain.

7. Examine the part of the body involved once a day and be sure that the skin is covered with a single layer of sheet or towel. Watch for skin necrosis at parts where there is pressure from thermal blankets.

8. If the blanket tubing should break, turn off the machine, disconnect the blanket and replace it with another blanket.

Care of the Machine After Use

1. Turn *off* both switches.

2. Disconnect blankets from machine, holding the connection above the level of the machine to minimize loss of Ethanol, which is expensive. Let them drain into bottles provided.

3. Make sure that all switches are OFF. Place drainage tube in collection bottles and allow Ethanol in tank to empty completely.

4. Turn all valves open or on (pressure valve to low level).

5. Empty blankets of alcohol by holding one side and tipping one end and then the other to run alcohol out of the blankets.

6. Wash blankets with solution of green soap. Dry thoroughly and then dust powder on them.

7. Store blankets *flat*. *Do not bend*. It is better not to roll them unless special containers are provided.

8. Be sure that the tank of the machine is dry and empty before storing.

NURSING TECHNICS

GRAVITY DRAINAGE

This is the withdrawal of fluids and discharges from a wound or cavity through the effect of gravity.

Equipment

Glass connecting tube—sterile, s.o.s.
Connecting tubing—q.s. sterile, s.o.s.
Drainage bottle—graduated if possible
Wire basket to hold drainage bottle (should have a hook to permit it to hang at bedside)
Metal clip or safety pin

Procedure

1. Connect catheter or drain to connecting tubing with glass tube.
2. Place open end of tubing in drainage bottle.
3. Secure tubing to bottom covers of bed with clip or safety pin.
4. Observe character of drainage frequently.
5. Measure the drainage at least every 12 hours. Record, including description of its character and color.

NOTE: Ambulatory patients should be instructed to keep the drainage bottle below the part being drained.

HYPODERMIC INJECTION

METHOD 1

Equipment

TRAY: Container (covered) with sterile cotton balls or gauze sponges. Another container (covered) for syringes and needles (needles may be kept in a separate container).

NOTE: Syringes and needles may be autoclaved in individual wrappers or tubes in which case the container need not be covered. A larger container usually is necessary.*

---

* If disposable needles and/or syringes are used, they should be broken before discarding.

Wide mouth jar or cylinder containing antiseptic solution (i.e., Aqueous Zephiran 1:1,000).

Thumb forceps 5½ in. long.

ADDITIONAL EQUIPMENT

Solutions for skin preparation (i.e., Zephiran Tr. 1:1,000).

Metal file

Receptacle for disposal of waste

Receptacle for used wrappers or tubes, s.o.s.

Prescribed medication

Procedure

PREPARATION OF MEDICATION

1. If drug comes in a bottle with a rubber cap, remove a sponge from the jar (using forceps), wet sponge with Zephiran Tr. 1:1,000, or other disinfectant, and wipe off rubber cap thoroughly. Discard sponge.

2. If an ampul is to be used, collect all of solution in body of ampul by shaking with a vigorous downward motion or by snapping tip of ampul with nails of the thumb and middle finger. With the file make a visible scratch on the neck of ampul. Cover with a sponge and break off top by bending it backward, using pressure above and below scratch.

3. Using forceps, remove syringe and needle from sterile jar. Attach needle to syringe and tighten with forceps. Check condition of needle point with tip of forceps. (Discard needle if hooked, rough or bent.)

4. Draw medication into syringe and expel all air bubbles.

5. Cover needle with sponge wet with solution to be used in preparing patient's skin.

INJECTION

1. Expose the site of injection and prepare, using sponge covering the needle.

2. Check dose in syringe.

3. With skin stretched taut between thumb and forefinger of left hand, grasp arm firmly at either side of site of injection; lift tissues up to form a cushion.

4. With a quick thrust, insert needle at an angle of

45° to a depth of about ½ in. (at least ⅛ in. of needle should be visible above surface of skin).

5. Inject medication slowly.

6. Withdraw needle gently but quickly, keeping needle covered with sponge.

7. Massage area gently with a circular motion.

AFTER-CARE

1. Rinse syringe and needle thoroughly.

2. Sterilize.

NOTE: Sterile equipment on tray should be resterilized every other day.

METHOD 2

Equipment

    Small tray
    Hypodermic set
    Tablets
    Bottle of alcohol; bottle of sterile water
    Alcohol lamp and matches
    Dessert spoon
    Sterile sponges

Procedure

1. Remove stopper from the alcohol bottle, fill the syringe with alcohol several times and leave partially filled in the alcohol bottle.

2. Light the lamp. Fill the dessert spoon with water, place it over the lamp and when the water is boiling put the needle in the spoon and boil it for 1 minute. Put out the lamp.

3. Expel the alcohol from the syringe. Draw up a little sterile water from the spoon and rinse the syringe. Draw up the remainder of the sterile water into the syringe and place it on a sterile sponge.

4. Turn the needle onto the sterile sponge. Put the tablet into the spoon, expel the water in the syringe over it and, when the tablet is dissolved, draw the solution into the syringe. Attach the needle. Expel the air and place the syringe in the fold of the sterile sponge.

5. Continue as in Method 1.

6. Rinse syringe and needle with cold water.

HYPODERMOCLYSIS

Introduction of an isotonic solution into the subcutaneous tissue is called hypodermoclysis.

Equipment
Commercially prepared set
Sterile needles
Skin preparation tray
Sterile hypodermic syringe and needles for procaine
Sterile solution—as ordered
Irrigating pole
Bath blanket

Procedure
1. Drape the patient, exposing the area about the mid-thighs.

2. Assist the doctor in preparing the skin and assembling the equipment.

3. Adhesive tape may be necessary to secure the needles in position.

NOTE: If the fluid collects in the tissue, gently massage the periphery of the swelling and change the patient's position to make him comfortable. Solutions of hyaluronidase added to the fluid being administered greatly reduce the discomfort that sometimes accompanies this procedure.

Hypodermoclyses are used frequently to administer a comparatively small amount of fluid to an infant when an intravenous infusion is not indicated. The preferred sites are each side of the back, and the needles are inserted at a point about 2 fingers to the left and the right of the mid-line and just under the tip of the scapula. If any type of chest surgery is to be performed, these sites should not be used, and the clysis can be given into the thighs. In premature infants, the doctor gives the clysis by syringe. A clysis for an infant or a small child should not run for more than one-half hour, and a nurse should stay at the bedside to ensure the protection of the patient as well as to regulate the flow of the solution.

NURSING TECHNICS

ICECAP OR COLLAR

Equipment

Icecap or collar
Ice; spoon or scoop for handling
Cover, cloth or gauze

Procedure

1. See that the cap or collar is in good condition.
2. Place ice in bag (from one third to one half full).
3. Compress bag to expel the air. Secure the cap.
4. Dry the bag and put on the cover.
5. Apply to prescribed area.
6. After use, the bag should be emptied, dried inside and out, inflated with air and hung in a cool, dry place.

NOTE: When ice is applied over a period of time, care must be taken to avoid "ice burns."

INDWELLING CATHETER

Equipment

As for catheterization
  Catheter—Special retention type may be used.
    Foley—male or female patients
    Mushroom—female
  For Foley catheter
    Luer syringe—20 cc.
    Sterile water or saline
    Elastic band
  Adhesive: 1 in. and ½ in.
  Gravity drainage set
    Sterile tubing and connecting tube
    Drainage bottle
    Clip or safety pin

Procedure

NOTE: Shave thigh, s.o.s.

1. Catheterize the patient

NOTE: If a Foley catheter is used, select as for any other catheter (sizes 12 to 30 French). Size of balloon may be ordered by the doctor—5 cc. is average.

Insert catheter gently until posterior bladder wall is felt, then withdraw catheter slightly.

Inflate balloon by injecting 5 cc. (or amount indicated on catheter) of sterile water or saline with the Luer syringe.

Fold over "balloon end" of catheter and secure with an elastic band.

2. Leaving the catheter in place, attach tubing to catheter with connecting tube.

3. Place open end of tubing in drainage bottle.

4. Secure tubing to bottom sheet to avoid tension on it.

5. Secure catheter to thigh with adhesive.

INHALATIONS, STEAM

This is the administration of moist heat by inhalation of the steam arising from plain or medicated boiling water.

INTERMITTENT INHALATIONS

Purposes

To relieve congestion in the upper respiratory passages. To provide moisture.

Equipment

Pitcher or wide-mouthed container
Large towel or stiff paper
Safety pins
Solution—tap water
Medication added as ordered—usually 1 teaspoon to a quart of water.

Benzoin Tincture
Pine oil
Menthol, etc.

NOTE: If Benzoin Tincture is used, the sides of the container should be coated with milk of magnesia before preparing the solution.

Procedure

1. Wrap the towel or stiff paper around the container so that it will direct the steam toward the patient.

2. Prepare the solution in the pitcher or container.

3. Make patient comfortable in sitting position.

4. Arrange the inhaler in a convenient position.

5. Instruct and assist the patient to inhale the steam.

NURSING TECHNICS

NOTE: It is important to prevent the patient from being burned by the solution and to instruct him in ways to avoid this.

6. The treatment should be continued until steam no longer is rising.

7. The patient's position then may be adjusted. Cold dry air from open windows, etc., should be minimized during the period that inhalations are indicated.

8. The container should be washed. The wrapping material may be used repeatedly until the treatment is canceled.

NOTE: If the container is stained with Benzoin Tincture, acetone (nail polish remover) usually will remove the stain.

CONTINUOUS INHALATIONS

Purpose
To warm and moisten the inhaled air.

Equipment
FOR BOILING WATER: Specially designed inhalers—electric; or electric plate with pitcher or container (tea kettle); or electric coffee percolator.

PROVISION FOR CONFINING STEAM: Small room; or screens to fit around head of bed and covered with:

1. Absorbent material: flannel or terry cloth (Turkish toweling)

NOTE: Woolen blankets must not be used, since they will shrink because of the steam.

2. Cone of stiff paper to direct the steam into the "tent."

Specially constructed frame with tight-fitting covers that may be attached to the head of the bed.

Umbrella—adequately draped. (This is not completely satisfactory, as the condensed steam will drip from the umbrella after a period of time.)

Procedure
1. Assemble the equipment selected.
2. Direct the steam to the back of the tent.
3. Be sure that the patient is not overly confined within the "tent."

4. Be sure that there is a continuous supply of water in the container.

5. Arrange the heating unit to avoid burning the patient.

INTRADERMAL INJECTION

NOTE: Equipment and preparation of medication as for hypodermic injection.

Procedure

1. Cleanse the area (usually the inner aspect of the forearm).

2. Hold skin taut.

3. Insert the needle shallowly under the skin until the bevel of the needle is under the skin.

4. Inject enough solution to form a small welt (like a mosquito bite).

5. Remove the needle and again cleanse area.

INTRAMUSCULAR INJECTION

Equipment

(*See* Hypodermic Injection, p. 64.)
Syringe, 2 to 5 cc.—sterile
Needle—1½ × 22
Medication—as prescribed

Procedure

1. As for preparation of a hypodermic injection.

2. The injection is given best in the upper outer quadrant of the buttock, although the deltoid muscle may be used. In young children the anterior or lateral aspects of the thigh may be the site of choice to avoid injury to the sciatic nerve.

3. Assist the patient so that the site of the injection is exposed.

4. Cleanse the area.

5. Compress the skin around the area so that it is taut or pick up the muscle and hold it tightly.

6. Insert the needle quickly and directly into the muscle.

7. Draw back the plunger of the syringe. (If blood appears, reinsert the needle.)

8. Inject the solution slowly.

9. Remove the needle quickly and massage the area gently with the sponge.

INTRATHECAL INJECTION

Equipment

Add to lumbar puncture tray—syringe (from 20 to 30 cc.) 6-in. tubing with needle adapter
Medication—as ordered
Basin—with warm water

Procedure

(After lumbar puncture, including the removal of spinal fluid.)

1. Warm medication by placing container in basin of warm water. (This is not always considered necessary.)

2. Pour medication into barrel of syringe.

3. Allow the drug to flow through the tubing to expel the air.

4. Attach the tubing to the needle and allow the medication to flow into the subarachnoid space by gravity.

5. Manometric readings may be made again.

6. Continue as for lumbar puncture.

INTRAVENOUS INFUSION

Equipment

Commercially prepared set
Sterile needles—No. 18 or No. 20
Skin preparation tray
Towel—with protecting sheet
Irrigating standard
Sterile solution—as ordered
Arm splint and bandage, s.o.s.

Procedure

To assist the doctor:

1. Collect equipment—check label of flask with the order.

2. Place protecting sheet and towel under the part to

be injected. (Remove patient's arm from sleeve of gown if the arm is to be used.)

3. Check the label on the flask with the doctor.

4. Pour solutions for the preparation of the skin.

5. Open the set.

6. Recheck label on the flask and prepare for use.

7. After the vent tube has been inserted in the bushing, arrange flask on irrigating pole.

8. Cut 2 pieces of adhesive to secure the needle.

9. Watch the rate of flow, position of the needle and condition of the patient during the treatment.

NOTE: Fluids administered to infants are computed very carefully and must be administered at an exact rate per hour. Restraints should be applied so that the needle is not pulled out. The baby's position should be changed at intervals. If he is getting no fluids by mouth, his need to suck should be satisfied.

IRRIGATION

BLADDER

Equipment

As for a catheterization, plus:
Irrigating set—sterile towel containing:
    Graduate—500 cc.
    Asepto syringe—60 cc.
    Solution cup—30 cc.
    Emesis basin—12 in. × 3½ in.
Sterile irrigating solution about 105° F.—500 cc.
Solution for instillation, s.o.s.

Preparation of Equipment

1. As for catheterization.

2. Open sterile package on end of tray.

3. Using handling forceps, remove syringe bulb and solution cup from graduate and place on sterile towel.

4. Pour irrigating solution into graduate (500 cc. unless otherwise ordered).

5. Pour instillation solution into cup—if instillation is not ordered remove cup from tray.

6. Cover irrigating set with the fold of sterile towel.

NURSING TECHNICS

Procedure

1. Catheterize the patient.
2. Pinch off the catheter and hold in left hand.
3. Remove basin containing urine and replace with clean large emesis basin.
4. With the Asepto syringe inject 60 cc. (2 oz.) of irrigating solution slowly through the catheter (count 30 during injection).
5. Remove syringe from catheter and allow solution to return into the emesis basin.
6. Repeat steps 4 and 5 until entire amount of solution has been used.
7. Instill medication, if ordered. (Pinch catheter and remove, allowing medication to remain in bladder.)
8. Continue as for catheterization.
9. Note and record:
   The character and amount of urine obtained
   The irrigating solution used
   The character of the returns from the irrigation
10. Thoroughly wash and rinse equipment.
11. Sterilize equipment and reset tray. (*See* Equipment, Cleaning and Sterilization of.)

BLADDER-INDWELLING CATHETER

Equipment

Sterile reservoir for solution
Sterile Asepto syringe—60 cc.
Large emesis basin—unsterile

Procedure

1. Disconnect drainage tubing from the catheter.
2. Irrigate the bladder through this catheter—as for any bladder irrigation.
3. Reassemble the catheter and tubing.
4. Remove other equipment.
5. Wash and rinse equipment thoroughly and sterilize. (*See* Equipment, Cleaning and Sterilization of.)

COLON (2-TUBE METHOD)

A colon irrigation is an injection of fluid into the colon in a steady stream under low pressure, providing for immediate return of all that has not been absorbed.

Purpose

	TEMPERATURE
1. To cleanse the colon	105°-110° F.
2. To supply stimulation by heat	110°-118° F.
3. To reduce body temperature	85°- 95° F.
4. To supply fluid to the body	100°-105° F.

Equipment

TRAY

2 towels
Protecting sheet 18 × 36 in.
Half sheet
Catheter No. 18 or No. 20 French ⎤
   marked 3 in. from tip.   ⎬ Inflow tube
Connecting tubing—24 in.   ⎟
Irrigating tip   ⎦
Catheter No. 36 or No. 38 French ⎤
   marked 7 in. from tip.   ⎬ Outflow tube
Straight glass connecting tip   ⎟
Tubing—4 in.   ⎦
Irrigation can
Large emesis basin
Large clip or safety pin
Toilet tissue
Small basin

ADDITIONAL EQUIPMENT

Lubricant
Irrigating pole
Stool
Pail with bedpan cover
Bedpan with cover

Procedure

1. Arrange protecting sheet and half sheets under the patient.

2. Assist the patient into a left Sims' position (preferred, but any position may be used).

3. See that the patient is comfortable and adequately draped.

4. Insert the small catheter into the second hole of

75

the large catheter. Allow solution to flow through the catheter to expel the air.

5. Lubricate both catheters and insert gently until the 3-in. mark on the small catheter is reached. Advance large catheter until the 2 markings meet.

6. Start the flow of solution.

7. If there is difficulty in obtaining the return flow, move the colon tube up or down. It may be necessary to remove and cleanse it.

8. Secure tubes to the sheet with the clip or pin.

9. Stay with the patient until you are certain that the treatment is proceeding as desired.

10. Add fluid as necessary.

11. When the desired effect has been attained remove the tubes gently; cleanse the patient and remove all the equipment.

12. Chart pertinent facts as usual. Include the amount of solution retained.

COLOSTOMY

A colostomy irrigation is the injection and the return of a fluid through an artificial opening into the large intestine for the purpose of evacuating the colon.

NOTE: Careful instruction given by the nurse to the patient concurrent with his convalescence will ensure intelligent managing of the colostomy following his discharge from the hospital.

Equipment

TRAY

Towels (for setting up tray)

2-qt. irrigating can with rubber tubing and glass connecting tube

Catheter—No. 24 French

Compresses 4 × 8 in.

2 large emesis basins

Toilet tissue with lubricant

Half sheet and protecting sheet

Irrigating stand

Mild soap solution for irrigation—110° F.

Procedure

1. Fold spread and blanket to patient's mid-thighs and top sheet to groin. Roll gown out of way. Arrange protecting sheets.

2. Turn patient on his left side and support with pillow at back.

3. Tuck large emesis basin at patient's side for collection of return flow.

4. Place large compress over colostomy opening to aid in directing return flow into basin.

5. Expel air from tubing and lubricate catheter.

6. Insert catheter gently allowing fluid to flow as catheter is advanced from 6 to 7 in.

7. When desired amount of solution has been administered remove the catheter.

8. When sufficient time has elapsed to ensure complete evacuation, cleanse the area about the colostomy opening and apply necessary dressing.

9. Chart amount and character of returns, etc., as for other treatments.

10. Wash equipment thoroughly. Sterilize, s.o.s. (*See* Equipment, Cleaning and Sterilization of.)

NOTE:

1. If obstruction is encountered as the catheter is passed, wait a few seconds and again attempt to advance the catheter. Never force the catheter against resistance.

2. If the patient has a "double-barreled" colostomy, the nurse is responsible for ascertaining which loop is the distal loop and what the doctor's orders are concerning its care.

EAR

METHOD 1

Purpose

To dislodge excess and impacted cerumen of the canal; to dislodge foreign bodies in the external canal (not beans or peas)

Equipment

Rubber ear bulb

NURSING TECHNICS

Solution cup containing tap water or ordered solution at 100° to 110° F.
Absorbent cotton
Emesis basin
Towel and treatment sheet or bib
Wooden clothes pin (towel clip), s.o.s.

Procedure

1. Have the patient sit up. Protect his neck and shoulders with towel and treatment sheet or bib.

2. Pull the auricle upward and backward to straighten the canal in an adult; downward and back for a small child. Expel the air from the bulb. Fill it with the solution and use moderate force in irrigating. Have the patient hold the emesis basin close to his neck below the ear.

3. Continue the irrigation until the solution returns clear and the patient notes the ear is clear.

4. Tip head to allow all solution to drain out and dry the canal and the outer ear with cotton and leave a small plug of cotton in the ear.

NOTE: When both ears are to be irrigated a different bulb must be used for each ear.

METHOD 2

Equipment

High irrigation stand
Large irrigating can with 4 ft. of rubber tubing and a metal clamp.
Medicine dropper, its bulb removed and its tip covered with fine rubber tubing 2 in. long.
Toothpick swabs
2 emesis basins
1 qt. of normal saline or prescribed solution at 105° to 110° F.
Protecting towel and sheet or bib.

Procedure

1. Prepare the solution in the can. The surface of the solution should be only 6 to 12 in. above the patient's ear.

2. Attach the medicine dropper to the tubing of the irrigating can.

3. Make the patient comfortable in a sitting position if possible. This may be done in bed or on a chair. If a recumbent position is necessary, assist the patient to turn his head toward the affected side.

4. Protect the patient's shoulders with the towel and sheet or bib.

5. If the patient is able, have him hold the basin close to his neck below the ear.

6. Run a little of the solution through the tubing to expel the air.

7. Pull the auricle upward and backward with one hand; with the other, rotate the tip of the irrigator in the external part of the canal.

8. Continue the irrigation until the return flow is clear, or until about 1 qt. of the solution has been used.

9. Wipe the ear perfectly dry with the cotton swabs.

NOTE: If both ears are to be irrigated, a different irrigating tip must be used for each ear.

NASAL

A nasal irrigation is the directing of a stream of water or medicated solution into the nasal cavity under low pressure.

Equipment

TRAY

 2 patient's face towels
 Metal nasal syringe or rubber ear bulb
 Treatment sheet and towel or bib
 500-cc. enamel graduate
 Tissues—q.s.

Procedure

1. Assist the patient into a sitting position—preferably in a chair—with his head over a sink or basin.

2. Arrange treatment sheet and towel or bib around neck.

3. Instruct the patient to hold the basin under his chin with his head lowered.

4. Inject the solution up one nostril, allowing it to return through the other nostril. Have patient say "k k k" while fluid is being injected.

5. Remove syringe and place finger over nostril, instructing patient to bow into emesis basin. Repeat this procedure with the other nostril.

6. Chart amount of solution used, character of the returns and the patient's reaction to the treatment.

THROAT

A throat irrigation is an application of a hot solution to the mucous lining of the throat.

Equipment

TRAY

2 towels—tray covers
2-qt. irrigating can
Rubber tubing (about 12 in.)
1 glass drinking tube or irrigating tip
2 large emesis basins
Bib
Mouth wipes—q.s.
1 tongue depressor and flashlight, s.o.s.

Preparation of Equipment

Prepare ordered solution or tap water in the irrigating can. Temperature from 115° to 118° F. or as hot as can be tolerated by the patient.

Procedure

1. Assist patient into sitting position.

2. Protect patient's gown with bib.

3. Instruct patient to hold basin under chin with left hand. His head should be bent slightly forward.

4. Either the nurse or patient may direct the flow of hot solution to the affected areas.

5. Flow should be interrupted frequently to allow patient to "catch his breath."

6. Outflow basin should be changed when half of the solution has been used.

7. After completing the treatment see that the patient is comfortable.

8. Remove equipment. Wash. Sterilize. (*See* Equipment, Cleaning and Sterilization of.)

NOTE:

1. If the patient is unable to sit up, the treatment may be done with the patient lying on his side.

2. The treatment usually is more effective if the patient directs the flow of solution.

3. "Gagging" may be avoided if the patient is instructed to hold his breath while the solution is flowing.

VAGINAL, OR DOUCHE

Equipment

TRAY

2 towels—tray covers
Half sheet
Treatment sheet, 18 × 36 in.
2-qt. irrigating can
Connecting tubings: 1 about 28 in. long
                       1 about 18 in. long
Glass connecting tube
Glass douche tip in dressing towel
Clamp (optional)
Emesis basin
Small round basin
5 large or 10 small cotton balls

ADDITIONAL EQUIPMENT

Douche pan with bedpan cover
Unsterile dressing towel
Equipment for draping the patient
Irrigating stand
Standing lamp
Solution—as ordered, or tap water
Bath blanket—in patient's unit

Procedure

1. Explain procedure to patient; secure privacy.

2. Place protecting sheets under the patient's buttocks.

3. Drape patient in dorsal recumbent position.

4. Pad douche pan with towel and place under the patient's buttocks.

5. Cleanse vulva, using moist cotton balls.

6. Separate labia and insert douche tip into vagina, allowing solution to run in as tip is inserted.

NURSING TECHNICS

7. Rotate douche tip and move it back and forth gently in order to ensure thorough cleansing.

8. Dry patient with cotton balls.

9. Make patient comfortable.

10. Remove equipment. Wash. Sterilize. (*See* Equipment, Cleaning and Sterilization of.)

11. Chart character of returns.

NOTE: Good lighting is essential to effectiveness of treatment. Douche tip should be inspected carefully before use for cracks, chips, etc. Nurse should wear protective goggles if patient has gonorrheal vaginitis.

LAVAGE
AUTOMATIC

Equipment

2 drinking glasses
1 or 2 large emesis basins
Towel or bib; tissues
Lavaging solution
Mouthwash

Procedure

1. Prepare lavaging solution in glasses.
2. Instruct the patient to:
   A. Take several deep breaths.
   B. Hold his breath.
   C. While holding his breath drink the 2 glasses of solution as quickly as possible.
3. Arrange the towel or bib to protect the patient's clothing.
4. Assist the patient to drink the solution.
5. Assist the patient with the emesis basin, etc., as vomiting occurs.
6. Assist the patient to rinse his mouth with the mouthwash.
7. Note the character of the vomitus; save if indicated.
8. Wash and rinse the equipment. Sterilize. (*See* Equipment, Cleaning and Sterilization of.)

COLON

A colon lavage is an injection of fluid, slowly and by

gravity, into the colon and the immediate siphoning back of the fluid.

Equipment

TRAY

    2 towels—tray covers

    Protecting sheet and half sheet

    Catheter, 36 or 38 French (marked 7 in. from the end)

    Rubber tubing—8 in.

    Funnel—500 cc.

    Large glass connecting tube

    Toilet tissue with lubricant

    Large emesis basin

    Small round basin—for cleansing perineal area

    Covered output pail—on stool at bedside

    Bedpan with cover

    5-qt. pitcher of solution at desired temperature

NOTE:

  85° to 95° F.—cooling

 105° to 110° F.—cleansing

 110° to 118° F.—heat

Procedure

1. Place protecting sheets under the patient.

2. Assist patient to turn on her side with her buttocks near the edge of the bed.

3. Expel air from tubing and lubricate catheter.

4. Insert catheter to 7-in. mark and allow funnel of solution to run in (funnel 12 in. above anus).

5. Lower the funnel to siphon back the fluid and pour returns into output pail.

6. Repeat this procedure until desired effects have been obtained. Avoid tiring the patient.

7. If patient so requests, assist her onto a bedpan.

8. Cleanse patient—remove protecting sheet.

9. Wash and rinse equipment. Sterilize.

10. Record treatment, noting *particularly* amount of flatus and fecal fluid returned.

GASTRIC

A gastric lavage is the administration and siphoning

back of a solution through a catheter passed into the stomach.

Equipment

DEEP TRAY

  2 towels—tray covers
  Solution bowl
  2 emesis basins
  Waterproof bib
  Tongue depressor
  Mouth wipes—q.s.
  Lubricant
  Catheter No. 32 (stomach tube)
  Asepto syringe, 60 cc. ⎱
  Crump bulb   ⎰ One of these according
  Asepto syringe, 120 cc. ⎰ to doctor's choice
  Funnel, 500 cc.   ⎰
  Solution as ordered

Procedure

1. Support the patient in a sitting position.
2. Protect patient's gown with bib.
3. Assist doctor in lubricating and inserting tube.
4. Instruct patient to take deep breaths and swallow as directed while catheter is passed.
5. Assist with lavage as necessary.
6. Offer patient mouthwash after treatment.
7. Measure residual.
8. Chart pertinent facts as usual.
9. Wash and rinse equipment.
10. Sterilize equipment. (*See* Equipment, Cleaning and Sterilization of.)

NOTE: The rubber tube is made less unpleasant to the taste and easier to insert if it is iced for from 15 to 30 minutes before the treatment.

LEVARTERENOL (LEVOPHED) DRIP

Equipment

As for intravenous infusion.

Solution—5 per cent dextrose in water or 5 per cent dextrose in saline.

Levarterenol bitartrate as ordered—usually 4 cc. of a 0.2 per cent solution to 1,000 cc. of dextrose

Sphygmomanometer and stethoscope

Procedure

1. As for any infusion.
2. Adjust flow to 2 to 3 cc. per minute.
3. Take patient's blood pressure *immediately*.
4. Adjust the rate of flow to the desired blood pressure (i.e., normotension). Average maintenance dose—0.5 to 1.0 cc. per minute.
5. Check blood pressure every 2 or 3 minutes until desired pressure is obtained, then check it every 5 minutes for the duration of the treatment.

NOTE: 1. Treatment usually is continued until the patient is able to maintain adequate blood pressure without therapy.

2. Care should be taken to avoid extravasation of the levarterenol bitartrate into the tissues, as local necrosis might ensue due to the vasoconstrictive action of the drug.

Action

See Levarterenol *under* Drugs to Treat Hypotension and Cardiac Collapse *in* Pharmacology.

LOCAL APPLICATION OF DRUGS
LOTIONS

Lotions are suspensions of powders in watery preparations.

Equipment

Shallow dish, clean varnish brush, prescribed lotion

Procedure

1. Wash area gently with water or light mineral oil.
2. Pour medication into shallow dish.
3. Apply lotion, using brush, or apply by hand.

NOTE: Once every 24 hours, the residual lotion should be removed from the skin. This is done gently with moistened gauze sponges soaked in oil, warm water, boric acid or other cleansing agents.

OINTMENTS

Both the equipment and the procedure are the same as for pastes, below.

PASTES

Pastes are mixtures of absorbent powders in a solid or semisolid fat.

Equipment

Soft muslin—q.s.
Tongue depressors or a spatula
Ordered paste
Bandage, roller or fine-mesh tubular bandage

Procedure

1. Cleanse the affected areas with warm oil to remove crusts.
2. Apply paste by rubbing and then spread on as a thin layer.
3. Cover with a single layer of soft muslin that has been "buttered" with the paste.
4. Secure muslin with bandage. Be sure to separate all skin surfaces.
5. Change dressing every 6 to 8 hours.
6. Cleanse lesions with warm oil before each application of paste.

WET DRESSINGS

Types

1. Open—fluid allowed to evaporate. As evaporation occurs, the drug concentrates, which may be dangerous.
2. Closed—covered to prevent loss of heat and moisture.

Equipment

Soft muslin—q.s.
Soft towels—absorbent
Bandage or safety pins to secure dressing

Prescribed solution
Vegetable oil
Oiled silk or rubberized sheeting—for closed dressing only.

Procedure

1. Fold muslin into compresses, from 6 to 8 ply.

2. Immerse in medicated solution.

3. Spread smoothly over involved areas. Remove all wrinkles or folds.

4. Moisten towels with medicated solution and place over compresses.

5. Cover with oiled silk or rubberized sheeting, if a closed dressing.

6. Moisten compresses every half hour by removing and wetting the towels. Pour solution over compresses as well, s.o.s.

7. Change dressing completely at least every 2 hours, preferably every 15-20 min.

8. Apply vegetable oil to surrounding normal skin surfaces, between each dressing.

NOTE: No more than one third of the body surface should be covered with wet compresses at one time. Soiled compresses may be laundered and reused. Wet dressing must be kept *wet*.

USEFUL MATERIALS

1. *To remove pastes and ointments*—discarded soft bed or table linen and oil (mineral, cottonseed, peanut or olive).

2. *For dressings*—discarded soft bed or table linen. Gauze, if used, should always be washed first as this removes the stiffening present in new gauze, which may be irritating and abrasive.

3. *To hold dressings in place*—stockinette, Surgitube, bandages, sleeves cut from old white cotton shirts, women's white cotton stockings and white cotton gloves.

4. *To protect clothing of the ambulatory patient*—loose cotton underwear.

5. *To protect the mattress from oils and ointments*—a full-length quilted bed pad placed directly on the mat-

tress, and/or an oil-resistant and waterproof mattress cover.

6. *To prevent the staining of new linen*—use old linen, which is very acceptable because of its softness, or purchase a supply of linen that can be kept for these patients alone. (Colored linen, e.g., light gray, would help in keeping these two supplies separate.)

NOTE: "Absorbent cotton" should not be used.

LUMBAR PUNCTURE

Equipment
3 dressing towels
Compresses—2 (4 × 4 in.)
5-cc. syringe
Needles: 1 No. 24 hypodermic
        1 No. 22 intramuscular
3-way stopcock
Manometer (2 sections)
Equipment for skin preparation

Procedure
1. Place patient on side very near edge of bed, head toward knees, knees flexed on thighs and brought up toward head.

2. Protect bed directly beneath lumbar area with towel and rubber.

3. Assist doctor with treatment as necessary.

4. Observe the patient carefully throughout the treatment.

5. Assist with manometric readings if requested.
    Initial pressure—first level reading
    Light compression—instantaneous light pressure to jugular veins
    Deep compression—heavier pressure to both jugular veins for 10 seconds
    Abdominal strain—patient instructed to breathe deeply and strain for 10 seconds

6. Assist in collecting and labeling of specimens.

NOTE: The patient may be instructed to lie flat in bed for from 8 to 24 hours following the procedure. Shock blocks are used to elevate the foot of the bed as ordered.

MEDICAL ASEPTIC TECHNIC
PRECAUTIONS

NOMENCLATURE AND PROCEDURE	DISEASES	DURATION OF ISOLATION
Simple Respiratory Precautions		
Red card (Bed-chart)	Influenza	
Mask—recommended		3 days after temperature is normal
Wash hands		
Patient to remain in own unit	Pneumococcus pneumonia	
Complete Respiratory Precautions		
Red card (Bed-chart)	Acute streptococcal throat including scarlet fever	
Mask	Acute encephalitis	
Gown	Pneumonia: influenza, streptococcus, virus	
Wash hands		
Care of:	Meningococcus infections	3 days after temperature is normal
Linen	Diphtheria	
Dishes		
Patient to remain in own unit	Measles	
	Pertussis	
	Psittacosis	
	Pulmonary tuberculosis	
G.I. Precautions		
Red card (Bed-chart)	Typhoid fever	10 days after temperature remains normal and 2 negative stools 48 hours apart
Mask—(poliomyelitis only)	Paratyphoid	
	Amebic dysentery	
Gown		
Wash hands		
Care of:	Bacillary dysentery	After adequate treatment and subsidence of symptoms. Food handlers—3 negative stools, 24 hours apart
Linen		
Dishes		
Food		
Feces*		
Urine		
Fluid and solid waste	Infectious hepatitis	7 days after temperature is normal
Nets in fly season	Poliomyelitis	7 days after temperature is normal
Patient to remain in own unit (Carriers as above unless otherwise ordered by the doctor)		
Contact Precautions		
Red card (Bed-chart)	Acute gonorrhea	Until no longer likely to infect others, depending on dark-field examinations, etc.
Roll sleeves	Epidermic infections	
Wash hands	Conjunctivitis	
	Keratoconjunctivitis	

* See No. 3 *under* Care of Equipment, *below.*

MEDICAL ASEPTIC TECHNIC (Cont.)

NOMENCLATURE AND PROCEDURE	DISEASES	DURATION OF ISOLATION
Contact Precautions (Cont.) Care of:		
Linen	Open syphilis	
Dishes	Trachoma	
Patient to remain in own unit unless otherwise ordered by the doctor.	Tuberculosis— surgical Urinary tract tuberculosis	
Gloves—open syphilis		
Goggles—gonorrhea, s.o.s.		
Gown—infants		

IMPORTANT NOTES

Visitors to wear gowns and masks as indicated under precautions in effect for patient.

When it is necessary to move a patient on precautions from his own unit, viz., x-ray, etc., the technic should be maintained as far as is practical, i.e., patients on respiratory precautions should be masked or those in immediate contact with patient should be masked, i.e., infant. It is also recommended that the patient, if his condition permits, wear a mask when in contact with visitors or personnel.

Care of Equipment

1. Care must be taken to see that the contaminated equipment does not contaminate anything else before it is sterilized.

2. All equipment may be washed and sterilized in the usual manner. (*See* Equipment, Cleaning and Sterilization of.)

EXCEPTION

Equipment that cannot be sterilized otherwise should be aired in the sun for 6 to 8 hours.

When precautions are being taken against sporebearing organisms (i.e., acute tetanus infections) the equipment must be autoclaved or sterilized fractionally.

    A. Wash equipment and rinse thoroughly (wear gloves).

B. Boil for 20 minutes.

C. Allow to stand unused for 24 hours.

D. Repeat steps 2 and 3 on two consecutive days.
(Total boiling—3 times.)

3. When required by the local board of health, waste disposed of through the sewage system must be disinfected with 5 per cent chloride of lime for 2 hours. (Sometimes required for enteric infections.)

NOTE: It is convenient to determine the capacity of the vessel to be used for disinfecting this waste and to place the necessary amount of chloride of lime in it so that when it is filled it may simply be allowed to stand for 2 hours. Fecal material should be disinfected at once and discarded.

4. Food, other solid waste and receptacles containing nose and throat discharges should be burned.

5. Dishes and other eating utensils should be boiled for 10 minutes.

6. Linen should be boiled for 20 minutes unless being laundered in a hospital laundry. (Hospitals usually provide special laundry hampers for such linen. This helps to protect laundry personnel by identifying the linen as contaminated.)

7. Woolen blankets should be aired in the sun for 6 to 8 hours and then laundered or dry cleaned as any other woolen blanket if grossly soiled.

8. Terminal disinfection usually is not necessary.

A. Exception—on termination of isolation following:

Enteric infections

Tuberculosis

Condition caused by spore-bearing organisms

B. Procedure:

1. All equipment sterilized or discarded.

2. Patient given a bath and shampoo.

3. Place patient in a clean unit.

4. Furniture and walls should be washed and allowed to air for 24 hours.

NOTE: Fumigation is not necessary unless required by the local board of health.

MILLER-ABBOTT TUBE TREATMENT

Purpose

1. To relieve pressure caused by an accumulation of gas or fluid in the small intestine in the presence of an intestinal obstruction and to restore normal intestinal movement.

2. To aspirate material from the site of an intestinal obstruction for study.

3. To make possible an x-ray study of the location and nature of an intestinal obstruction by the use of barium injected through the tube.

4. To prevent or relieve postoperative distention.

Equipment

CARRIED TO BEDSIDE IN BASKET

Miller-Abbott tube
Nasal speculum
Applicator and cotton
2 per cent cocaine spray
10 per cent cocaine solution
Tongue depressors-wipes
Glass drinking tube
K-Y jelly
One half inch adhesive (roll)
20-cc. Luer syringe
Emesis basin
Small and large elastic bands
Large safety pins
Suction apparatus
Rubber sheet and towel or waterproof bib

TO BE LEFT AT BEDSIDE AFTER INTUBATION

TRAY—small
Bowl or cup—for irrigating solution
Syringe—20-cc. Luer
Emesis basin
2 towels
Albolene or similar nose drops

Preparation of Patient

1. Omit solid food 6 hours before treatment.

2. Explain treatment to patient.

3. Elevate head of bed and have patient in a sitting position.

4. Place protective covering about patient's neck.

Procedure for Insertion

1. Nose and throat cocainized.

2. Tube passed through nose-pharynx and into stomach to the 60-cm. mark.

3. While tube is being passed by doctor, nurse may assist patient in drinking water to facilitate passage.

4. Stomach contents aspirated.

5. Two or 3 cc. of metallic mercury injected into the deflated balloon.

6. Bed lowered and patient placed flat in bed and turned on right side.

7. Tube inserted slowly to 75-cm. mark and fastened to patient's nose with adhesive.

8. Tube is connected to suction apparatus.

NOTE: The tube should be secured with adhesive only where so ordered by the doctor.

Subsequent Treatment

1. Irrigate and aspirate from *Suction Side* of Miller-Abbott tube as ordered. (*Do not touch balloon side of tube. Mark this side distinctly.*)

2. Record accurately all intake and output and chart character of material aspirated.

3. Encourage patient to take clear fluids as ordered.

4. Carry out frequent mouth cleansing.

5. Report throat discomfort to doctor.

6. Make sure that nasal passage is kept lubricated.

Care of Patient While Tube Is in Place

Encourage him. Try to lessen the discomfort of the tube by helping him to keep in mind the importance of the treatment.

Irrigation of the Tube

EQUIPMENT

Tray or bowl with towel acting as lining and cover
20-cc. Luer syringe with irrigating adapter

NURSING TECHNICS

1 small emesis basin
1 small solution cup with tap water
1 dressing towel in tray

PROCEDURE

1. Turn off suction machine, disconnect the Miller-Abbott tube and aspirate it, using 20-cc. syringe and emesis basin.

2. Instill ordered amount of water (usually 120 cc.) in 40-cc. series, aspirating *after each 40 cc.*

3. When all possible fluid has been aspirated, reconnect the Miller-Abbott tube to suction machine. *Turn on suction machine.*

4. Measure amount of return, noting its character. Wash emesis basin and return to tray at bedside.

5. Record:
   Time of irrigation
   Total amount of water instilled
   Total amount of fluid aspirated
   Description of returns

Removal of the Tube

USUAL INDICATIONS FOR

No vomiting
No distention
Passage of flatus
No recurrence of symptoms after tube has been clamped off for 24 to 48 hours
Obviously a doctor's order is necessary.

PROCEDURE

1. Withdraw tube slowly—for a distance of 6 in.

2. Tape the tube to patient's nose or cheek to prevent its slipping back.

3. Repeat steps 1 and 2 until the 75-cm. mark is reached. It may be assumed then that the tube is in the patient's stomach.

4. Attach a syringe to the balloon end of the tube and remove the air from the balloon. Continue to aspirate until all air is removed.

NOTE: The mercury in the balloon will not hinder the removal of the air.

5. Completely withdraw the tube as for any naso-gastric tube.

Care of Tubes After Treatment

1. Keep balloon side closed so that the mercury is not lost. Do not inject water into the balloon.
2. Remove all adhesive marks on tubes with benzine.
3. Soak in soap and water for 20 minutes.
4. Inject soap and water through tube with syringe.
5. Rinse.
6. Additional cleansing depending on the nature of the tube.

MURPHY DRIP

The Murphy drip is used to increase body fluids.

Solutions Used

Warm water or normal saline, half strength

Temperature

95° to 100° F.

Duration of Treatment

Length of treatment is prescribed by the doctor: usually 20 to 40 drops per minute for 2 hours; a rest period of 2 hours; treatment for 2 hours; etc.

Equipment

Catheter No. 18
Irrigation can or Kolinsky flask
Murphy drip bulb
Rubber tubing—2 pieces
Glass irrigating tip
Hoffman clamp
Lubricant
Emesis basin
Half sheet and protecting material
Irrigation stand

Procedure

1. Protect the bed.
2. Connect the irrigating can to the proper end of the Murphy drip bulb by means of a 12-in. piece of rubber

tubing. Connect the free end of the bulb to the catheter by means of tubing and the glass irrigating tip. Before connecting the tubing and bulb slip the Hoffman clamp in place.

3. Place the irrigating can on the stand. Expel the air from the tubing by allowing the solution to run through it. Regulate the number of drops per minute by means of the clamp and bulb. Lubricate the catheter and insert it into the rectum about 3 in.

4. Record the amount of solution retained in 12 hours, any expulsion of flatus and feces and any unusual symptoms.

5. A hot-water bag may be placed over the tubing near the rectum to maintain the proper temperature. This is believed by many to be unnecessary, since a solution flowing so slowly can again cool before it enters the rectum and the amount administered per minute is so small that it will at once take on the body temperature and not produce any irritation or discomfort.

Important Points

1. Care must be taken to prevent the backing up of the solution.

2. Flatus or feces in the rectum will prevent proper absorption. This may be relieved by a small enema. (A doctor's order is necessary for this.)

MUSTARD PASTE

Equipment

The amount of ingredients used will depend on the area to be covered. The proportions of flour and mustard vary according to the patient's age, sensitiveness of the patient's skin and the number of applications already given.

Average Proportions

Adult—1 part mustard to 4 to 6 parts flour
Child—1 part mustard to 5 to 8 parts flour
Infant—1 part mustard to 1 to 12 parts flour
Dry mustard (powder)
Flour

Tepid water

Spoon and bowl

Muslin or heavy paper—twice the size of the area to be covered.

Towel

Hot-water bag—or other means of warming the paste

Procedure

1. Mix the desired amount of flour and mustard.
2. Add tepid water to form a thick paste.
3. Spread mixture on one half of the muslin or paper. Fold other half to enclose the paste.
4. Warm the paste to make it more comfortable for the patient.
5. Wrap in towel to retain warmth until it is applied.
6. Apply paste to the prescribed area. Cover with towel to protect the patient's gown and bedding.
7. Observe the area every 5 to 10 minutes. Remove when skin is reddened or after one half hour.
8. Wash the area to remove the oily deposit on the skin.

NOTE: A fresh paste must be prepared for each application.

NASOGASTRIC TUBE

Equipment

As for Miller-Abbott tube

Nasogastric tube No. 18 French

Tray or bowl arranged with a towel as lining and a cover for equipment

Luer syringe—20 cc. with irrigating adapter

Small solution cup with tap water

Emesis basin

Suction machine or wall suction outlets, s.o.s.

Procedure

INSERTION OF THE TUBE

1. Support the patient in a sitting position.
2. Protect patient's gown with bib.

3. Assist doctor in lubricating and inserting tube.

4. Instruct patient to take deep breaths and swallow as directed while catheter is passed. Sips of water may help the patient to swallow the tube.

5. Secure tubing to patient's nose and forehead or cheek. Keep tube out of patient's line of vision.

6. Fold over end of tube and secure with an elastic band or attach to suction if ordered.

IRRIGATION OF THE TUBE

1. Turn off suction machine, disconnect the nasogastric tube and aspirate it using 20-cc. syringe and emesis basin.

NOTE: If patient has just had an esophageal or gastric operation, irrigation should be *very* gentle. Notify the doctor if there is an unusual return or no return after the irrigation.

2. Instill ordered amount of water in 20-cc. parts, aspirating all possible fluid after each 20-cc. instillation (the total amount ordered usually is 60 cc.).

3. When all possible fluid has been aspirated, reconnect the nasogastric tube to suction machine. *Turn on suction machine.*

4. Measure the amount of return, noting its character. Wash emesis basin and return to tray at the bedside.

5. Record the following on the "Irrigation Slip" attached to the over-the-bed table.

Time of irrigation
Total amount of water instilled
Total amount of fluid aspirated
Description of returns.

NEBULIZER, ADMINISTRATION OF MEDICATION BY

A nebulizer is used to administer medication in the form of a fine spray which, when inhaled, deposits particles of solutions upon the mucous membranes of the respiratory tract.

Equipment

Bronchodilators (Vaponefrin, Neo-Synephrine, etc.)
    Medication as ordered
    2-cc. syringe
    No. 22 needle
    Nebulizer with drug
    Y-tube
    $\frac{3}{16}$-in. to $\frac{3}{32}$-in. rubber tubing, 2 lengths
        1—12 in.
        1—3$\frac{1}{2}$ to 4 ft.
Oxygen regulator or flowmeter
Oxygen piping outlet or oxygen cylinder
Regulator wrench
Antibiotics (penicillin, streptomycin, etc.)
  Same as above, but add the following, if saline rinse is ordered.
    2-cc. syringe
    Isotonic saline 0.5 cc.
    Mouthpiece
    Rubber connector
    Rebreathing bag

Preparation of Equipment

1. Draw up ordered amount of medication
2. Draw up 0.5 cc. saline in second syringe if saline rinse is ordered
3. Connect equipment
   A. Bronchodilators, as shown in Diagram 1

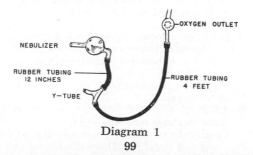

Diagram 1

NURSING TECHNICS

B. Antibiotics, as shown in Diagram 1. If rebreathing bag is ordered, follow Diagram 2

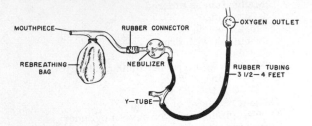

Procedure

1. Have patient assume a comfortable position, sitting preferably.
2. Remove both corks from nebulizer.
3. Place medication in nebulizer.
4. Turn on oxygen at rate of 5 to 8 L. per minute.
5. Create spray by placing thumb over open end of Y-tube.
6. Discontinue spray by releasing thumb.
7. Instruct patient in technic of nebulization.
    A. Bronchodilators
    Breathe out normally
    Place nebulizer tip in mouth just inside the teeth
    Place thumb over open end of Y-tube
    Inhale slowly through mouth more deeply than
        normally
    Remove thumb from open end of Y-tube
    Hold inspiration for a moment
    Exhale
    Continue alternating inhalation and exhalation
        —thumb on open end of Y-tube for inhalation;
        off for exhalation—until medication is used
        completely
    Stop for a few minutes if dizzy or tired
    Force cough
    B. Antibiotics
    Same as above for steps 1 to 9
    Be alert to signs of hypersensitivity, e.g., wheezing and coughing. Discontinue and call doctor
    Nebulize 0.5 cc. of saline (if ordered)

Assist patient to rinse his mouth and gargle with tap water

Give patient a drink of water

After-care of Equipment

1. Concurrent
   A. Wash nebulizer (mouthpiece and rebreathing bag if used) in warm soapy water.
   B. Rinse thoroughly in warm tap water.
2. Terminal
   A. Same as above including the tubing
   B. Soak nebulizer and mouthpiece in benzalkonium chloride 1:1,000 for 1 hour

Recording of Treatment

1. Record medication and time of initial treatment.
2. Record patient's reactions.
3. Indicate patient's ability to perform the treatment by himself.

NOSE DROPS

Administration

The passages of the nasal tract are so complicated that unless nasal medication is administered properly it may not reach the area where it is needed most.

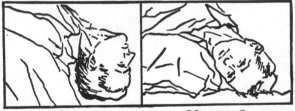

METHOD 1   METHOD 2

Procedure

METHOD 1. Lie on back with head hanging far down over side of bed, as shown in illustration above (*left*). Insert drops in both nostrils. Stay in this position for 5 minutes, turning head slowly from side to side as far as possible. (This should not be practiced with children.) Then sit up and lower head forward and down, eyes facing floor. Maintain position about 30 seconds (to keep drops from running down throat too soon).

METHOD 2. Lie on side, with large pillow supporting lower shoulder, head as shown in illustration above. Insert drops in *lower* nostril. Stay in this position about 5 minutes, breathing through mouth only. Complete by turning head to face downward, maintaining position for several minutes. Lie on other side and repeat in *other* nostril.

ORAL HYGIENE

GENERAL CARE

The nurse's responsibility is one of health teaching and, in the instance of caring for a patient confined to bed, making the equipment for adequate care available to the patient and assisting the patient as necessary.

Equipment

Toothbrush—usually with "medium" bristles: line of the bristles straight; bristles spaced to allow for proper cleaning of the brush.

Dentifrice—very mildly abrasive, flavored to the patient's taste.

NOTE: Salt and soda or oxygen-liberating preparations, such as sodium perborate, should be used only on the recommendation of the physician.

Mouthwash—according to the patient's taste.

NOTE: A normal salt solution or salt and soda makes an inexpensive, acceptable mouthwash.

Face towel

Emesis basin

Drinking tube, s.o.s.

Procedure

1. Arrange patient comfortably, place the towel under his chin, squeeze the paste out on the brush and give this and the cup of water to patient.

2. Allow patient to cleanse his mouth (teeth, gums, tongue, etc.).

3. Assist him by holding the emesis basin in place and relieving him of the articles as used.

4. Have him rinse his mouth with the clear water or an acceptable mouthwash.

5. When the patient is unable to brush his teeth, the nurse should not hesitate to assume this respon-

sibility. Brushing probably affords the most effective care.

6. The patient should be offered this care at least twice a day and oftener, if his condition indicates. A patient with very little appetite for food and fluids may be encouraged to take both if his mouth is cleansed before and after he is offered these.

SPECIAL CARE

When Indicated

1. When lesions or inflammation in the patient's mouth make general care impossible, for example following mouth surgery, carcinoma of the tongue, stomatitis, gingivitis, etc.

2. When a patient is unable to co-operate in any way with the procedure.

3. When a patient's facial muscles are to be kept as quiet as possible, for example following plastic surgery or eye surgery.

Equipment

A small tray or bowl should be kept at the bedside. This should contain glasses for the solution, lubricant, mouth wipes, toothpick swabs, drinking tube, tongue depressors and emesis basin.

Procedure

1. Use mouth wipes to cleanse the teeth, the gums and the roof of the mouth. Remove particles of food with the toothpick swabs. Pad a tongue depressor with gauze and use to cleanse the tongue, or hold the tongue with one hand, and use the wipes to remove the secretions.

2. Padded tongue depressors saturated with a rinsing solution may be pressed gently against the cheeks or gums. The patient's head should be turned to one side and the solution allowed to flow into an emesis basin.

NOTE: A syringe, with a short piece of rubber tubing attached, often is useful in rinsing the patient's mouth.

3. Cold cream or a lubricant of some kind applied to the patient's lips is often very acceptable.

4. If a patient's mouth is dry and he is breathing through his mouth, a moistened piece of gauze placed over his lips is comfortable.

REMOVABLE DENTURES

General Consideration

1. Any sensitiveness the patient may feel regarding removable dentures should be appreciated by the nurse.

2. The same diligent care must be given to removable dentures as to teeth.

3. The patient's mouth, gums, tongue, etc., must be cared for as usual.

4. If possible, the patient should wear the dentures for some part of every day to maintain the proper condition and contour of his gums and cheeks.

5. Provision must be made for keeping the dentures moist and safe when they are not in the patient's mouth.

Equipment

Toothbrush

Dentifrice—carefully selected (certain chemicals are injurious to the composition holding the teeth or may cause discoloration of the teeth)

An acceptable mouthwash

Emesis basin or a basin of water

Towel and drinking tube, s.o.s.

Covered jar—preferably glass, with water or mouthwash

Procedure

1. Provide the necessary equipment and assist the patient as necessary.

2. When the nurse brushes the teeth:

A. They should be held over a basin of water to reduce any damage that may be done if they are dropped accidentally.

B. Give special care to the inner surface of any clips used to hold a bridge in place.

C. Rinse the teeth thoroughly before returning them to the patient.

3. See that the dentures are properly cared for when they are not in the patient's mouth.

NOTE: A transparent container is recommended for this purpose because it allows the nurse to observe, unobtrusively, the condition of the dentures.

OXYGEN THERAPY

Purpose

To administer a sufficiently high concentration of oxygen to overcome or relieve the patient's symptoms of oxygen want. To maintain the temperature and humidity at comfortable levels in an oxygen tent. To administer positive pressure on expiration with a positive pressure mask in certain clinical conditions as pulmonary edema, obstructive dyspnea and asthma. To administer a high relative humidity with a Croupette in certain clinical conditions as croup or following a tracheotomy. To enable a patient to inhale aerosolized medications for action directly on the respiratory tract.

Preparation of Patient

When oxygen is to be administered, it is important to gain the patient's co-operation by explaining carefully what is going to be done and, thus, calm any fear or anxiety that may exist. Only in this way can the maximum effectiveness of the treatment be obtained.

A doctor's order is necessary for all oxygen therapy.

Source of Oxygen Supply

	CYLINDER OF OXYGEN	PIPING SYSTEM OUTLET VALVE
Equipment needed to use oxygen	Cylinder strap or stand Oxygen regulator Regulator wrench Caution signs	Flowmeter Piping system wrench Caution signs
Procedure to use oxygen supply	Crack cylinder outside of patient's room Stabilize cylinder Attach regulator Close regulator handscrew by making it loose (turn counterclockwise) Slowly open cylinder valve completely Adjust desired rate of flow by turning regulator handscrew clockwise (tighten)	Remove dust cap from wall outlet valve Connect flowmeter and tighten with wrench Flowmeter must be exactly vertical and valve must be closed Turn top nut counterclockwise on outlet valve with finger until fully open Adjust desired rate of flow by turning flowmeter handwheel counterclockwise
NOTE: *Follow procedure specific to method of oxygen administration ordered*		
Discontinuing use of oxygen supply	Close cylinder valve Close regulator handscrew by making it loose Remove regulator	Close outlet valve by turning clockwise Close flowmeter by turning handwheel clockwise Remove flowmeter Replace dustcap on outlet valve

NURSING TECHNICS

General Precautions

When therapeutic gases and equipment are used, safety precautions are necessary for the following reasons:

1. Oxygen supports combustion. Material that burns slowly in air, flares up and burns with great rapidity in an atmosphere high in oxygen.

2. Flammable materials, such as oil, grease, mineral oil and petrolatum, may undergo spontaneous combustion with oxygen under high pressure, and the heat from such combustion may cause spread of the fire and melting of the metal, permitting escape of the oxygen.

3. The high pressure in an oxygen cylinder itself warrants proper control by a suitable regulator.

4. The weight of the cylinder is considerable; therefore, damage to equipment and injury to personnel or patients may occur if a cylinder is tipped over.

Precautions Regarding Cylinders and Equipment

1. Inspect the label on the cylinder to ascertain its contents.

2. Keep cylinders away from all sources of flame, sparks, combustible substances, such as oil, grease and paint and all flammable materials.

3. Keep cylinders in a dry place, away from hot radiators and steam pipes.

4. Transport cylinders only on cylinder carrier.

5. Arrange cylinder in use so that it cannot be tipped over accidentally. Fasten to bed with strap, use cylinder stand or place in corner or wall recess.

6. Always crack cylinder valve outside patient's room before attaching regulator.

7. Never use a cylinder without a regulator.

8. Never use oil or grease on cylinders, piping outlets, regulators or flowmeters.

9. Wash oily or greasy hands before handling oxygen equipment or connections.

Precautions Regarding Patients and Oxygen Administration

All persons who come in contact with a patient receiving oxygen (nurses, doctors, patients, visitors, technicians, etc.) should be made aware of the following precautions:

1. *No Smoking!* Remove all tobacco, cigarettes, pipes and matches from patient; repeat inspection after visitors leave.

2. Warn patient and other occupants of the room against smoking and of the fire hazard.

3. Warn visitors against smoking and providing smoking supplies to the patient.

4. Prohibit use of devices such as switches, cautery, signal light switches, heating lamps, alcohol lamps and heating pads.

5. Prohibit use of x-ray, EKG and physical therapy equipment unless the oxygen concentration is reduced to atmospheric level.

6. Do not give oil or alcohol rubs or use readily ignitible substances while the patient is in a tent.

7. Do not allow oxygen to flow when a patient is not using equipment.

Suggested Oxygen Flows in Liters per Minute for Oxygen Administration

OXYGEN TENT, MOTOR DRIVEN, ICE OR ICELESS

For Adults: Start and continue with 12 L./min. No flushing will be necessary when 50 per cent oxygen concentration is desired.

For Children 6 to 12 Years: Start and continue with 10 L./min. oxygen flow. No flushing will be necessary when 50 per cent oxygen concentration is desired.

HEAD TENT, CLOSED TOP

For Adults: Use concentration meter set at 50 per cent and 8 to 12 L./min. oxygen flow. No flushing is necessary.

For Children up to 6 Years: Use concentration meter set at 50 per cent and 4 to 6 L./min. oxygen flow. No flushing is necessary.

CROUPETTE, FOR CHILDREN OR ADULTS: Start and continue with 8 L./min. No flushing necessary.

NURSING TECHNICS

OXYGEN INCUBATORS (ISOLETTE, ARMSTRONG-ROBERTS): Follow directions of manufacturer. Usually, flush at 6 to 8 L./min. for 20 minutes, then turn back to setting for desired concentration.

METER MASK, REGULAR OR POSITIVE PRESSURE: Liter flow is determined and adjusted according to the inflation and deflation of the reservoir bag. The reservoir bag should collapse partially but never completely during inspiration. Always use a concentration meter.

NASAL CATHETER, OROPHARYNGEAL OR DEEP CATHETER TECHNIC

Approximate Concentration	Small Patient	Medium Patient	Large Patient
35%	4 L./min.	5 L./min.	6 L./min.
40%	5 L./min.	6 L./min.	7 L./min.
42 to 45%	6 L./min.	7 L./min.	8 L./min.

NASAL CATHETER, NASOPHARYNGEAL OR SHALLOW TECHNIC

Approximate Concentration	Small Patient	Medium Patient	Large Patient
28%	2 L./min.	3 L./min.	4 L./min.
33%	4 L./min.	5 L./min.	6 L./min.
38%	6 L./min.	7 L./min.	8 L./min.
42%	8 L./min.	9 L./min.	10 L./min.

DOUBLE BENT NASAL CANNULA

Approximate Concentration	Oxygen Flow	
26%	2 L./min.	
28%	4 L./min.	
33%	6 L./min.	Average size adult
38%	8 L./min.	
40%	9 L./min.	

FACE TENT: Use concentration meter set at 50 per cent and 6 to 8 L./min. oxygen flow.

AEROSOL (FOR ANTIBIOTICS, VASOCONSTRICTORS, ETC.): Use 5 to 8 L./min. oxygen flow.

METHODS OF OXYGEN ADMINISTRATION

	ICELESS TENT	HOOD TENT	CROUPETTE
Equipment needed	Oxygen supply Oxygen tent with canopy Pressure tubing	Oxygen supply Complete head tent Concentration meter Tubing for water waste Small size ice Basin or pail	Oxygen supply Complete Croupette Tubing for oxygen Tubing for water waste Distilled water Basin or pail Small size ice
To start treatment	Bring all equipment to bedside. Connect tubing to regulator or flowmeter and inlet on tent. Start motor and oxygen flowing at 12 L./min. Place canopy over patient Cover entire bed, tuck adequately under mattress Adjust temperature to patient's comfort by setting thermostat	Bring all equipment to bedside. Fill ice chamber three fourths full. Attach concentration meter to regulator or flowmeter and preset at prescribed concentration. Connect tubing. Place tent over patient's head, with oxygen flowing at 6 to 8 L./min. for children; 8 to 12 L./min. for adults. Place basin under drainage tubing	Bring all equipment to bedside. Fill ice chamber three fourths full. Fill water jar. Start oxygen flow at 8 L./min. Attach tubing. Place tent over patient's head. Place basin under drainage tubing
Continuation of treatment	No flushing is necessary Do not use less than 12 L./min. because carbon dioxide will accumulate. Check oxygen supply frequently. Empty drain basin in back of tent Remove canopy for alcohol or oil rubs. Wash hands after any rub. Turn canopy infrequently. Turn motor off when opening canopy	No flushing is necessary Do not use tent in drafty room. Replace ice frequently. Tubing should not be kinked or pinched Check oxygen supply frequently	No flushing is necessary Always start oxygen flow before connecting tubing. Adjust damper valve on top of stand pipe to control humidity. Keep water jar full. Check oxygen supply frequently. Replace used ice frequently
Discontinuation of treatment and after-care of equipment	Remove canopy from patient Disconnect all attachments Wash outside of canopy Turn canopy inside out, wash with soap and water Dry. Replace equipment neatly, ready for future use	Remove tent from patient. Disconnect all attachments. Empty ice chamber Wash entire tent with soap, and dry. Replace equipment neatly, ready for future use	Remove Croupette from patient. Disconnect all attachments. Empty ice chamber and water jar. Wash entire tent with soap and water. Dry. Replace equipment neatly, ready for future use. Do not use alcohol on this tent.

METHODS OF OXYGEN ADMINISTRATION (Continued)

	Nasal Catheter or Cannula	Regular Meter Mask	Positive Pressure Mask
Equipment needed	Oxygen supply Humidifier Proper size tubing Straight glass connector No. 10 or 12 French catheter with extra holes at end Lubricant (water soluble) Narrow adhesive tape Safety pin, large	Oxygen supply Complete meter mask Concentration meter Large bore rubber tubing (Complete meter mask consists of facepiece, expiratory valve, inspiratory valve, reservoir bag and headstrap)	Oxygen supply Complete pressure mask Concentration meter Large bore rubber tubing (Complete pressure mask consists of facepiece, pressure disk in place of expiratory valve, reservoir bag and 2 sets of headstraps)
To start treatment	Bring all equipment to bedside Fill humidifier one half full with water Attach humidifier to regulator or flowmeter, tubing to humidifier, and catheter to tubing with glass connection Determine depth catheter is to be inserted by measuring distance from external nostril to tragus of ear Mark distance on catheter Start oxygen flow as prescribed Lubricate catheter tip sparingly Test in a glass of water Insert catheter slowly through nose into oropharynx. Check position by observing patient's mouth whether catheter tip is opposite uvula Adjust oxygen flow as per doctor's order	Bring all equipment to bedside Attach concentration meter to regulator or flowmeter. Set at prescribed oxygen concentration Attach tubing to concentration meter and inspiratory valve of mask Start oxygen at 8 L./min. Adjust mask to patient's face Gradually adjust liter flow to a sufficient rate so that reservoir bag partially, collapses at depth of inspiration regardless of prescribed oxygen concentration The liter flow will vary with the pulmonary ventilation of each patient	*Caution:* do not use in shock or Peripheral Vascular Failure Positive pressure requires presence of a doctor Procedure is same as regular mask Set prescribed pressure by rotating calibrated disk on facepiece until hole corresponding to the pressure is at the top

METHODS OF OXYGEN ADMINISTRATION (Concluded)

	Nasal Catheter or Cannula	Regular Meter Mask	Positive Pressure Mask
Continuation of treatment	Change catheter q. 8 h. and insert in alternate nostril Check oxygen supply frequently Maintain one half full water level in humidifier Check for oxygen leaks at humidifier top and tubing connections	Mask should fit snugly against face. Reservoir bag should be partially inflated at all times Remove mask q. 2 h. to wash patient's face Do not tape or remove expiratory flutter valve on facepiece	Same as for regular meter mask Check position of mask, leaks and oxygen supply
Discontinuation of treatment and care of equipment	Remove catheter Disconnect all attachments Wash catheter with soap and water, rinse and boil for 5 minutes	Wash facepiece, bag and inspiratory valve with soap and water, rinse and wrap in gauze. Boil for 5 minutes. Dry. Lightly powder facepiece and reservoir bag Put away neatly	Decrease pressure 1 cm. gradually until no pressure is obtained Same as for regular meter mask

[111]

PACK, SEDATIVE

A sedative pack is a prolonged application of wet sheets to body surfaces. It is used for a sedative effect.

Equipment

4 cotton blankets
2 large sheets—fanfolded
3 half-sheets if needed for restraint
Large water-repellent sheet
Patient's gown
Face towel, bath towel
Ice bag with cover
Blanket roll, p.r.n.
Bottle olive oil with roll of cotton, or a jar of cold cream
Bottle 60 per cent alcohol
Shaker of talcum
Foot tub

Procedure

1. Immerse fanfolded sheets and 1 half-sheet in water of from 50° to 70° F. in foot tub. Wring fairly dry.

2. Place wet sheets and the half-sheet on bottom of empty foot tub, protecting sheet next, then dry blankets. Fill ice bag and place in foot tub along with other equipment.

3. Carry all equipment to bedside.

4. Explain the treatment and reassure the patient.

5. Have the patient void.

6. Remove the patient's clothing. Oil his skin if indicated.

7. Wrap the patient in dry blanket.

8. Fanfold bed clothing to foot of bed.

9. Place protecting sheet on bed.

10. Place cotton blanket over protecting sheet.

11. Place pack blanket over protecting sheet. Arrange the blanket so that one third of it lies in the center of bed, two thirds to right.

12. Arrange second pack blanket so that one third of it lies in center of bed, two thirds to left.

13. Arrange third blanket, folded in thirds, at foot of bed.

14. Place wet sheets on pack blankets in same manner as above.

15. Fold back 6 in. of upper hem of pack sheets.

16. (Place half-sheet, folded in half, in center of bed if restraint is indicated.)

17. Arrange the patient in center of sheets.

18. Loosen blanket that has been wrapped around patient, so that it acts purely as a draping blanket.

19. Draw wet sheets across patient's trunk under the armpit and place between the legs.

20. Remove the draping blanket and turn the patient to side.

21. Smooth sheet under back and legs. (The sheet should end at patient's legs.)

22. Roll the patient onto his back and place arms straight at sides.

23. Draw second wet sheet across patient's trunk, the upper border of the sheet being grasped with the right hand (the upper border is drawn at right angles to the clavicle downward).

24. Fold the border at right angles, tuck under opposite shoulder and draw sheet smoothly over trunk and legs.

25. Turn patient to side, smooth sheets under back and legs and drape sheet loosely over feet.

26. Apply blankets in same manner as the second wet sheet

27. Drape foot blanket, anchoring under calves of legs.

28. Place pillow under shoulders and head.

29. Place blanket roll under knees for 10° flexion, or raise foot of bed to 10° flexion and dorsiflex the feet.

(If the patient is not under constant observation, side rails must be applied to the bed, padded as indicated. If restraining sheets are needed, use 2 half-sheets over the pack, one over chest, one over thighs. If necessary, with a doctor's order, bed restraint may be applied.)

30. Place spread over the patient. (Spread already on bed may be used.)

31. Place towel on spread under chin and place ice bag at nape of neck or on forehead.

32. Groom patient as attractively as possible.

33. Darken room, maintain quiet and remove unnecessary equipment.

34. Determine temporal pulse, respiration. Note color, shivering, violent chill, restlessness, degree of sedation, talking, etc.

NOTE: Note and record above observations every 15 minutes. When patient falls asleep, omit check of pulse if it is disturbing and is not otherwise indicated. Shivering is a normal initial reaction and may last for 5 minutes.

The patient should be removed from the pack immediately if:

>He soils the bed

>He is unduly restless

>He shows excessive fear (claustrophobia)

There are untoward vasomotor signs (marked change in pulse rate, pallor, cold clammy skin)

The usual length of treatment is 4 hours, unless otherwise ordered by the physician or otherwise indicated.

Termination of the Treatment

1. Warm the alcohol; have draping blanket, bath towel, clean gown in readiness.

2. Loosen the blankets, remove first wet sheet.

3. Place draping blanket over patient, remove second wet sheet and damp blanket next to it, leaving the patient on dry treatment blanket.

4. Pat the patient dry; give alcohol rub.

5. Observe the skin for pressure areas, abrasions. There should be a generalized pink glow to the skin.

6. Assist the patient into a gown.

7. Remove blankets and rubber sheet used for treatment.

8. Draw up bed covers.

9. Remove equipment from bedside.

10. Permit the patient to rest.

PARACENTESIS

Withdrawal of fluid from the peritoneal cavity is called paracentesis.

Equipment

STERILE TRAY

3 towels—tray covers (4 if tray is kept set up)
4 compresses, 4×4 in.
5-cc. syringe
4 needles:
    1—No. 24 hypodermic
    1—No. 20 or No. 22 intramuscular
    1 curved ⎰
    1 straight ⎱ suture needles
Bard Parker handle No. 3 and blade No. 11
2 trocars and cannulae; 1 curved, 1 straight
Probe
Artery clamp
Mouse-tooth forceps
Needle holder
Scissors
Tube No. 000 catgut
Black silk on wheel, q.s.
Large metal funnel
Rubber tubing with glass connecting tube, q.s.

ADDITIONAL EQUIPMENT

Pair laparotomy stockings or trousers
Sheet, protecting sheet, half-sheet
3 stools or chairs
Pail or 4-pt. bottle
Equipment for skin preparation
Dakin's pad—sterile
Abdominal binder
Safety pins, q.s.

Procedure

1. Arrange the equipment so that it can be used conveniently.

2. Arrange the patient comfortably in a sitting position with his feet resting on a chair or stool.

3. Drape patient's thighs with protecting sheet and half-sheet.

4. Assist doctor with treatment as indicated.

5. Secure dressing and apply an abdominal binder.

NURSING TECHNICS

NOTE:

1. Have patient void before procedure to avoid injury to urinary bladder.

2. Observe the patient's color and vital signs carefully throughout the procedure.

3. Maintain strict aseptic technic.

PEDICULOSIS, TREATMENT OF

Equipment

Towel, smooth-surface
Combs—plain and fine-toothed
Cup or similar container for medication
Absorbent cotton
Towel or material for turban
Safety pins, s.o.s.
Medication: Cuprex, DDT, larkspur tincture, kerosene, etc.

Procedure

1. Comb hair carefully to remove snarls.

2. Part hair into small sections.

3. Apply solution lavishly to small sections of the hair and scalp.

4. Secure hair within a turban.

5. Follow directions for particular medication used. If larkspur tr. is used, give shampoo after 8 hours. Hot vinegar may be applied to assist in the removal of the nits. Watch patient closely for the appearance of more pediculi.

PERICARDIUM, ASPIRATION OF

Equipment

STERILE TRAY

Aspirating needles—2
Luer syringe—50 cc.
Hypodermic syringe with needle
Solution glass
Sponges and compresses

UNSTERILE

Equipment for skin preparation.

Important Points

1. The patient must be in the most comfortable position.

2. Any discomfort, any change in pulse or color, or any coughing must be noted.

3. The nurse prepares the tray, cares for the patient and assists the doctor.

PHLEBOTOMY

Phlebotomy is the removal of blood by opening a vein.

Equipment

STERILE

Deep tray
Dressing towel
Syringes: 2 cc. and 20 cc.
Needles: 1 No. 24, 2 No. 15
Bard Parker handle No. 3
Bard Parker blade No. 11
Tubing: 1 length 12 in.; 1 length 10 in., narrow lumen
2 connecting tubes, glass (bent)
Hose to Luer adapter—glass
Rubber stopper—2 hole
Hoffman clamp
Compress—for dressing
Muslin envelope

ADDITIONAL EQUIPMENT

Aspirating pump
Unsterile graduated bottle
Tray for skin preparation

Procedure

1. Explain treatment to patient and take equipment to bedside.

117

2. Protect bed with water-repellent sheet and towel—put tourniquet in place.

3. Assist doctor in preparing the skin.

4. Open sterile tray.

5. After doctor has placed stopper in graduated bottle, close Hoffman clamp on collecting tube.

6. Attach aspirating pump to other tube and make a vacuum in the bottle.

7. When adapter has been attached to needle and clamp released, pump as necessary until desired amount of blood has been removed.

8. Watch patient's pulse, color and general condition.

9. At completion of treatment see that the patient is comfortable. Remove equipment from bedside.

NOTE: 1. If blood collected is to be used for a transfusion, the collecting bottle must be sterile and contain an anticoagulant.

2. Commercially prepared, disposable "donor sets" (blood donor) may be used for this procedure.

POSITIONS FOR EXAMINATION AND TREATMENT

Dorsal Recumbent

Place the patient flat on her back with one pillow under the head and her knees flexed and separated (feet flat on the bed).

METHOD OF DRAPING. Replace the bed covers with a sheet that is crosswise of the bed. Gather the center of the sheet up between the patient's legs and place the fullness above the pubes. The lower edge of the sheet covers the inner aspects of the thighs and the corners are draped about the feet and fastened about the ankles. Place a towel under the buttocks.

NOTE: Large triangular-shaped leggings may be used —the long end covering the pubic area.

Sims's Position

Place the patient on her left side with the buttocks at the edge of the mattress. Incline the body forward, draw the left arm back under the patient and place the right arm forward. Flex both legs, the right over the left with the knee touching the mattress.

METHOD OF DRAPING. Replace the bed covers with a sheet that is crosswise of the bed. Assist the patient into position. Gather up the center of the sheet and place the fullness near the lumbar region. Drape the lower edge of the sheet about the legs and feet. Place a folded towel under the buttocks.

Lithotomy Position

Place the patient on her back across the bed with the buttocks slightly beyond the edge of the mattress. Flex the thighs on the abdomen and separate the knees. Have 2 assistants support the legs or support them by means of a sheet folded diagonally and passed under the knees and around the neck and tied over one shoulder.

NOTE: The patient should wear stockings or leggings.

Knee-chest Position

Place the patient in the prone position. Assist the patient to kneel so that her weight rests on her chest and knees. Turn her head to one side and flex her arms at the elbows, extending them on the bed in front of her. Be sure that the thighs are perpendicular.

METHOD OF DRAPING. Replace the bed covers with a sheet that is crosswise of the bed. Cover the lower part of the patient's body with the draping sheet, selvage edge at her waist. Pin the 2 upper corners of the sheet together at the center of the patient's back. The circle of sheet thus created should be arranged to expose the perineal area. The remainder of the sheet may be used to cover the legs and the feet.

See also MATERNITY NURSING

POSTMORTEM CARE*

Equipment
Brush and comb
Muslin

---

* Commercial packs are available. Directions for their use are supplied with the packs.

NURSING TECHNICS

Shroud
Muslin bandage; gauze bandage—2 in.
Absorbent cotton
Tags and safety pins
Paper bag
Equipment for bathing patient

Procedure

1. As soon as possible after the patient ceases to breathe and the doctor has pronounced the patient dead, the body should be straightened (pillows, shock blocks, etc., removed). Close the eyelids gently, using pieces of moistened cotton to keep the lids down if necessary.

2. Remove jewelry and place for safekeeping.

3. Wash patient's face with soap and water. Replace false teeth or eyes if these have been removed.

4. Cut a piece of muslin bandage long enough to go under the chin and tie on top of the head. Cut a 4-in. slit in the bandage for the chin. Divide the ends of the bandage in two. Tie the 2 lower pieces on top of the head and the upper pieces at the back of the neck.

5. Usually catheters, i.e., nasogastric, indwelling bladder catheters, etc., may be removed. However, it is wise to ascertain a doctor's or institution's practice in this regard as well as to the removal of drains or tubes in wounds.

6. Wash the entire body. Apply a fresh dressing if indicated.

7. Cut a muslin square to make a double-thickness diaper. Secure with safety pins as a diaper.

8. Place arms across chest and tie wrists with gauze bandage. Pad with cotton to prevent discoloration due to pressure. Tie an identifying tag on the bandage.

9. Place shroud diagonally over body bringing the corner at the top over the head and down to the middle of the back. Bring the opposite corner over the feet similarly to the back of the knees.

10. Tuck the corner nearest the head under the opposite arm, turn body on one side and push the remainder of the shroud under the body. Turn body on other side and bring the remaining corner to the ankles.

Fasten here with gauze bandage and attach second tag. Tie another bandage around the neck of the body.

11. Cover body with top sheet until mortuary stretcher arrives.

POSTURAL DRAINAGE

Gravity is used to facilitate drainage of bronchial secretions.

Equipment
Bedside chair
2 large emesis basins
Tooth mug with mouthwash and small emesis basin
Celluwipes, q.s.

Procedure
1. Explain procedure and its purpose to patient.
2. Put the bedside chair facing and close to the side of the bed, with one large emesis basin on the seat.
3. Draw the curtains, assist the patient to lean far over the edge of the bed, head hanging down and palms on the seat of the chair.
4. Instruct the patient to cough and expectorate into the large emesis basin for 10 to 15 minutes. (Watch for signs of weakness or fatigue.) When the lungs and bronchial tree are considerably higher than the mouth, the law of gravity is utilized and the patient may produce 100 to 400 cc. of sputum.
5. Assist the patient into a comfortable position following the treatment and offer the mouthwash to rinse the mouth.
6. Arrange the unit and remove equipment.
7. Measure amount of sputum collected, note the color and consistency and *record*.

POULTICE, FLAXSEED

A poultice is used to apply moist heat to the skin by means of a hot, moist paste.

Equipment
Flaxseed meal and water
Saucepan; cup or tablespoon

NURSING TECHNICS

Spatula or long spoon
Sodium bicarbonate
Towel, abdominal pad or Turkish towel
Oiled paper
Old muslin
Gauze or cheesecloth 4 in. larger in all dimensions than the muslin.

Procedure

1. Cut muslin 2 in. larger in all directions than area to be covered. If gauze or cheesecloth is not used, cut muslin twice the size of area to be covered—use as an envelope.

2. Cut abdominal pad and oiled paper the size of area to be covered.

3. Open the towel, on it place the pad, the oiled paper and the muslin in that order. These items should be arranged one on top of the other.

4. Place water in saucepan (1 qt. for large abdominal poultice). Boil.

5. Add flaxseed meal slowly, stirring constantly.

6. When mixture is of semisolid consistency (will drop from spatula or spoon), remove mixture from fire.

7. Add 1 tsp. soda bicarbonate.

8. Beat.

9. Spread mixture on muslin leaving a 1½ to 2 in. margin on all sides.

10. Fold edges over paste (as a hem).

11. Cover with gauze or cheesecloth and tuck gauze under poultice.

12. Arrange poultice, oiled paper, pad and towel so that they may be carried easily.

13. Expose the area to which poultice is to be applied. (Dressings may be left in place.)

14. Apply poultice slowly. Raise frequently for patient's comfort and to prevent burning.

15. Watch the area carefully for signs of too great heat. Burns from poultices may be very severe.

16. When the poultice has cooled it may be removed.

NOTE: A new poultice must be made each time but the pad and the towel may be saved for subsequent use for the same patient.

PRESSURE AREAS AND DECUBITI, CARE OF

Prophylaxis

1. Keep the patient's skin clean and dry.
2. Turn the patient at least every 2 hours.
3. Rub patient's back with alcohol or a light oil, as indicated, at least 3 times a day.
4. Give special attention to areas over bony prominences and points of greatest pressure, such as the lower back.
5. Apply cold cream or cocoa butter to dry areas such as patient's heels and elbows, s.o.s.
6. If the patient is incontinent, wash the skin with soap and water and dry thoroughly after each incontinence.

NOTE: Treatment of decubiti is dependent upon the orders of a physician. However, the above-mentioned care also should be given.

SPECIAL MATTRESS (ALTERNATING PRESSURE)

The mattress is composed of 45 tubes, 1¼ in. in diameter, which are alternately inflated and deflated approximately every 5 minutes. This is accomplished by an attached electric pump. The cycle is slow and barely perceptible to the patient. By this means the pressure points under the body are being changed constantly.

How to Install Mattress

1. Place the alternating pressure mattress on the regular mattress, with the air inlet tubes at the foot of the bed.
2. Place the mattress skirt between the regular mattress and the springs at the head of the bed. This feature permits the bed to be raised without allowing the alternating-pressure mattress to slide.
3. Attach the tubing to the pump and connect the pump to the electrical circuit.
4. Allow the mattress to fill before making the bed.

NURSING TECHNICS

Be careful to see that the tubing is not kinked or pinched.

5. For installation in Emerson or Drinker respirators, follow the same procedure as above, except that the air inlet tubing should be at the head of the respirator. A special attachment is provided for entrance of the tubing through the respirator shell.

Cleaning and Sterilizing

1. The mattress cannot be autoclaved.
2. Use soap and warm water to clean the mattress.

How to Repair Leaks in Mattress

1. A "Use No Pins" sign is provided with each unit and should be placed in a conspicuous location so that the conventional nursing practice of pinning items to the mattress will be avoided.

2. A bottle of special pin-hole sealer is provided in the event that a small puncture occurs. Deflate the mattress and apply a small quantity of the pin-hole sealer over the hole with the applicator. Allow to dry 4 hours before inflating.

3. The mattress is guaranteed against seam splitting. In the event that a seam comes open, return the mattress and it will be reheat-sealed and returned as early as possible.

Care of the Pump

The only oiling point required on the pumping unit is at the motor. Add 2 or 3 drops of SAE No. 30 oil to each oil cup every month. At the same time add 2 or 3 drops of the oil through the oil holes in the alternator motor. Every 6 months add 10 to 15 drops through the oil hole in the alternator body (removing the screw exposes the oil hole).

PRINCIPLES OF CARE OF PATIENTS REQUIRING ARTIFICIAL RESPIRATION

1. *Acquaint yourselves with the mechanics of the equipment you are using.* However, remember that the patient, his appearance and reactions are the best indicators of the efficiency of your machine.

2. *Maintain a clear airway.* In order to provide for free exchange of air and carbon dioxide it is imperative that the respiratory tract be clear of obstructions from the mouth to the alveoli of the lungs. The tongue must be in a forward position so that it does not occlude the airway, and the neck must be in good alignment. All food and mucus must be removed from the patient's mouth and nasopharynx mechanically or by suction if the patient is not able to do this for himself. The tracheobronchial tree can be cleared best by having the patient cough if possible, by mechanical cough stimulation or by deep suction. Postural drainage and frequent turning are also necessary to promote drainage of secretions.

Possible agents of respiratory infection should not be allowed near the patient and it is good practice for all who have contact with the patient to wear masks as prophylaxis.

3. *Provide for adequate nutrition and fluid intake in the diet.* Modifications may be necessary if the patient is weak or has loss or weakening of gag reflex. Baby food or liquids may be offered with nasogastric or intravenous fluids as indicated. The patient must be watched carefully for evidence of aspiration.

4. *Provide for integrity of skin, muscles, joints.* Pressure areas may be avoided by frequent lubrication of the skin and change of position and by padding areas which may be subject to considerable pressure. The body must be maintained in a neutral position; foam rubber pads and towel rolls may be used for support if indicated. To be kept supple and free from deformity, the patient is encouraged to move extremities freely and put joints through the range of motion. This is done by the nurse if the patient is incapacitated. It is suggested that the arms be supported on pillows to lessen the energy needed to maintain position and to avoid pressure on the chest wall.

5. *Provide for elimination.* It is extremely important that proper bowel and bladder elimination be provided for, since distention of either type may seriously compromise the patient's vital capacity.

6. *Provide emotional support.* For the patient who

must labor for the "breath of life" someone on whom he can depend is a necessity. The patient is never left alone, and some means of communication must be provided for him. The atmosphere must be as calm as possible, and this can occur only if the nurse knows her technic and her patient. Much co-operation can be gained if the patient is acquainted with the machine used.

The patient's family can assist in this area if they are given adequate information to understand the problems at hand.

Diversion in keeping with the patient's condition should be planned by the nurse in such a way that it will not fatigue him.

RESPIRATOR

The respirator is a means of artificial respiration. The patient's body, with the exception of the head, is inserted into a hollow cylinder. The pressure within the cylinder is decreased below the atmospheric pressure and returned to the atmospheric pressure by the movements of a diaphragm attached to an electric motor.

When the diaphragm moves inward, the air within the tank is compressed, and the pressure is increased. Since the patient's diaphragm is forced upward, the patient exhales.

When the diaphragm moves outward, the air expands, the pressure is reduced; consequently, the patient's diaphragm moves downward. The atmospheric pressure forces the air into the air sacs of the lungs. The negative pressure usually is 15 to 20.

Usually only negative pressure is used. When removal of mucus is desired, positive pressure may be employed under the direction of a physician only. Hyperventilation may be a complicating factor when positive pressure is used, since the patient's reflex control of respiration is interrupted by positive pressure. The positive pressure usually is 5 to 10. (Reflex control is interrupted by negative pressure, also.)

Respirator

1. Head-rest adjuster
2. Bed adjuster
3. Opening for infusions
4. Pressure gauge (shown in negative position)
5. Screw head
6. Hydraulic jack
7. Driving belt (#B42)
8. Motor
9. Respiratory rate adjuster
10. Emergency lever for hand power
11. Cord
12. Pressure adjuster
13. Switch for motor
14. Electric light switch
15. Plugs
16. Pressure adjuster (shown open for negative; to be closed for positive)

NURSING TECHNICS

Warning

1. Too great pressure may cause emphysema, hemorrhages, alkalosis and death.

2. Too rapid a respiratory rate may cause hyperventilation and death.

NOTE: Doctor's order should include rate of respiration, amount of pressure (both negative and positive) when the patient is placed in the respirator.

Equipment

RESPIRATOR

Sponges in all openings except door for inserting large objects.

Leather collar straps at cervical opening if sponge rubber collar is used.

Spare driving belt for the motor.

Bag containing: extra strap, airway, mouth gag, tongue clamp, extra collar and cuffs, neck protector, double plug, towel roll, hand bell

Sponge rubber mattress, plastic-covered

3 half-sheets

Foot support

Small pillow with rubber or plastic cover

Cotton blanket

Electric bulb with wire shield.

UNIT

Powder

Petroleum jelly and applicator

Nasal oxygen equipment

Container of water

Equipment for posturing

Wall outlet free for respirator attachment

Auxiliary continuous suction

Bedside stand for vital signs sheet, fluid slip, mouth-care tray, blood pressure apparatus, thermometer

PREPARATION OF EQUIPMENT

1. Obtain a respirator. (Refer to illustration, p. 127.)
2. Prepare stockinette collar to protect patient's neck.

3. Place respirator to far side of room, bellows away from door.

4. Attach respirator motor to wall outlet.

5. Tightly close plastic collar.

6. Close all openings except the small opening No. 16 labeled "close for positive."

7. Turn on motor.

8. Turn valve No. 12 toward "increase" until the pressure reading is neg. 10 on gauge. No. 4.

9. Count the number of times in a full minute that the diaphragm moves inward (this is the respiratory rate.)

10. Turn wheel No. 9 toward DEC or INC until the rate is 12 to 18.

11. Turn off the motor.

12. Roll the collar backward by pulling back the straps as far as possible, attaching each to the related steel peg or open the plastic collar if it is in use.

13. Open door hasps.

14. Pull out the stretcher.

15. Add linen.

16. Adjust foot support as indicated.

Insertion of the Patient

WARNING: In cases of cervical and suboccipital lesions, *do not flex the neck toward the chest.* Severe complications or death may ensue.

1. Physician and nurse must reassure the patient that the machine will give him needed rest, that it is a temporary measure, that he must relax and let the machine breathe for him, the he will never be left alone and that he can call by prearranged signal.

2. Assemble at least 4 assistants (including physician, anesthetist and engineer) if possible. Have stretcher at the lowest possible level.

3. Transfer the patient to the respirator stretcher by any of the accepted methods. Do not flex the patient's neck.

DRAWING THE HEAD THROUGH THE CERVICAL SPONGE OR PLASTIC COLLAR

1. Assistant at head places one hand over patient's

nose and under patient's head. Patient's nose is in line with the angle of the collar.

2. On count of 3, the patient's trunk is drawn toward the head board.

3. The assistant at the head guides patient's head through. (If there is no suboccipital or cervical lesion, the head can be turned to one side and flexed toward chest.)

4. Place the stockinette collar around patient's neck.

5. Release sponge or plastic collar so that it fits snugly about neck.

NOTE: A soft vinyl plastic collar provides a perfect air seal for all neck sizes. A 10-in. opening facilitates passage of the patient's head. The collar closes to zero, which is an advantage if the nurse wishes to check the pressure readings of the gauge on the respirator before inserting the patient into the respirator. The patient's neck is protected with 1 or 2 layers of stockinette.

TO CLOSE THE COLLAR

1. Loosen the wing nuts "C."

2. Grasp the handles of the collar, turn right or left.

3. Avoid pressure on the patient's carotid arteries and jugular veins by too tight a collar. Check the degree of snugness about the patient's neck with your finger. At times a better fit may be obtained by adjusting the level of the stretcher.

4. An extra layer of stockinette can be used if leaks are a problem.

5. The collar is disposable after use.

AT THE SAME TIME

1. Patient's arms are folded on his chest.

2. The stretcher is pushed into the tank.

3. Door hasps are secured.

4. The motor is turned on.

5. The doctor adjusts the respiratory rate and negative pressure to the patient's individual needs.

6. Patient is taught that when his chest is moving out he is breathing in; when air is pushed out past his neck, he is breathing out.

7. The level of the head is adjusted by wheel "1."

8. The patient's trunk and extremities are postured in neutral alignment.

9. Reassure the patient by suggestion and efficient care.

    A. Tell patient to relax—let machine do the work.

    B. Tell patient he will have difficulty talking because of involuntary respirations.

    C. If allowed fluid by mouth, teach patient to swallow as he breathes out.

Care of the Patient While in the Respirator

The patient is on direct relief—*never left alone.*

All contacts wear masks so as to protect the patient from possible infection. It is suggested that no persons with upper respiratory infections be allowed near patient.

The graduate nurse adjusts the pressure and respiratory controls only as needed to maintain the rate and the pressure set by the physician and/or the anesthetist.

The nurse suctions the patient as indicated.

Whenever anything is done for the patient check all handles on portholes to make certain that they are tight.

OBSERVATIONS:

1. Report to physician any irregularity of excursion of chest wall (may indicate mucous plug in trachea).

2. Use of alae nasa.

3. Accessory muscles of respiration.

4. Cyanosis

5. Choking

6. Diminishing amount of air coming through nose and mouth.

Patient's posture is changed at least every 2 hours, and exercise to the joints is given.

1. Bed can be tilted to right or left. See wheels No. 2.

2. Patient can be rotated to abdomen with permission of physician.

3. Dorsiflex feet with holster.

4. Flex knees 5° to 10° with a small towel or blanket roll.

5. Place support under lumbar curvature if needed.

6. Support arms on pillows, with towel roll to prevent wrist drop position.

7. Place towel rolls to side of legs to prevent outward rotation contractures.

8. Elevate heels from mattress with strip of foam rubber.

Pad sides of tank with pillows if patient is subject to seizures.

Infusions can be given via opening No. 3 on headboard. Prepare a foam rubber stopper to fit the opening in the tank. Make a slit along the radius at one point. Slip the tubing through this slit.

Bath water, linen, bedpans, thermometers, hypodermic syringes, enema equipment are inserted into the large door opening.

1. To give bath: occasionally, patient can be removed from tank. If 3 or 4 helpers are available and equipment is at hand, bath can be given in 2 minutes, and the stretcher moved back into tank. Doctor's order is necessary.

2. If, when working through arm ports, pressure is decreased, it may be necessary to increase the pressure temporarily to maintain the patient's comfort.

3. Enemas can be given in the tank with the funnel method or by the enema-can method. The can is adjusted on the standard at the head of the respirator. The tubing is elongated and put through the infusion opening.

4. If the patient is permitted feedings by mouth, instruct him to swallow as he breathes out; choking on food or fluid is a sign of aspiration and is extremely dangerous.

IF MOTOR STOPS:

1. Open valve No. 12. Turn it all the way to increase pressure.

2. Rotate pressure gauge to face foot of respirator.

3. Push down emergency lever No. 10. Operate diaphragm by handle by hand.

4. Have someone check driving belt. Replace, if broken, No. 7.

5. Have assistant notify engineer.

To ELEVATE FOOT OF RESPIRATOR:

1. Fit the slit end of the jack handle on the small screw head.

2. Turn handle to right (this closes release valve).

3. Insert handle in socket above small valve at foot of jack.

4. Move handle up and down to pump up jack.

To REPLACE DRIVING BELT:

1. Remove belt from motor pulley first.

2. Replace belt on motor pulley last.

Removal of Patient from Respirator

INSTRUCTION TO PATIENT

1. He may feel weight on chest and have forgotten how to breathe; he needs re-education in breathing.

2. He will be left on stretcher for a time under continuous observation.

3. He may become tired and go back into tank for a rest.

PROCEDURE

1. Gradually decrease the negative or positive pressure deviations.

2. Open a port.

3. Turn off motor.

4. Draw out stretcher.

5. Observe patient closely for depth and regularity of respirations and color and signs of anxiety.

6. Then, if removal is permanent:

A. Place bed with foot at right angles to head of respirator.

B. Attach cervical collar straps to related pegs or open plastic collar.

C. Tell patient he will be drawn through opening.

D. Place hand over patient's nose.

E. Nurse at head places hand under patient's head.

F. Assistants at sides draw patient down with the lifting sheet.

G. Assistants stand side by side with the respirator next to bed.

H. Hands are gently placed under patient's hips, shoulders, head.

I. Maintaining patient in neutral alignment, assistants move backward, drawing patient out as they move.

J. Assistants move forward to bed, place patient on bed.

CHARTING

Time of the written order by physician.

Respiratory rate, pressure as set by physician and anesthesiologist.

Respiratory rate every 15 to 30 minutes. Record on vital signs sheet, also regularity and depth of respiration, pulse, temperature, blood pressure as ordered by physician.

Color of patient

How patient handles his secretions

Changes in level of consciousness

Patient's reaction to the respirator

Care of Respirator

Respirator should be cleaned with mild detergent solution. The interior may be washed after use.

Sponges on arm parts must be changed when worn in order to maintain proper pressure. This may be accomplished by having an assistant occlude the opening from within with a pillow or piece of cardboard while the sponge is replaced from the outside.

Plastic collars are easily perforated and should be examined for tears and repaired with adhesive or gummed tape. They can be replaced if the patient can tolerate removal from the respirator. The plastic collar must be replaced after every use.

Linen changed p.r.n.

Suction bottle cleaned, tubing sterilized.

The engineer must check the respirator while in use and at regular intervals in storage.

THE CUIRASS AND CHEST RESPIRATORS

There are portable respirators which operate on the same principle as the tank respirator. They are the chest and the more extensive chest-abdomen (cuirass) respirators, which are used in the less severe respiratory problems or to assist in "weaning" the patient from the tank. These devices consist of a shell of light material, such as plastic, which can be placed over the chest and the abdomen and by means of cuffs can be made relatively airtight. A base attachment connects this respirator with an electrically driven pump which can be regulated to provide sufficient negative pressure and the respiratory rate required by individual patients. The portable cuirass and the chest respirators may also be battery-powered for emergency situations or may be operated by manual pumping.

There are certain advantages to the cuirass and chest respirators which are rather obvious. They are much less cumbersome, and the patient is much more accessible for nursing care. He may be turned, positioned, given attention to skin and elimination with greater facility. In addition, more mobility of joints may be maintained. For the patient who must be in a respirator for a long period of time it is a more attractive device than the cumbersome tank.

Before applying the respirator, attention must be given to the selection of size, choosing the largest one which will fit the patient to provide for greater chest expansion. The skin should be examined for signs of irritation, then cleansed and lubricated. The patient can wear a light cotton "T" shirt to protect the skin, and bony prominences must be padded with foam rubber, cotton or felt.

Observation, care and charting are the same as for the tank respirator with a special emphasis on skin care necessitated by the snug fit of the cuirass and chest respirators. Another point is to check the position of the respirator when a tracheostomy is present so that it does not slip up and occlude the patient's airway.

If the smaller respirator is used as a step in weaning the patient from the "tank," it can be applied while the patient is on the respirator stretcher to ensure smooth operation in and out of the "tank" and to help prevent respiratory embarrassment.

After use, the equipment is cleansed with a mild

soap solution, thoroughly dried and stored ready for use.

RESTRAINT (PROTECTORS)

Restraints are mechanical devices used to prevent a patient from harming himself or others.

General Rules

Do not restrain a patient (except in extreme emergency) without a doctor's order.

Make restraint as inconspicuous as possible and use no more than is necessary.

Never leave a restrained patient unwatched.

Fasten the restraint so that the patient cannot reach the knots or buckles.

Guard against chafing by padding all appliances.

Avoid restraining a patient in an uncomfortable position.

Never restrain the feet unless the hands are also restrained; always restrain hands first.

Watch the circulation, pulse and general condition of the patient.

Types of Restraints

Sheet

1. A sheet may be folded in fourths, laid over the upper part of the patient's body and tucked firmly under the mattress. Another may be arranged in the same way over the legs. The sheet should not be high enough to embarrass the breathing and should reach well below the knees.

2. Fold a sheet diagonally and make it into a long strip about 16 in. wide. Place the center of this under the patient's shoulders, bring the 2 ends under the arms at the axillae, pass them over the shoulder, cross them and fasten them to the bars at the head of the bed. Have the knots well out of the patient's reach.

Gauze

Use 4 pieces of gauze each 1 yd. wide and 3 yds. long.

Make a figure-of-8 with both ends on top but extending in opposite directions. Put the loops together and pass them over a hand or foot. Protect the wrists and ankles with cotton and draw the ends of the gauze tightly enough to prevent the hands or feet from slipping through. About 12 in. from the hand or foot tie a knot and fasten the restraint to the bars of the bed on each side.

Gauze for the hands and feet and a sheet fastened securely over the body make an effective restraint for a moderately confused patient.

Leather Halters

Place patient in halter, lock and secure straps over the bar of the bed. The key should be carried or kept easily accessible so the restraint may be removed promptly, if necessary.

Leather Handcuffs and Wristlets

Pad the wrists and ankles, apply the cuffs, lock and secure the straps over the bar of the bed. Keep the key easily accessible to the nurse so the restraint may be removed promptly if necessary.

Restraining Sheet

This consists of a heavy canvas sheet that extends over the bed and is laced to it with heavy cord. Provision is made for further restraint of the arms and legs.

Side Boards

Boards 1 in. thick, 12 to 18 in. high and as long as the bed are used. These may be clamped or tied on to the head and foot of the bed.

NOTE: Side rails—similar to crib sides—are available for purchase and are much more acceptable to patients and nurses.

RESTRAINT OF YOUNG CHILDREN

Restraining young children is often necessary (1) to prevent accidents and (2) to carry out necessary procedures that the child would instinctively resist. Before

NURSING TECHNICS

applying any type of restraint, the nurse should explain what she is going to do and why it is necessary, if the child is old enough to understand.

Mechanical Restraint

Mummy: used for treatments involving the head, such as infusion in scalp vein, drawing blood from jugular vein, ventricular tap, duodenal drainage. Also in examination of the ears, eyes, nose and throat.

A sheet or a light blanket large enough to tuck each end beneath the child and to reach from the back of the neck to the feet. Place the patient on his back in the middle of the sheet, shoulders about 4 inches down from the top. Bring one end down over the shoulder (arm should be at side); miter just below the shoulder; bring across the body and, leaving the second arm free, tuck beneath the patient. Repeat with the second end, tucking beneath the body as anchor.

If the neck and the shoulders are to be exposed, slip the sheet down below the shoulder line (after removing dress and shirt) and pull ends straight across the body and tuck; remember to restrain only one arm at a time.

Always remove restraints as soon as possible.

Jacket: used to prevent the child from climbing over the side of the crib; also it should be used when any child is put into a baby carriage, if he is old enough to be able to pull himself up. When applied in the crib, freedom of movement is allowed if the strings are fastened to the vertical bars of the crib. When used in a carriage or a wheel chair, care should be taken to fasten the strings securely so that it is not possible for the child to fall.

Elbow cuffs: used to prevent flexion of the elbow and so to make it impossible for a child to get his hand to his head for any reason, i.e., eczema, cleft lip and palate repair, plastic surgery to head, mastoid dressing. Elbow cuffs consist of muslin with pockets containing tongue depressors. For a young baby, satisfactory elbow cuffs can be made with a small paper bag, tongue depressors, Scotch tape and twilled tape. When applying the elbow cuffs, the child should be wearing a shirt or pajamas

138

with long sleeves; otherwise, the cuffs are likely to slip out of place. The cuff is put on center over the elbow, and first the center tie is tied. The flap of the cuff is at the top and inside. All ties should be tied snugly; then fold the shirt or pajama sleeve back over the bottom of the cuff and pin so that it will not slide or slip.

Be sure that the cuffs are removed when the child is served his meal. At regular intervals during the day, the cuffs should be removed for a short time while a nurse

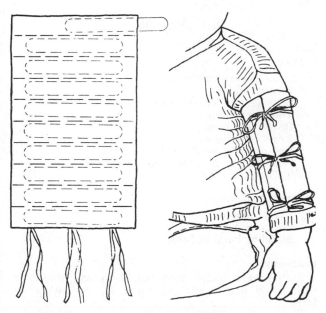

Elbow cuff restraint. (*Left*) Elbow cuff for use in treatment of eczema. (*Right*) Elbow cuff applied. (Jeans, P. C., Wright, F. H., and Blake, F. G.: Essentials of Pediatrics, ed. 6, Philadelphia, Lippincott)

stays with a child, observing him closely so that he does not get his hands to his head.

Flannel straps: from a roll of canton flannel, make a strap 2 to 3 inches wide, depending on size of the child, and long enough to pin around wrists or ankle, then tie under the mattress to the springs of the crib. If pinned snugly around the wrist or the ankle, the strap will not slip off, but care should be taken to see that it is not pinned too tightly. This type of restraint is useful in keeping the child's hands away from an infusion, or some other type of tube; also, in preventing a child with eczema from scratching himself.

SHAVING

Equipment
TRAY

2 towels—tray covers
3 round basins
Solution cup—30 cc., s.o.s.   } For abdominal
Toothpick swabs—q.s., s.o.s.   }   preparation only
Razor with blade
2 or 3 compresses
Emesis basin, medium-sized—or paper bag
Half-sheet or towel with protecting sheet
Toilet tissue—q.s.

ADDITIONAL EQUIPMENT

Liquid soap or shaving cream*
Cottonseed oil—abdominal preparation
Standing lamp or flashlight

Procedure

1. Prepare 2 basins with hot water and the third with liquid soap. (Add hot water for patient's comfort.)

---

* NOTE: When soaps containing hexachlorophene are used, a slightly different technic often is followed. This should be determined from the doctor or institution. These preparations are not used (ordinarily) preceding plastic surgery.

2. Place a compress in a basin of water and one in the soap solution.

3. For abdominal preparation—pour cottonseed oil into 30-cc. cup.

4. Protect the bed under the part to be shaved.

5. See that the patient is in a comfortable and convenient position. Drape patient as necessary.

6. Be sure to have an adequate amount of light.

7. Using the compress in the soap solution, make a lather over the part to be shaved.

NOTE: Before shaving the abdomen apply cottonseed oil to the umbilicus with toothpick swabs. After shaving the abdomen remove the oil and cleanse the umbilicus with soap and water.

8. Hold the skin taut, using toilet tissue, and shave in the direction in which the hair grows. Repeat steps 7 and 8 as necessary until the entire area has been shaved clean.

9. Rinse the area and dry with the patient's hand or bath towel.

10. Remove the protecting sheets or towels and see that the patient is comfortable.

11. Wash equipment and boil emesis basin, round basins and razor 10 minutes.

12. Discard razor blade.

13. Shake towels to remove all hairs and discard towels in laundry.

14. Reset tray.

LANE PREPARATION

Equipment

STERILE TRAY

> 2 or 3 towels
> Sponges—q.s.
> Small cup—liquid soap
> Small cup—alcohol 70 per cent
> Clamp—Kelly
> Emesis basin

UNSTERILE

> Half-sheet and water-repellent material

NURSING TECHNICS

Bandage
Stockinette to fit part
Bottle of ether

Procedure

1. Shave area as ordered by surgeon.
2. Arrange sterile tray.
3. Wash hands thoroughly.
4. Have assistant hold extremity during preparation, s.o.s.
5. Scrub part 2 or more times with liquid soap, starting from area of incision and working outward.
6. Wash thoroughly with alcohol, 70 per cent.
7. Clean off with ether.
8. Apply sterile towels (2 thicknesses) and stockinette over area; hold with gauze bandage, s.o.s. (no adhesive!).
9. After 24 hours, repeat procedure, except shaving.

SHAVING AREAS

PART TO BE SHAVED	EXTENT
Scalp Preparation For intracranial and plastic operations	Shave entire head. (Be sure proper explanation of this procedure is made to the patient or his family before procedure is done.)
For scalp wounds	Shave area at least 1 inch around wound or as specified.
Mastoid Preparation *(Right or left)* For mastoid, ear and plastic operations For certain neck operations	Shave 2-in. area around ear.
Trigeminal Preparation *(Right or left)* For neurosurgical operations	Shave 2 in. in front of ear. Extend upward to

PART TO BE SHAVED	EXTENT
	about 1 in. from midline. Shave face of male patients and of female patients if specified.
Neck Preparation For thyroid and other neck operations	Shave male patients from ears, including neck, chest to nipple line, and over shoulders. Do not shave female patient unless specified.
Thoracic Preparation *(Right or left)* For chest, breast and heart operations	Shave the anterior and posterior chest, on the operative side, from the shoulder to the waist. This area should be extended laterally to the nipple line anteriorly and to the vertebral column posteriorly. The axilla and the area from shoulder to elbow on the operative side should be included. Smaller areas only when specified.
Kidney Preparation *(Right or left)* For kidney and ureteral operations	Shave horizontally from a little beyond anterior mid-line on the opposite side to just beyond midline in back, and vertically from xiphoid process to include the pubis, and from the lower edge of scapula to sacrum.

NURSING TECHNICS

Part to Be Shaved	Extent
Abdominal Preparation	
For abdominal and pelvic operations	Shave from nipple line to mid-thighs. Remove pubic hair visible when thighs are together.
Back Preparation (Upper, lower and complete) (For neurosurgical procedures, low back operations and combined with perineal preparation for some perirectal, rectal or orthopedic operations)	
Upper Back	Shave from top of shoulders to iliac crests.
Lower Back	Shave from iliac crests to below buttocks, including perineum and anus.
Complete Back	Combine steps of upper back and lower back.
Back Preparation for Cervical Laminectomy	Shave from crown of head to middle of back.
Thoracic and Lumbar Spine Preparation	Combine steps of upper back and lower back.
Perineal Preparation	
For hemorrhoidectomy or other rectal, vaginal or perineal operations	Shave abdomen below umbilicus, the pubes, external genitalia and surrounding parts including anus and at least 6 in. of the inner aspect of thighs.
Upper Extremity Preparation	
Forearm Preparation	Shave hand and completely around arm to above elbow.

144

PART TO BE SHAVED	EXTENT
Arm Preparation	Shave completely around arm from below elbow to base of neck and well over shoulder, including axilla.
Elbow Preparation	Shave from wrist to axilla completely around arm.
Upper Extremity (Complete)	Combine steps of forearm and arm, *above.*

Lower Extremity Preparation (Right or left)

Hip Preparation	Shave lower abdomen, including pubic area, and entire thigh. Posteriorly shave from waist to popliteal space.
Thigh Preparation	Shave from umbilicus to knee, including pubis and completely around thigh.
Leg Preparation	Shave completely around leg and foot from above patella.
Knee Preparation	Shave completely around leg from ankle to groin.
Lower Extremity Preparation (Complete)	Combine hip and leg, above.

SMEARS

Equipment
Slide, clean and dry
Sterile applicator or swab
Covering slide

Procedure
1. Visualize the part from which the smear is to be taken.

NURSING TECHNICS

2. Gently rub the swab over the area (care must be taken not to touch any other part with the swab).

3. Roll the swab over the glass slide several times (always in the same direction).

4. Cover with cover slide.

NOTE: An elastic band wound around either end of the cover slide will separate the 2 slides, and the 2 may be secured together with a third elastic.

SOAKS

Equipment
Large tray
Arm or foot tub and cover
Bath towel
Hand towel or hot-water bag
Bath blanket
Safety pins
Pitcher
Large emesis basin
Towel for drying part-sterile, s.o.s.
Suitable dressing, s.o.s.

Solutions Used
Normal salt solution
Tap water
Others as ordered

Duration
As ordered.

Temperature
To apply heat—110° to 118° F.
For a soothing bath—100° to 110° F.

HAND SOAK

Procedure
1. Arrange the pillows and the head of the bed so that the patient is in a comfortable position sitting near the edge of the bed.

2. Prepare the prescribed solution.

3. Invert the tray on the bedside stand and place it close to the bed. On this place the arm tub and arrange the equipment so that the patient may be relaxed and comfortable and the arm well covered with the solution.

4. Remove the dressing and, supporting the hand at the wrist and elbow, lower it gently into the tub.

5. Protect the patient's arm by putting a folded towel over the edge of the tub or by using a partially inflated hot-water bag.

6. Place the cover on the tub and over it put a folded bath blanket.

7. If the soak is to be continued longer than half an hour, add hot water to keep the temperature constant.

8. Carefully and slowly lift the hand out of the tub.

9. Dry the arm and the hand and apply the dressing. Use sterile technic if indicated.

FOOT SOAK

Additional Equipment

Half-sheet
Treatment sheet

Procedure

1. Loosen the upper bedclothes at the foot of the bed. Turn them back to facilitate the removal of devices used to protect or support the foot.

2. Fold the bath blanket in half and place over the foot of the bed. Tuck one edge under the bottom of the mattress. Hold the other edge of the bath blanket and bring the blanket up over the leg as you fold back the top covers.

3. Slip the half-sheet and treatment sheet under the affected foot and over the other foot.

4. Prepare the solution in the tub.

5. Fold back the bath blanket to expose the affected foot. Place the tub parallel with the foot, remove the dressing and, supporting the foot above and below the wound or behind the knee and ankle, steadily lower it into the tub.

6. Cover the tub as for the hand soak. Pull down the upper covers even with the foot of the bed.

7. Prepare the sterile dressing, s.o.s.

8. Fold back the covers again. Fold the bath blanket to one side and remove the cover of the tub.

9. Carefully lift the foot out of the tub.

10. Dry the foot. Use sterile technic if indicated. Apply the prescribed dressing.

11. Replace supporting devices and readjust the covers.

12. Adjust the position of the leg and foot to assure comfort, proper alignment and elevation if it is ordered.

NOTE: 1. If the dressing has adhered to the wound, remove the outer layers and allow the remainder to loosen in the soak.

2. The tub should be scrubbed thoroughly and sterilized in the utensil sterilizer or filled with water and placed over the gas heater until the water boils for 10 minutes.

3. If the skin is not broken, this procedure need not be a sterile one.

STAIN REMOVAL

Procedure

1. Remove immediately to prevent fixation.

2. Cold or tepid water or milk will not fix a stain.

3. Soap sets a stain; therefore, the stain should be removed before the article is washed.

4. When boiling water is used, stretch the stained part over a bowl and pour the boiling water over with force until the stain disappears.

5. When using an acid, stretch the stained part over a bowl of boiling water. Apply the acid with a medicine dropper or old toothbrush, dipping the stain occasionally into the hot water and again applying the acid.

6. Rinse out acids or bleaches thoroughly.

STAIN	AGENT
Argyrol	Fresh stain—salt and ammonia Old stain—soak in potassium iodide 5 per cent
Benzoin tincture	Acetone—ether or alcohol
Bichloride of mercury	Chlorine water or oxalic acid, neutralize with ammonia
Blood	Tepid water and ammonia Old stain—hydrogen peroxide Unwashable material—starch and water in a paste—dry in the sun—steam to remove ring if necessary
Bluing (aniline dye)	Wash in boiling water with vinegar or javelle water
Castor oil	Alcohol—wash with ammonia and water
Chewing gum	Washable material—soften with egg white then wash Unwashable material—turpentine, carbon tetrachloride
Chocolate	Washable material—apply borax and cold water then boiling water Unwashable material — benzine — carbon tetrachloride
Cod-liver oil	Carbon tetrachloride—wash
Coffee	Pour boiling water from a height On silk or wool—use tepid water
Egg	Unwashable material — allow to stand until dry—then—benzine or carbon tetrachloride
Fruit	Same as for coffee—borax aids in removing stubborn stains Woolens—borax and ammonia
Gentian violet	Fresh stain—alcohol or chloroform
Glue	Warm water and soap — sponge with vinegar
Grass	Wash in cold water—molasses—let stand—wash

STAIN	AGENT
Grease or oil	Carbon tetrachloride — chloroform or gasoline
	Unwashable material—a paste made with the solvent and French chalk or magnesia—allow to dry—brush off
Ink	White material—salt and lemon—chlorine water
	Colored material—stand in milk a day or two
	Dilute solution of oxalic acid and ammonia alternately
Iodine	Wash, soap with water and ammonia, starch paste or 1 tbsp. of sodium thiosulphate to a pint of water
Iron rust	Salt and lemon juice—dry in the sun—concentrated solution of ammonia—acid fluoride or a saturated solution of oxalic acid
Mercurochrome	Old stain—alternate with cold potassium permanganate and warm sodium hydrosulphite
Mildew	Lemon juice and salt—allow to dry in the sun or soak in sour milk 10 to 12 hrs. or in a 10 per cent oxalic acid solution
Nail polish	Ether—acetone
Paint	Turpentine or carbon tetrachloride —boil in solution containing 3 tbsp. sodium carbonate to 1 gal. water
Perspiration	Cotton or linen—wash—add javelle water or ammonia
	Silk or woolens—dilute solution of sodium thiosulphate
	Old stains—sponge with vinegar
Peruvian balsam	Ether or kerosene

STAIN	AGENT
Picric acid	Ammonia—if possible boil in a strong solution of sodium hydroxide for 30 minutes then apply javelle water
Potassium permanganate	Oxalic acid
Scorch	White fabric—dampen a white cloth with hydrogen peroxide and place over stain. Place a clean dry cloth over this and iron with a medium iron. Replace top cloth if peroxide soaks through — repeat if necessary
Silver preparations	Ammonia 10 per cent or a solution of 3 Gm. of ammonia chloride and 3 Gm. of uncolored mercuric chloride in an ounce of distilled water
Tea	As for coffee
	On cotton or linen—soak in borax solution 1 tsp. to a cup of water
Urine	Warm solution of salt and hydrogen peroxide
Wax	Remove large pieces—apply lard or oil then turpentine or carbon tetrachloride—wash
Wine	Sponge with wood alcohol or acetic acid 80 per cent, s.o.s.

STUPES, ABDOMINAL

Equipment

TRAY

Stupe flannels—2

Stupe wringer

Abdominal pad, oiled paper, towel

Medicine glass containing oil and turpentine (proportions determined according to the sensitivity of patient's skin, 2 to 1, 3 to 1 or 4 to 1)

151

NURSING TECHNICS

Swab (tongue depressor padded with gauze)
Small protecting sheet
Rectal tube, urinal, lubricant

AT THE BEDSIDE

Shawl or bath blanket
Electric stove
Basin with boiling water

Procedure

1. Keep the basin of water boiling and in it put the wringer and 1 stupe flannel.

2. Arrange the patient:

A. Place the treatment protective sheeting for bed protection between the patient's hips and chest.

B. Insert rectal tube. Place open end in urinal.

C. Turn the covers down to the groin.

D. Protect the upper part of the body with the bath blanket and roll up the gown. Place the towel over the edge of the covers and on it place the pad and oiled paper.

3. Apply the oil and turpentine to the abdomen with the swab.

4. Wring out the flannel, shake it, and spread it smoothly and gradually over the abdomen. Raise as necessary to prevent burning the patient. Turn the towel, the pad and the paper over the flannel. Draw up the bedclothes.

5. Wring out the second flannel, shake it, turn back the bedclothes, the pad, etc., and spread the second flannel over the first. Draw out the first flannel and cover abdomen with the pad and covers.

6. Swab the abdomen with oil and turpentine after every third stupe or as indicated.

7. Continue the treatment for the time ordered: usually 10 to 20 minutes.

8. Wash and dry the abdomen and leave the abdominal pad in place.

SUPPOSITORIES, ADMINISTRATION OF

Equipment

Suppository—as prescribed

Rubber finger cot or glove
Lubricant, s.o.s.

Procedure

1. Assist the patient onto his side.
2. Expose the anus.
3. Introduce the suppository gently into the rectum and advance it as far as possible. (Use glove or finger cot.)
4. If the patient has difficulty retaining the suppository compression of the buttocks may assist in relieving the desire to defecate.

THORACENTESIS

Thoracentesis is the surgical withdrawal of fluid from the pleural cavity.

Equipment

STERILE TRAY

3 towels—tray covers (4 towels if tray is to be kept set up)
2 compresses, 4 × 4 in.
2 syringes, 5 cc. and 50 cc.
5 needles
1 No. 24, 1 No. 22
1 No. 19, 1 No. 18, 1 No. 15—blunt tips
Bard-Parker handle No. 3 and blade No. 11
3-way stopcock, syringe to Luer with hose connection
Wing adapter
Connecting tube, straight glass
3-ft. rubber tubing

ADDITIONAL EQUIPMENT

4-pt. bottle, graduated
Equipment for skin preparation
(Adrenalin, hypodermic syringe and needle should be readily available)

Procedure

1. Arrange the equipment so that it can be used conveniently.

2. Assist the patient into the position requested by the doctor.

3. Assist doctor with procedure as indicated.

NOTE: 1. Observe the patient's color and vital signs carefully throughout the procedure.

2. Maintain strict aseptic technic.

TIDAL DRAINAGE

Equipment

IRRIGATION SET (assemble in order listed)

1. Solution bottle adapter with an air vent
2. 4-in. tubing (5 mm. internal diameter)
3. Clamp—preferably a C-clamp—to regulate flow
4. Murphy drip bulb
5. 15-in. tubing (5 mm. internal diameter)
6. 1 ½-in. No. 20 needle—insert into one side of tubing as an air vent for siphon
7. Glass Y-tube—(5 mm. internal diameter)
8. 41-in. tubing (5 mm. internal diameter)
9. 2-in. glass connecting tube
10. Foley catheter

SIPHON

45-in. tubing (5 mm. internal diameter)

Stopper or adapter for drainage bottle (5 mm. opening)

NOTE: The above equipment may be autoclaved or boiled for 10 minutes

ADDITIONAL EQUIPMENT

Solution as ordered

Adjustable irrigating standard

Fisher clamps: 3 small and 1 large

Meter ruler

Calibrated drainage bottle—air vent on adapter, cap or stopper (unless already in siphon set)

A label to read—"Symphysis Pubis" (make from adhesive or masking tape)

Sterile catheterization set with appropriate Foley catheter

Procedure

INITIAL

1. Hold meter ruler horizontally from the patient's pubis to the irrigation standard. Indicate this point on the standard with the prepared label.

2. Attach meter ruler along the length of the irrigation standard.

3. Attach adapter to solution bottle.

4. Close clamp above Murphy drip bulb.

5. Fasten tubing 8 in. below level of symphysis pubis by a Fisher clamp.

6. Hang solution bottle on standard (adjust height of standard by screw adjuster or by using twill tape to suspend bottle).

7. Hold the 2 ends of tubing below the level of the drip bulb.

8. Open the clamp above the drip bulb.

9. Allow the solution to force air out of the tubing.

10. Close the clamp above the drip bulb.

11. Catheterize the patient using a Foley catheter.

12. Leave catheter in place.

13. Attach the tubing from the irrigating system (tube extending from the base of the Y-tube) to the patient's catheter.

14. Attach the tubing from the long arm of the siphon to the drainage bottle.

15. Secure tubing extending from Y-tube to the bed with a clamp so *that there is no lag between the bed surface and the Y-tube.*

NOTE: The doctor will determine the height of the siphon arc by cystometrics. The height of the siphon arc is related directly to the strength of the emptying contractions of the individual patient's bladder and the capacity of the bladder.

16. Regulate the flow of the irrigation solution at 15 gtts. per minute until specific orders are written by the physician.

17. Record the order and the following data:
   Name the doctor who regulated the flow
   Rate of flow per minute

NURSING TECHNICS

Amount and character of urine obtained

Difficulties encountered if any

NOTE: Care for catheterization equipment in the usual manner.

DAILY CARE

1. Maintain level of the siphon arc. Adjust level of the Y-tube if bed level is changed.

2. Urge and *record* fluids taken by mouth—200 cc. per hour unless contraindicated during the day.

3. Record the replacement of a bottle of solution.

4. Measure, record and compare intake and output, b.i.d. Urine output equals the total output (drainage bottle) minus the amount of solution used.

5. Flush entire system with 200 cc. of solution daily when solution is changed or whenever necessary because of sediment.

TO PERMIT AMBULATION

Equipment

2 gauze squares 2 × 2 in.—sterile and in a sterile towel

Emesis basin

Measuring graduate

Rubber bands—small—q.s.

2 adhesive strips—3 in. in length

Procedure

1. Pull screens and drape the patient.

2. Close clamp above drip bulb.

3. Open towel on side of bed and place connecting tube across one corner. Disconnect catheter.

4. Collect urine in basin and also any fluid in other length of tubing. (Record the amount.)

5. Cover each end of tubing with sterile compress and fasten with elastic bands. (Catheter corks may be used with physician's order.)

6. Tape catheter to patient's leg.

7. Secure other length of tubing to standard.

8. Ambulate the patient.

9. Observe patient for bladder distention. Release catheter p.r.n.—usually q. 3 h.

WEEKLY CARE (Change catheter—sterilize set)

To Discontinue:

1. Close clamp above drip bulb.
2. Disconnect catheter, empty bladder.
3. Release fluid from balloon of Foley catheter.
4. Gently remove catheter.
5. Remove equipment from the bedside.

Care of Equipment:

1. Fill solution bottle with tap water and permit to run through entire set.
2. Remove set from the standard.
3. Remove Bakelite adapters from the solution bottle and the rubber tubing.
4. *Do not detach the other tubing and connections.*
5. With an Asepto syringe, flush soapy water through the tubing. Repeat process using clear tap water until the set is clean. *Never soak the tubing.*
6. Replace Bakelite top.
7. Boil complete set for 10 minutes or autoclave.
8. Re-establish drainage with this or another set.

TOURNIQUETS, ROTATION OF

Equipment

4 tourniquets
Paper for scheduling of rotation

Procedure

1. Place 1 tourniquet under each extremity (above the elbow and above the knees).
2. Apply tourniquets to *3* extremities firmly enough to impair venous return but *not* arterial flow to the part. The pulse rate should be felt after applying the tourniquets. Changes in skin color distal to the tourniquet due to venous stasis are expected.
3. Leave tourniquets in place for length of time ordered by the doctor, e.g., rotate every 15 or 20 minutes.
4. At the end of designated time, release 1 tourniquet and apply the free one, rotating them clockwise.

NURSING TECHNICS

Recording

1. Make a list of extremities on the slip of paper for rotation; head this column "Part to be Free."

2. Make a list of time intervals in the next column opposite the list of extremities in first column. This second column to be headed "Time Interval," the time listed, of course, will start when tourniquets are first applied and the following ones at the interval ordered.

3. Cross off the time periods as the extremity is left free and the tourniquet rotated. The following is a typical example:

PART TO BE FREE	TIME INTERVAL (Q. 15 MIN.)
~~left arm~~	~~9:30 A.M.~~
~~left leg~~	~~9:45 A.M.~~
right leg	10:00 A.M.
right arm	10:15 A.M.
etc.	etc.

4. Record when started and observations of the condition and appearance of extremities as well as the nature of the patient's respirations, etc.

TRACHEAL SUCTION

Equipment

Suction machine—with motor preferred
Syringe
Catheter, 8 to 14 French, in towel
Bowl with water
Gauze compresses or muslin

Procedure

1. Attach catheter to suction machine or syringe and test its patency by sucking water through it.

2. Insert catheter through patient's nose or mouth.

3. Turn on suction machine and move catheter gently back and forth. (If a syringe is used, detach from catheter after each aspiration and expel contents. Repeat as necessary.)

4. Remove catheter and wipe free of mucus as necessary.

5. Draw water through the catheter to rinse it.

6. Place catheter in towel at bedside.

NOTE: The same procedure may be followed when the patient has a tracheotomy; the catheter is inserted through the tracheostomy tube.

TRACHEOSTOMY CARE

Equipment

SUCTION

Suction machine or waste bottle and tubing for water suction

Catheter: No. 8 Robinson or whistle tip preferred

Pitcher or other container for normal saline

Muslin bag or towel for catheter

TRAY

Gauze—q.s.—6 × 6 in. (wipes)

Small basin for soda bicarbonate solution—5 per cent

Thumb forceps

ADDITIONAL EQUIPMENT

"Magic" slate and pencil, or other writing material

Tissue wipes

Mirror

Bell or signal

Paper bag—waste

EMERGENCY EQUIPMENT (IMMEDIATELY AVAILABLE)

Trousseau dilator or Kelly clamp

Duplicate tracheostomy tube and dressing set

Procedure

GENERAL

1. Connect suction equipment and test.

2. Arrange other equipment at the bedside. (If a

muslin bag is used for the catheter this may be attached to the bed.)

3. Assist the patient to understand his present circumstances.

4. Show the patient the equipment to be used in his care and explain the procedure to him.

5. See that the patient understands the methods of communication that are available, i.e., by writing, covering the lumen of the tube to talk, ringing the bell, etc. (The extent to which steps 3, 4 and 5 can be carried out will depend, of course, on the immediate circumstances and the preoperative preparation that has been possible.) Constant care will be necessary immediately following surgery.

To Suction

1. Have the patient cough deeply.

2. Test patency of the catheter by drawing saline through it.

3. Insert catheter, after inner tube has been removed, to a distance of about 1 inch below tube.

4. Rotate catheter and withdraw quickly.

5. Allow patient to rest.

6. Repeat steps 2, 3 and 4 as often as necessary to keep airway passage clear.

7. Suction water through catheter until clear.

8. Wipe outside of catheter and replace in muslin bag or towel.

Care of Inner Cannula

1. Suction mucus from inner cannula.

2. Remove inner cannula only.

  A. Support the outer cannula with thumb and forefinger.

  B. Unclasp the safety catch.

  C. Slide inner cannula out.

NOTE: Undue jarring of the outer cannula will result in discomfort to the patient. Be gentle, but give firm support to the outer cannula.

3. Place inner cannula in sodium bicarbonate solution and cleanse by pulling gauze or pipe stem cleaner, for smaller size tubes, through the cannula with a forcep.

4. Suction mucus from outer cannula.

5. Inspect and reinsert inner cannula and reclasp safety clasp.

6. Clean inner cannula as often as necessary. (Remain with patient as long as inner cannula is out.)

CHANGE OF DRESSING

1. Assemble the following equipment:
   Sterile scissors
   2 forceps
   Keyhole dressing
   2 × 2 in. compresses for cleansing skin area
   Aqueous Zephiran
   Basin for waste
2. Support the outer cannula while changing dressing.
3. Clip and remove soiled dressing.
4. Cleanse skin area.
5. Apply keyhole dressing.

CARE OF OUTER CANNULA (AFTER DOCTOR HAS CHANGED OUTER CANNULA)

1. Remove the soiled tapes. These may be soaked in sodium bicarbonate.
2. Clean and polish cannula.
3. Apply fresh tape.
4. Boil tube for 10 minutes—or autoclave.
5. Place in sterile tube and label.

CARE AND OBSERVATION OF THE PATIENT

Attend the patient constantly for the first 24 hours or longer as indicated.

Observe patient closely to determine necessity of repetition of process of suctioning and changing dressing. NOTE:

   Color

   Respirations—sound, rate and depth
   Bleeding, swelling or inflammation around tube
   Twisting of tube away from mid-line
   Amount and type of drainage from tube

Keep writing material and call bell always within reach of patient.

Give patient mouth care at frequent intervals.

Record

Restlessness
Emotional reaction of patient
Time and frequency of treatment
Character and amount of mucus, dyspnea, cyanosis, diaphoresis
Response of patient to treatment
Inflammation, swelling or bleeding around cannula
Whether or not patient is coughing deeply

Patient Teaching

1. Teach patient how to sponge away quickly any mucus that appears at opening of cannula before it is redrawn into tube.

2. Demonstrate and explain suction while patient observes in mirror; then help him to suction cannula.

3. Assist the patient until he acquires self-confidence in his own ability to perform this activity and until his technic is satisfactory.

4. When one aspect of self-care has been learned, introduce another according to the interest and needs of patient; namely:

Methods of communication
Suctioning and wiping away of mucus
Mouth hygiene
Remove, cleansing and replacing inner cannula

5. Mouth hygiene is very important. The patient should assume responsibility of thorough toothbrushing at least 3 times daily.

6. Use terminology that the patient can understand; e.g.; *suction* instead of "aspirate," *suction tip* instead of "catheter," *salt solution* instead of "saline."

Suggest use of mirror as when shaving.

7. Adjust the teaching to meet individual needs of patient. If he seems to have undue anxiety, review the demonstration and practice with him without introducing any new information or responsibilities. Encourage him to verbalize about himself, and his success or failure at self-care, to aid his psychological acceptance of his condition and to indicate where further help may be needed.

Points To Be Emphasized

1. Never remove the outer cannula.

2. The patient must be watched closely and suctioned according to his needs.

3. Be sure the inner cannula and obturator fit the outer cannula.

4. Always lock the inner cannula when replacing it.

5. The procedure must be adapted to the individual patient.

6. Should the patient expel the outer cannula from the opening, medical help should be obtained at once. *Do Not Leave the Patient Alone!* If necessary maintain the airway through the tracheostomy with the tracheal dilator.

7. Do not keep the catheter in the cannula for a long period of time.

8. Keep the tape securely tied in a square knot so that the outer cannula will not slip out. The tie should be tight enough so that the tube will not ride in and out as the patient breathes or coughs, yet not tight enough to be constricting.

9. Remember the patient cannot talk.

10. Avoid dressings with cotton fillers and the use of power at the patient's bedside, to prevent aspiration of foreign material.

URINE SPECIMENS

To Obtain Single Specimen of Urine

Have patient void into a clean bedpan.

(Obtain the specimen from the first voiding in the morning, if possible.)

Fill a specimen jar with the urine and cover it.

Attach the laboratory slip on which is written the required information.

To Obtain a Single Sterile Specimen of Urine

Catheterize the patient, allowing the urine to flow into a sterile test tube. Flame the tube after removing the stopper and before returning it to the tube. Fill out the laboratory slip as above and attach it to the test tube.

NURSING TECHNICS

To Obtain a 24-hour Specimen of Urine

PROCEDURE. Have a clean 5-pt. bottle tagged with the patient's name. Have the patient void at 7 A.M. Throw this voiding away; that is, start with an empty bladder at 7 A.M. Save all urine until 7 A.M. the next morning, and at this time have the patient void again and add this urine to the amount already collected.

To Obtain Many Specimens

To obtain partitioned or 3-part or 4-part specimens for glucose, acetone and diacetic acid (G.A.D.) use 3 or 4 clean 5-pt. bottles. Label bottles indicating the time period during which each specimen is to be collected, e.g., 7 A.M. to 11 A.M., 11 A.M. to 3 P.M., etc. Collect urine in the appropriate bottle.

To Obtain Urine Specimens from an Infant

For collecting a urine specimen from an infant or a toddler who is untrained, a satisfactory method is the use of a special commercial plastic bag which has an adhesive surface with a round opening that fits over the genitalia. The ankles should be restrained to prevent the bag from being dislodged. If the child is old enough to have normal exploratory tendencies, wrist restraints should also be used until the speciman is obtained.

WET DRESSINGS

Equipment

Basin

Prescribed solution at desired temperature

Dressing as indicated (Sterile, s.o.s.)

    Compresses

    Gauze—5-yd. roll

    Muslin—cut to size desired

2 forceps or clamps for sterile dressing

NOTE: If these are not available arrange a wash cloth or suitable piece of material to act as a wringer.

Towel or other material (sterile, s.o.s.) if dressing is to be left in place

Water-repellent material—for closed dressing

Lamp or other heating device if dressing is to be kept warm

Paper bag or other receptacle for waste, s.o.s.

Procedure

1. Immerse dressing in solution.
2. Wring out the dressing and straighten it.
3. Apply over affected part.
4. Apply towel or other covering, s.o.s.
5. If constant hot application is desired change as dressing cools. Continue for about 20 minutes every 3 hours or as ordered.
6. When external heat is to be applied take special precautions to avoid burning the patient or creating fire hazards.

NOTE: When wet dressings are to be continued over a period of time, protect the surrounding unaffected skin with petroleum jelly or a similar substance.

Section 2
Medical and Surgical Nursing

Part I. Physical States

CARE OF THE ACUTELY ILL

Ministration to the acutely ill patient requires skillful, thoughtful and well-planned nursing care. In caring for these patients, the nurse should recognize that modifications of basic nursing care often are essential to meet their needs.

Observation is of primary consideration—both with respect to obvious signs and symptoms and to slight changes in the condition of the patient. The entire welfare of the acutely ill patient depends upon early recognition of minute changes. Alert observation and accurate reporting are essential for planning care that will meet all his needs.

The plan for care should provide for nursing care, for examination and treatment of the patient by the doctor, for carrying out new orders and for the greatly needed rest periods of the patient himself. Plans should be flexible enough to include meeting such unexpected developments as sleepless nights, necessitating postponement of planned morning care; gastrointestinal disturbances, such as nausea and vomiting, which may mean interruption of previously made plans; or exacerbation of the patient's symptoms requiring further medicine and treatment with skillful observation.

It should be realized that all aspects of nursing care will be more demanding of nursing time; and that care and treatment can be performed only as a patient can accept them without being unduly fatigued.

During this acute episode in the patient's life, great concern is expressed by his close friends and members of his family. All are looking eagerly for something to do that can be helpful in the situation. Recognition of this fact cannot be overlooked by the nurse. She must consider the welfare of both the patient and his family. Where possible, provision can be made for some member of the family to participate in the patient's care. Often, however, the nurse must use a great deal of ingenuity and tact in providing support for the family while not depriving the patient of his needed rest and care.

Since modern therapy has done much to lessen the time of the acute period in many conditions, the focus of all care may be placed on meeting the immediate needs imposed by the disease. Therefore, treatments, medications or rest may be the main concern, often at the sacrifice of personal hygienic measures.

The posturing of the seriously ill patient is of great importance since it is recognized that to maintain any one position for a long time not only is uncomfortable and fatiguing but it also may be dangerous. Therefore, when the patient either is helpless or too ill to move about freely, the nurse must plan for a regular change and variation in his position at least every 2 hours. Sandbags, pillows, footboards, etc., may be used to help maintain normal physiologic alignment.

Nutritional needs often are met by food substitutes given parenterally until the patient can tolerate adequate amounts of food. The nurse then must help the individual to develop an appetite. This may be accomplished by understanding the patient's nutritional requirements, considering his likes and dislikes and using imagination and tact in helping him to regain his appetite.

During this acute illness, often there is impairment of bowel function, usually resulting from lack of exercise, limited dietary intake and the use of highly constipating drugs such as opium and its derivatives. If rectal treatments are ordered, an irrigation (or siphon enema) usually is administered, for even the most gentle treatment can be exhausting to the patient.

When urinary retention occurs such measures as increasing fluid intake, creating the sound of running water or pouring warm water over the external genitalia may be used to relieve this situation. Catheterization may be required (*See:* Technics).

Personal hygiene measures, of course, play a great role, especially if the acute phase is to be a long period. Modifications in its approach may be necessary with the seriously ill patients, and often the nurse must use her own judgment and initiative in providing it with the least amount of strain to the patient. (*See:* Technics *for* Special Care of Skin, Teeth, etc.)

CARE OF THE DYING AND THE DEAD

Between the time the patient shows signs of impending death and the cessation of life occurs, much of the care of the patient is specifically nursing and the interpretation of the doctor's orders. The nursing care essential for any acutely ill patient must be continued with the aim of maintaining the patient's comfort and preserving his strength. Oral administration of fluid must be guarded, lest undue collection should occur in the stomach; or lest aspiration should occur as a result of loss of the swallowing reflex. Distention of the bladder may cause undue restlessness of the patient. Sedatives and narcotics should be given as indicated for relief of general discomfort and pain. Moist, noisy respirations resulting from accumulation of secretions in bronchi and trachea may be relieved by turning the patient on his side or by medications, such as atropine, and by oral and nasal suction. The room should be kept light, and one often will notice that the patient will turn toward the source of light, whether it be a window, a lamp, etc.

Whatever the patient's attitude toward death, the consolation he may receive from the religious advisor of his faith cannot be overestimated. For Catholic patients in particular, a visit from the priest under these circumstances to hear the patient's confession or to administer last rites may be of utmost importance. The priest should be summoned before the patient loses consciousness.

The ability of the patient to hear what is said and done around him often continues when his appearance and other symptoms would suggest the contrary. Care must be taken by all of those close to the patient to say nothing that they would not wish the patient to hear.

In this period, the consideration and the understanding that the nurse may extend to the patient's family is of inestimable value. Much thought and tact are necessary in order to give the patient's family the feeling that watchful care is being given to the patient without at the same time arousing alarm and concern in the family. The nurse must remember, however, that any specific information regarding the patient's condition should be given by the patient's physician.

When death has been pronounced by the physician, the nurse can be of great assistance to the family by offering reassurance. If any member of the family is very upset emotionally, she can administer a bromide to him if a doctor's order is available.

Care of the patient's body is directed toward cleanliness and maintenance of natural expression and posture. Artificial dentures should be replaced, and the eyelids and the jaws should be closed. Drains and tubes, etc., should be removed, and clean dressings applied to the wound. If the patient is hospitalized, the nurse should check the policy of the hospital before attempting to remove drains, etc. Then the body is bathed in the usual manner.

If the patient died in the hospital, the body usually is wrapped in a shroud and is tagged carefully to maintain its identity. Patient's belongings should be listed and signed for by the nurse and the person who removes them from the hospital.

CONVALESCENCE

The period of a patient's illness, between the cessation of the acute phase and the patient's resumption of his usual activities, has many implications for nursing.

The aim of the convalescent period is to help the individual regain his own independence within the limitations imposed by his particular illness. Maintaining adequate nutrition and providing for sufficient periods of exercise and rest are important in helping the patient to make maximum progress during this time.

Because, for many conditions, current medical practice has reduced greatly the need for long periods of bed rest and its subsequent debilitating effect on the patient, the time for the convalescent period has been reduced. However, there still are diseases for which long periods of bed rest are prescribed, and for patients with these conditions a carefully planned convalescence must be considered.

Emotional support is most essential for any patient. This is especially important for the individual who has experienced a long illness where progress has been slow. Motivation of these people to get well and to take on their usual activities as soon as possible is of prime importance. Occupational therapy offers much in helping them to develop interests and in relieving the monotony. Physical therapy also has a significant role in helping the individual regain muscle tone. Contacts with friends and family also play an important role in helping the individual keep up with interests—a motivation toward the time when he will be able to resume his usual relationships with them.

The nurse must assume the role of interpreter and teacher as she helps the patient to regain his health. Whether the patient is in the hospital or at home, the nurse must be sure that she understands correctly the recommendations of the doctor, that he knows how to carry them out and that he intends to do so. Also, it is advisable that the nurse discuss these points with members of the family so that all concerned will know what is expected. In some instances it may be advisable for a patient to go to a convalescent home. In this situation, the nurse can help in interpreting its purpose to the patient and also in interpreting the patient's needs to those who will be responsible for his care.

Many diseases present special problems in the convalescent period, and the individual must be taught how to adjust to his limitations resulting from the illness. Special measures will be discussed in the section on rehabilitation.

MEDICAL AND SURGICAL

REHABILITATION

Rehabilitation, the so-called third phase of medical practice, is concerned with assisting the patient to achieve his ultimate goal—resumption of a contributing role in society—as soon as possible.

The true impact of this phase was realized during World War II and now is an integral part of modern medicine. The success of this aspect depends upon close co-operation between all concerned with patient care—the doctor, the nutritionist, the physical therapist, the occupational therapist, the nurse, the psychiatrist, the social worker, the family and, by no means least of all, the patient himself. Because the nurse's role brings her into close contact with the patient and his family, she is in a unique position to make a valuable contribution by her interpretation of the patient's needs to all concerned, as well as by her interpretation to the patient of the various measures devised for his care.

Rehabilitation does not limit itself to the more dramatic situations, such as loss of a limb or one of the senses, but rather it concerns any individual who has had an illness. It is an integral part of the convalescent period, although some aspects may begin even while the patient is in the acute phase. For example, special emphasis on posturing the patient in the acute phase of a cerebral vascular accident will contribute greatly to the return of function of his limbs during his convalescent period.

The ability of the individual to carry on his own daily activities is considered as the major aspect in rehabilitation. Special devices to help the patient achieve this are available on the market, but, even more important, many devices can be made by the family, the nurse or others. Padding the handles of eating utensils, toothbrushes, combs, etc., will help the individual with limited hand motion to care for many of his personal needs. This in itself will raise the morale of the individual.

Exercise by itself can be very tedious, but by combining it with diversional therapies such as weaving, leatherwork, knitting, etc., its effectiveness can be realized, and the patient experiences a sense of accomplishment in making a product. Sometimes modifications must be made to enable a patient to enjoy recreational therapy, such as building up the knobs on a television set or a radio, making a rack to support a book or distinguishing checkers from one another by using different shapes to represent colors for the benefit of the blind patient.

In all aspects of rehabilitation the family should take a part so its members are aware of the progress made by the patient and of his ability to function within his own limitations. This co-operative approach adds much toward providing a positive environment in which the patient can function and contributes toward the emotional well being of all.

After a satisfactory convalescence, many patients may return to their former type of employment, whereas others may need to find new work that is consistent with the limitations imposed by their illness. Community resources offer much to the individual facing the need for change of employment. Many states have job replacement services for the handicapped, and in some communities private institutions offer much in this area. The nurse should be aware of the facilities available so that she can plan with the other members of the team for the patient's future.

Community resources also play a great role in helping the individual to live within the limits of his illness or to teach him how to adjust to mechanical devices such as braces, artificial limbs, etc. Other facilities are available for those needing speech therapy or adjustment to impairment of the sense organs such as hearing, seeing, etc. The nurse's unique position with the patient and his family affords her an excellent opportunity to interpret these resources and to encourage their use, thereby offering the patient a source of hope in his efforts to become independent.

The nurse must meet the challenge offered by this phase of medical practice. Her own positive attitude and sincere interest in understanding the patient and his problems on becoming an independent person are significant factors in making his rehabilitation a satisfying experience. Patience, empathy and the ability to inspire confidence are most important traits in the nurse. Her contributions toward the program of rehabilitation are not limited only to the patients under her care. She can do much toward helping those in a community understand the importance of rehabilitation, regardless of the degree, by encouraging those who need assistance to seek the help of the facilities available, by teaching those who need help in adjusting to their limitations and by supporting efforts to encourage employers to utilize the manpower resources available in many of the handicapped group.

CARE OF THE SURGICAL PATIENT

The modern concept of surgical treatment has come to indicate not only the removal of diseased structure and the restoration of body function in so far as possible, but the treatment of the individual as well. The role of the nurse in surgery is equally important as that of the surgeon, for the success of any operative procedure depends largely upon the reliability of all those engaged in the care of the surgical patient. The importance of the personal relationship between the patient and the nurse must not be overlooked. The patient often needs reassurance, for he is separated from his home, his family and his everyday routine of living. Often he is in actual physical discomfort and his comfort and the maintenance of his morale depend largely upon the nurse.

The confidence of the patient is gained by a sincere interest in both his illness and the implications it carries with it. Reassurance concerning the progress of his condition is of utmost importance and is doubly important for the patient who finds it necessary to change his mode of living as the result of an injury or of a destructive diseased condition.

Preoperative and postoperative care of the patient concerns those measures designed to increase the patient's comfort and assure his safety while he is undergoing and recovering from any surgical treatment. Preoperative care is concerned with the evaluation of the patient and his illness; the treatment of both primary and associated disease; mental hygiene in relation to anesthesia and surgery as well as the meaning that the diseased condition holds for the patient; local and systemic measures of preparation of the field of operation and prophylaxic against respiratory complications, circulatory complications and infections.

PREOPERATIVE CARE

Mental Preparation

Much of the patient's anxiety of the surgical experience can be eliminated by thoughtful and purposeful care by the nurse. The nurse should be fully aware of any information the doctor has given to the patient, so that she may intelligently answer questions of the patient and his family.

During the preoperative period the teaching role of the nurse is most important. She must carefully interpret all preoperative measures to the patient and his family, considering their purpose, length of time involved and the expected role of the patient during the various procedures. If the hospital has a recovery room to which the patient will be sent following surgery, the patient must be prepared for waking in this different environment. Its purpose should be explained to the patient and to his family. Postoperative measures in the early period should be fully explained to the patient prior to surgery; so he will not be unduly alarmed when they occur. These measures include: use of oxygen tent or suction if indicated, intravenous therapy, frequent checking of vital signs (especially blood pressure), coughing, deep breathing, changes in position, and any other treatments which relate to the patient's particular problem. Good mental preoperative preparation greatly facilitates the ability of the patient and his family to manage the surgical experience.

Physical Preparation

The patient's general condition must be evaluated through a thorough history and physical examination as well as specified laboratory tests. The patient's general nutrition and fluid and electrolyte balance also must be evaluated and remedied as necessary.

Specific Preparation

FOOD AND FLUID INTAKE. The meal immediately preceding the time of operation should be omitted. If anesthesia is general, usually fluids are stopped by midnight prior to surgery.

PREPARATION OF THE BOWEL. A cleansing soap-suds or saline enema should be given to lessen postoperative discomfort due to distention or fecal incontinence during surgery. The enema should be effectual.

PREPARATION OF SKIN. An extensive area should be cleansed and shaved the night preceding operation in order to ensure a wide margin of safety from contamination.

PERMISSION FOR SURGERY. The operative permit must be signed by the patient or by his appointed legal guardian.

NOTIFICATION of time of operation must be submitted to the patient or a member of his family. The referring doctor also should be notified.

CARE OF VALUABLES. Removable dentures and prothesis should be stored in a safe place. Other possessions such as jewelry, money and the like should be handled as valuables.

PREMEDICATION AND IMMEDIATE PREOPERATIVE CARE. A sedative should be administered to ensure a restful night's sleep, thus lessening apprehension preoperatively. All necessary treatments should be carried out as efficiently and quietly as possible.

VOIDING. The patient should void before operation. If he is unable to empty his bladder completely a catheterization may be necessary. The amount and the time of voiding should be recorded.

PREANESTHETIC MEDICATION. Preanesthetic medication or basal anesthesia should be given after immediate preoperative preparation has been completed and, ideally, 1 hour before operation. This allows adequate time for absorption and optimum effect of the drug. Maintaining a quiet nonstimulating environment is essential.

TRANSFER OF PATIENT. The patient should be protected adequately against draft and cold. Laparotomy stockings, a short gown untied at the back and a muslin cap to confine the hair of female patients should be worn.

ANESTHESIA. In selecting an anesthetic agent the anesthetist evaluates the patient as a whole as well as the nature and the extent of surgery required. Frequently, the patient dreads the anesthetic more than the operation itself. In many instances, the anesthetist visits the patient the evening before the operation.

POSTOPERATIVE CARE

A marked degree of nursing skill is involved in caring efficiently for the patient returning from operation. The evaluation of the patient's condition and the anticipation of his needs are essential in making the patient's environment safe and conducive to a good recovery. All postoperative orders should be carried out as efficiently and accurately as possible. The postoperative unit should be placed conveniently for close observation.

The operative bed should be protected adequately with rubber sheeting which can be removed with little disturbance to the patient as soon as the need for protection ceases.

The transfer of the patient to his bed should be accomplished gently, and care should be taken to avoid unnecessary exposure. Sufficient assistance is necessary to avoid all strain on muscles and sutures and to minimize the possibility of hemorrhage.

POSITION

The patient is placed most frequently on his side with his knees flexed and with a pillow at his back for support until he has recovered from the anesthetic. Then he is placed in a Fowler's position unless otherwise indicated. The patient with general anesthesia never should be left alone while still unconscious.

EARLY OBSERVATION

The patient's temperature, pulse, respiration, blood pressure, color and condition of skin should be observed frequently. The dressing should be inspected for ooze or drainage, and the patient should be observed closely for the symptoms of shock or hemorrhage.

GENERAL CARE

The patient's personal hygienic care should be limited to the absolute essentials until he can tolerate details, to avoid unnecessary fatigue. The psychological care of the patient is as important as his physical care.

Pain should be controlled by means of drugs, as prescribed and by the adjustment of the patient's position as necessary.

Nausea and vomiting are not unusual following general anesthetic. Water should be withheld at least 1 or 2 hours after vomiting has ceased. Cracked ice is thought by many surgeons to contribute to marked gastric irritability and intestinal obstruction and should be avoided in so far as possible. Adequate mouth care and the frequent use of a refreshing mouthwash are essential.

DIET

Food and fluid should be administered in gradually increasing amounts, in accord with the surgeon's orders and the patient's tolerance of them. An accurate record of fluid intake and output should be charted.

ELIMINATION

With proper fluid balance the average patient will void within 8 to 12 hours following operation. If the bladder is distended and the patient is unable to void, all accepted nursing measures should be employed in an effort to stimulate voiding. Defecation usually is not expected within the first day or two following operation, but an effort should be made to assist the patient in reestablishing normal elimination. A postoperative urine specimen often is required for analysis.

EARLY AMBULATION

Early postoperative rising means walking within the first 24 or 48 hours after operation. Immediate postoperative activity of the patient in bed should be encouraged. He should be turned frequently, encouraged to breathe deeply, cough and move his extremities.

The procedure for early rising is a gradual transfer of the patient from the bed to a walking position. This should be done by assuming a position of "dangling" first and then increasing the patient's walking distance each day.

The advantages of early rising are an appreciable reduction in general postoperative complications and an expedition of recovery. Contraindications to early rising pertain largely to any associated conditions accompanying the patient's surgical procedure.

POSTOPERATIVE COMPLICATIONS

With the advances in medicine, surgery, anesthesia and nursing skills, postoperative complications have diminished markedly.

Constant observation of the postoperative patient in terms of potential changes in his condition and a thorough understanding of the significance of these changes are the most essential tools of the nurse.

Relatively minor disturbances, seemingly unimportant at the time, are often the forerunners of more serious postoperative complications. The more common complications are listed and discussed below.

In the postanesthetic period, the unconscious or disoriented patient may be subjected to such injuries as dislocations or fractures or to nerve injuries which result in wristdrop or footdrop.

Postoperative Shock

Primary shock usually appears within the first 12 hours and responds quickly to treatment if started without delay.

Secondary shock caused by more severe injury or a delay in treating early shock is frequently more serious and more difficult to treat. The following physiologic characteristics and signs are indicative of circulatory collapse:

    Reduction of blood volume

    Vasoconstriction

    Reduction in cardiac output

Stasis of circulation in periphery
Decreased venous return
Decrease in blood pressure
Irreversible capillary damage
Lack of oxygen in tissues
Fluid loss in tissues
Failure of myocardium, vasomotor center and respiratory center

SIGNS AND SYMPTOMS. The patient looks and feels seriously ill. He is extremely weak and experiences difficulty of orientation which may be accompanied by nausea and vomiting. His face is anxious, drawn and pinched in appearance; his skin is ashen-gray or cyanotic. He may be perspiring freely, and the surface temperature of his skin is lowered markedly. His pulse is rapid, weak, irregular and reduced in volume, his blood pressure is lowered gradually, and, as shock progresses, there is a gradual diminishing of all vital bodily functions. If not treated, the symptoms of extreme exhaustion and anoxemia develop, and the patient becomes comatose, which condition progresses into death.

PROMPT PROPHYLACTIC TREATMENT is indicated to forestall the development of clinical shock. The immediate therapeutic measures should include the restoration of blood volume and control of peripheral circulatory collapse, as well as treatment of any associated contributory factors.

The patient should be kept quiet and free from pain. He should be placed in shock position (head slightly lowered and feet elevated) to increase circulation to vital centers. External heat should be applied cautiously, since overheating will result in further fluid and salt loss. All vital signs should be observed frequently (every 10 to 15 minutes) to evaluate the patient's immediate condition.

Hemorrhage

The presence of profuse bleeding, arterial, venous or capillary, may be external or internal in origin.

Arterial bleeding is a spurting stream of bright red blood, venous bleeding is a steady, slow stream of dark red blood, while capillary bleeding is recognized as a sample of ooze, usually at the site of the wound.

The following symptoms are manifested by the site and the degree of bleeding. The patient is restless, apprehensive and experiences air hunger. His respirations are rapid and gasping; his pulse rapid, full, bounding; his skin is flushed, warm and dry; and he is extremely anxious. He usually complains of thirst. His blood pressure while normal at first gradually will become lowered.

TREATMENT. The nurse's ability to act quickly and calmly will do much in reassuring the patient. The surgeon should be notified immediately. The patient should be kept quiet and well protected from chilling. Emergency measures should include direct pressure, if the bleeding is external, and elevation of the part whenever possible.

Vital signs should be checked constantly. Sterile equipment should be within immediate reach for the control of bleeding. Most important is the replacement therapy in the form of blood, plasma or normal saline sufficient to restore blood volume.

Sedation is administered to control apprehension and restlessness.

The patient may be treated for shock if symptoms progress.

Pulmonary Complications May Include the Following

Aspiration

Asphyxia

Respiratory failure

Cough

Atelectasis

Massive collapse of lung

Pneumonia (aspiration pneumonia)

Bronchitis

Lung abscess

ATELECTASIS (Partial Lung Collapse). Caused by a mucous plug obstructing a large bronchus.

The symptoms are characteristic of a rapid shallow

respiration, cyanosis and, usually, a marked elevation of the patient's temperature.

Treatment. Have patient cough or suction the trachea in an effort to dislodge the plug.

Prophylactic Treatment: Have patient breathe deeply and cough up mucus frequently. Also, alter patient's position frequently following operation.

Cardiovascular Complications (Treatment discussed elsewhere when each condition is presented in detail

These are seen more commonly at the end of the first postoperative week and include the following:

Cardiac failure

Thrombophlebitis

Pulmonary embolism

Gastrointestinal Complications

Nausea and vomiting

Distention: (1. Acute gastric distention. 2. Paralytic ileus. 3. Large bowel distention.) May be slight flatulence or tense tympanites and marked uncomfortable type of both large and small bowel.

A temporary paresis of the intestine occurs after every abdominal operation and usually is manifested on about the 2nd day after operation.

TREATMENT. The general treatment ordered usually is the application of heat to the abdomen and the insertion of a No. 24 French rectal catheter to facilitate the expulsion of gas. Further therapy might include drugs to stimulate the intestinal musculature, enemata, colon lavage or the Miller-Abbott tube. Frequent change of position and early ambulation have aided greatly in reducing the amount of postoperative distention.

Urinary Complications

URINARY RETENTION. The inability to void occurs more frequently following perineal or pelvic surgery but is observed also following abdominal and other procedures. Prolonged spinal or general anesthesia also may be a cause. Apprehension and a horizontal position also may be the cause.

Treatment. All accepted nursing measures to induce

voluntary urination should be employed. These are: providing privacy, placing the patient in an upright comfortable position when possible, hearing the sound of running water, pouring warm water over external genitalia. If these measures fail, stimulating rectal treatments such as magnesium, glycerine and water enema, parenteral fluids and, finally, catheterization should be ordered.

KIDNEY FAILURE (URINARY SUPPRESSION)

URINARY TRACT INFECTION: (1. Cystitis. 2. Pyelitis.)

Wound-Healing Complications Include

Wound hematoma
Wound infection
Wound disruption (evisceration)
Peritonitis
Adhesions
Wound hernia

Nutrition and Fluid-Balance Complications Include

Dehydration
Deranged electrolyte balance
Acidosis
Alkalosis
Malnutrition. (1. Vitamin deficiency. 2. Hypoproteinemia.)

Other Complications

Decubitus ulcers
Hiccoughs
Parotitis
Delirium and psychosis

HICCOUGHS. The mechanism of onset is not always apparent but may result from such widely divergent causes as diaphragmatic irritation, as in pleurisy and subphrenic abscess, or dilatation of the stomach or retention of toxic products in the blood.

Physiologically, hiccough is a sudden spasmodic contraction of one or both sides of the diaphragm resulting in a sudden inspiration interrupted by a reflex closure of the glottis. This clonic twitching is continued at intervals of a few seconds uninterruptedly and may interfere with sleep, speech and the taking of food.

Treatment. Medications usually have little effect. Some of the time-honored remedies, such as holding the breath as long as possible or drinking a glass of water slowly, are methods of increasing the carbon dioxide content of the blood. However, actual administration of carbon dioxide (5 to 10%) for several minutes almost always will relieve spasm if there is no physical basis. If carbon dioxide apparatus is not available, permitting the patient to rebreathe into a 2-quart paper bag held tightly over the mouth and the nose may be effective. Gastric lavage may be performed with success. The correction of a deranged electrolyte balance or urinary retention by the administration of fluids or other therapy also may restore the normal function of the diaphragm.

ORAL SURGERY

Important Points in Nursing Care

To avoid disfigurement, all wounds about the face should heal by primary union. Therefore, infection of the wound should be avoided.

Watch for symptoms of paralysis or of loss of sensation about the face.

In operations on the mouth or the jaw it is difficult to avoid infection, owing to the presence of bacteria. Therefore, the mouth should be cleansed thoroughly every 2 hours. The nose also should be kept clean.

Nourishment usually is given by gavage in order to keep the mouth clean and the parts absolutely quiet.

When the patient is able to take fluids through a drinking tube, the fluid should enter the unaffected side, and the mouth should be rinsed carefully after each feeding.

Watch the patient's color and breathing. Operations on the tongue often cause swelling sufficient to obstruct breathing (edema of the glottis).

Watch for hemorrhage in operations about the nose, the mouth and the jaw. Use ice caps to prevent hemorrhage.

To assist drainage keep the head turned on the side after operation.

ACIDOSIS

Acidosis is a disturbance of the acid-base equilibrium by a decrease in the amount of fixed bases in the blood, i.e., an increase in the acid ions and a decrease in the alkali reserve of the body.

Occurrence

Diabetes mellitus
Starvation, diarrhea, vomiting
Anesthesia
Cyclic vomiting in children
Infectious diseases, especially respiratory
Pregnancy
Renal disaese

Symptoms

MILD. Fatigue, loss of appetite, frequent headaches, general malaise accompanied by the presence of sugar and ketone bodies in the urine. No recognizable symptomatology.

ACUTE. Nausea, vomiting, headache, epigastric pain, acetone or fruity breath, elevated temperature; face flushed, deeper respirations; followed by drowsiness, hyperpnea, low temperature; coma—lowered blood pressure, skin cold and clammy, rapid weak pulse, collapse.

DEHYDRATION SYMPTOMS. Softening of the eyeballs, dry skin, concentration of acids in body tissues.

BLOOD. W.B.C. may be as high as 25,000. (Normal, 10,000.)

CO_2 as low as 2 vol. per cent. (Normal, 50 to 70 vol. per cent.)

Sugar as high as 3 to 5 Gm. to the L. (Normal, 0.8 to 1.2 Gm. to the L.)

URINE. Glucose, acetone and diacetic acid—3+ and 4+.

Treatment of Acidosis

Bed rest
Force fluids
Physiologic saline solution to replace water and electrolyte losses

MEDICAL AND SURGICAL

Glucose to reduce protein breakdown and excessive ketone formation (5 to 10 per cent solution I.V. or P.O.)

Alkali (bicarbonate, lactate) to relieve hyperpnea

Stimulants, if severe shock occurs

ASPHYXIA

Asphyxia is a condition of unconsciousness due to suffocation or interference of any kind with the oxygen action of the blood.

Causes

Mechanical interference with the entrance of air to the lungs

Inflammation or swelling of the throat and larynx or the formation of a membrane as in diphtheria

Edema of the glottis

Foreign bodies in the respiratory tract

Pressure on the trachea or bronchi from goiter, tumor or aneurysm

Water and mucus, etc., in the respiratory tract, as in drowning

The inhalation of smoke or poisonous gases

Interference with the interchange of gases between the blood and air in the lungs as in carbon-monoxide poisoning or diseases of the heart or lungs

Failure of the lungs to expand in the newborn

Symptoms

FIRST STAGE

The breathing is more rapid, labored and distinctly audible.

The lips are blue, the face congested, the eyes prominent, and the expression anxious.

The blood pressure is raised. This stage lasts about 1 minute.

SECOND STAGE

Convulsions. This stage lasts less than 1 minute.

THIRD STAGE

Unconsciousness, flaccid muscles, dilated pupils.

Blood pressure falls, pulse becomes imperceptible.

Slow and sighing respirations.

Death results from gradual exhaustion and paralysis of the centers in the medulla from the prolonged action of venous blood. The third stage may last 3 minutes or more.

Treatment

Remove all obstruction to the free passage of air.

Intubation, tracheotomy or the pulmotor may be indicated for emergency treatment.

Establish natural respiration with the least possible delay.

Treat the patient for shock.

Loosen clothing about the throat, the neck and the chest.

The position of the patient should be such as to keep the air passage wide open for the admission of air.

If asphyxia is due to fluid in the lungs and the bronchi, as in drowning, the patient's clothing should be loosened about the neck, the waist and the chest.

Mouth-to-mouth resuscitation should begin at once.

CONSTIPATION

Definition

The passage of unduly hard and dry fecal material.

Atonic: without abdominal distress. *Hypertonic or spastic:* abdominal pain and discomfort are present.

Prevention

Take plenty of exercise daily. Practice good habits. Do not take cathartics or laxative drugs except on the special advice of a physician.

Make a habit of going to the toilet at the same time every day. A bowel movement every day is not necessary for all individuals, but it should be maintained if habit is physiologic to the individual.

Eat meals slowly at regular hours and masticate food thoroughly.

Be cheerful and happy at meals.

Diet—high cellulose (*see* Diet, p. 538).

Drink 6 to 8 glasses of water daily.

CONVULSIONS

A convulsion is an abnormal discharge of nervous energy to the muscles, resulting in involuntary muscular contractions and defects in the state of consciousness.

Causes

Idiopathic epilepsy.

Head injuries.

Organic brain lesions due to infections or tumors.

Toxic substances in the blood as in acute infectious diseases, alcoholism, uremia, and poisoning by certain drugs.

Hysteric convulsions may simulate those of epilepsy. They are rarely attended by complete unconsciousness, rigidity, biting the tongue or involuntary passage of urine. In hysteria, the movements are usually tonic or, if chronic, appear purposive. Pupils retain their reaction to light, the person seldom injures himself.

Phases

Tonic phase is a generalized stiffening or rigidity of the body.

Clonic phase follows the tonic phase and is characterized by alternate contraction and relaxation of body muscles giving the "jerking" appearance. Consciousness usually is lost before the tonic stage.

Treatment

Coolness, presence of mind, promptness in action.

The patient should be placed in a recumbent position in a place where he cannot hurt himself.

Movements should not be restrained but guided so as to prevent injury to the patient.

A gag should be placed quickly between the teeth to prevent biting the tongue—do not force jaw open.

The clothing should be loosened, and fresh air admitted freely.

Patient never should be left alone while in a convulsion.

The symptoms of the attack should be carefully noted and reported.

Further treatment will depend on the diagnosis.

Points to Observe

The time of the attack

The onset of the attack, whether sudden or preceded by a warning (aura) or by nervous or emotional disturbances

The character of the contractions (tonic or clonic)

The area involved

The muscles first affected and pattern of progression

The frequency and duration of the convulsions

Whether the patient is hypersensitive, conscious, semiconscious or totally unconscious

Relaxation of sphincter and involuntary movements of urine or stools

The appearance of the eyes—closed or open, fixed or squinting, pupils dilated, contracted or irregular

The appearance of frothing at the mouth

The change in pulse, respiration and the color and expression of the face

The condition of the patient following the convulsion

CONVULSIONS IN CHILDREN (*See* Pediatrics)

EPILEPSY

Epilepsy is a disease characterized by attacks of sudden disturbance of consciousness, either with or without convulsions. The majority of epileptics are of average or even of superior intelligence.

SYMPTOMS

Petit Mal (Minor Motor Attacks)

There may be a feeling of dizziness and temporary loss of consciousness with or without muscle spasm lasting from 3 to 5 seconds.

There may be slight muscular twitching, with momentary loss of consciousness, and the patient then proceeds with whatever he was doing.

Grand Mal (Major Motor Attack)

Convulsions may be severe, and the period of unconsciousness prolonged.

Attacks often are preceded by an "aura" or warning.

Injuries are frequent because in falling, the patient makes no attempt to protect himself.

The tonic stage begins immediately. The whole body becomes rigid, the jaws are fixed, the eyes open and staring or else rolled back, and the face becomes increasingly cyanotic.

The weird cry which is uttered by some patients at the beginning of the attack is due to forced expulsion of air past the vocal cords.

The tonic stage lasts from 15 to 30 seconds and is followed by the clonic stage, marked by convulsive action of the muscles.

The body relaxes, and the patient lies unconscious, breathing heavily, and frequently is "frothing at the mouth."

During the convulsion the tongue may be bitten. Urine and feces may be passed involuntarily.

On regaining consciousness there is muscular soreness, headache and confusion.

Psychomotor (Temporal Lobe Epilepsy)

Consciousness is lost and amnesia occurs but no convulsion ensues and activity which may seem normal may be continued. The individual may appear drowsy, intoxicated or violent, behave normally or engage in violent antisocial behavior.

The attack lasts for from 30 seconds to several minutes and is followed by a clouding of consciousness.

Patients may commit some misdemeanors or serious crimes during such an attack.

Status Epilepticus

This occurs when attacks occur so frequently that consciousness is not regained after one attack before another one begins. Death can result due to general physical exhaustion if the attacks are not stopped.

Intravenous administration of sodium phenobarbital or of paraldehyde is most frequently administered to effect cessation of status epilepticus.

MANAGEMENT OF CONVULSIONS

Remove the patient's glasses.
Loosen clothing about neck and waist.

Place a padded mouth gag, cork, or wadded handkerchief between the molars to protect the tongue. Do not force the jaw.

If the attack begins during mealtime or while the patient is eating, place the head as low as possible and to the side to prevent aspiration.

If the patient falls on the floor, make no attempt to move him, but remove all objects against which he might harm himself. Place a pillow under his head.

After the seizure is over, examine patient for signs of injury. Place him in bed and allow him to rest undisturbed.

Treatment

Anticonvulsant Drugs

Phenobarbital	Mesantoin
Dilantin sodium	Mebaral
Tridione	Mysoline
Milontine	Paradione

Dexedrine

(*See discussion in* Pharmacology.)

Nursing Measures

Due to social trauma, epileptics may be difficult to manage.

The present trend is to make the patient as self-sufficient and normal as possible. This may be accomplished by:

Vocational guidance to avoid occupational hazards.

Development of hobbies and diversions.

Teaching patient to be responsible for taking his own medications and reporting untoward effects.

Participation in sports and normal activities with safeguards for such sports as swimming, etc. Driving an automobile is contraindicated.

Advising marriage to a nonepileptic.

A well-balanced and normal diet.

Hygienic measures to keep patient in best physical and mental health.

Stressing importance of continued medical supervision and necessity of taking drugs as prescribed by the

MEDICAL AND SURGICAL

doctor. Status epilepticus can be precipitated by abrupt withdrawal of seizure medication.

HEADACHE (CEPHALALGIA)

One of the most common symptoms of the human race, usually resulting from some disturbance of the cranial vascular structures or a direct effect on the sensory nerves of the head. It involves muscles, tendons and fascia.

Etiology

Localized intracranial disease
Symptom of systemic illness
Trauma
Emotional conflicts
Excessive psychic pressure
Eyestrain

Diagnosis

Accurate history of patient, to include the type of pain, the location, the duration and the frequency
Thorough physical and neurologic examination
Routine blood and urine tests
Evaluation of emotional status of patient
Ophthalmoscopic examination
If lesion of skull or brain is suspected a roentgenogram, an electroencephalogram and/or a pneumoencephalogram are taken.

Classification of Headaches

ACUTE. Associated with febrile diseases, exposure to toxins, grave illness, acute ear or sinus infection and with cerebral or subarachnoid hemorrhage.

OCCASIONAL. Associated with fatigue, unusual eyestrain, emotional upsets, lack of sleep, overeating or excessive drinking.

RECURRENT, PERIODIC AND CHRONIC. Associated with hypertension and other vascular disease, trauma, brain tumor, migraine syndrome and psychogenic disturbances.

Treatment

Find underlying cause and attempt to eliminate it.

Analgesic. (*See detailed discussion in* Pharmacology.)

Vasoconstrictors: ergot derivatives. (*See detailed discussion in* Pharmacology.)

Mild sedative, phenobarbital, once or twice a day as a prophylaxis.

Psychotherapy.

Comfort measures, such as rest, quiet, dark environment, icecap to head, etc.

MIGRAINE HEADACHE

Incidence

Occurs in individuals who otherwise are well.

Characteristics

Dull, throbbing or piercing in type

Usually involves one side of head

Often starts over one eye and radiates backward; may start at back of head and radiate forward

Accompanied by visual symptoms

Often accompanied by nausea and vomiting

May be preceded by an aura, such as drowsiness, depression, feeling of nervousness, etc.

Etiology

Allergy

Endocrine changes

Metabolic changes

Psychological factors. Personality traits common to many who have this kind of headache include

Thinker rather than doer

Tense, nervous, worrisome

Overconscientious

Work hard, fatigue easily

Perfectionism

Subject to fears and doubts

Treatment

Shorten the attack by treating at the first indication of the approaching headache.

Analgesics accompanied by mild sedative or caffeine. (*See discussion in* Pharmacology.)

Ergotamine Tartrate. (*See discussion in* Pharmacology.)

MEDICAL AND SURGICAL

Dihydroergotamine. (*See discussion in* Pharmacology.)

Cafergot. (*See discussion in* Pharmacology.)

Supportive care.

Prevent attacks or prolong interval between them.

Remove underlying mechanisms; allergies, etc.

Help individual to see why he has attacks.

Eliminate undesirable environmental factors.

HEAT EXHAUSTION

Heat exhaustion is caused by exposure to excessive heat and by profuse perspiration.

Symptoms

Weakness and dizziness.

Some elevation of temperature.

As a rule the patient does not lose consciousness, but complete syncope may occur or there may be semi-consciousness with muttering delirium.

Suspension of urine.

Treatment

Rest in a cool place.

Administration of salt or sodium bicarbonate.

Administration of stimulants, such as spirits of ammonia.

HEAT STROKE AND SUNSTROKE

Heat stroke results from exposure to high external temperature from any source, resulting in failure of the heat-regulating mechanism.

Sunstroke results from exposure to the direct rays of the sun.

Symptoms

Headache, dizziness, nausea, malaise.

High fever 105° to 110° F., flushed face, dry skin, rapid pulse, stertorous breathing.

Later there may be convulsions, delirium or coma.

Treatment

Ice water to drink.

Ice-water bath, or packing body in ice.

Brisk rubbing to bring the hot blood to the skin.

Cold enemas.

Treatments are continued until the temperature drops to 102° F., then cool sponge baths may be given.

Patient lies quietly in bed, head slightly elevated, and covered with a sheet only.

Watch pulse for symptoms of collapse.

Careful nursing care after active symptoms subside.

HEMOPTYSIS

Hemoptysis is the coughing up or "spitting of blood" from the lungs.

Causes

Pulmonary tuberculosis

Diseases of the lungs, e.g., pneumonia, cancer, abscess, bronchiectasis, etc.

Ulceration of the bronchi, the trachea or the larynx

Mitral stenosis, pulmonary infarction

Aneurysm of the aorta

Hemorrhagic disorders, such as purpura, hemophilia, or leukemia

HEMATEMESIS	HEMOPTYSIS
Previous history points to gastric, hepatic or splenic disease.	Cough or signs of some pulmonary or cardiac disease precede the hemorrhage in many cases.
The blood is brought up by vomiting, prior to which the patient may experience a feeling of giddiness or faintness.	The blood is coughed up and usually is preceded by a sensation of tickling in the throat. If vomiting occurs, it follows the coughing.
The blood usually is clotted, mixed with particles of food and has "coffee-ground" appearance.	The blood is frothy, bright red in color, alkaline in reaction.
Subsequent to the attack the patient may pass tarry stools, and signs of disease of the abdominal viscera may be detected.	The cough persists, physical signs of local disease in the chest usually may be detected and the sputum may be tinged for many days.

MEDICAL AND SURGICAL

Treatment

Rest in bed and absolute quiet and relaxation. Reassure the patient.

Morphine usually is given to quiet the patient. Demerol or codeine as continuation.

Subdue cough with codeine, do not suppress cough reflex.

Turn patient on affected side to prevent aspiration of other side.

Support patient to help allay anxiety.

Antibiotic therapy (i.e., penicillin) to prevent pneumonia.

Oxygen therapy may be needed if aspiration occurs.

Suction out passages if aspiration occurs.

HEMORRHAGE

Hemorrhage is any profuse bleeding from a blood vessel.

Classification

According to type of vessel involved
　Arterial—spurting stream of bright red blood
　Venous—flows out quickly and is dark red in color
　Capillary—slow general ooze
According to site of hemorrhage
　Evident—that which is on the surface and can be seen.
　Concealed—that which cannot be seen as in the peritoneal cavity, brain, etc.
According to cause
　Primary
　　Result of trauma
　　At time of surgery
　Secondary
　　Slipping of ligature due to
　　　Infection
　　　Insecure tying
　　　Erosion of vessel by a drainage tube
　Blood dyscrasias such as, hemophilia, purpura, etc.

Eroding or rupture of a blood vessel as in ulcers, tuberculosis, etc.

Following the administration of anticoagulants, such as heparin, Dicumarol

Signs and Symptoms

Marked pallor

Marked thirst

Normal or slightly elevated temperature

Pulse is rapid; often thready

Respiration, deep, regular, rapid

Later, air hunger with gasping and irregularity

Blood pressure, low, decrease with small pulse pressure

Skin cold and clammy

Anxious, restless, alert, sense of impending danger

Patient goes into shock as a result of the circulatory collapse from loss of whole blood.

Treatment

Rest and quiet

Direct pressure if bleeding point is evident

Application of tourniquet if bleeding is in an extremity; use with caution and release every 30 minutes

Elevation of part where possible

Replacement therapy, whole blood; plasma, normal saline or dextran may be given to raise blood volume

Careful observation of vital signs

Keep patient from chilling

SHOCK

Shock can be described only as the clinical syndrome following such conditions as extensive trauma, blood loss, prolonged operations, burns and toxic absorption. It is characterized by a progressive reduction in cardiac output and in circulating blood volume, apparently due to many factors.

Classifications

There are two main clinical groupings of patients suffering from shock.

REVERSIBLE SHOCK which, by definition, implies that therapeutic measures are effective in reversing the chain of physiologic events leading to vascular collapse and death.

IRREVERSIBLE SHOCK, again by definition, implies a state of severe shock where therapeutic measures are of no value or are of temporary value in reversing the same chain of physiologic events.

Physiologic Characteristics

Reduction of blood volume
Vasoconstriction
Reduction in cardiac output
Stasis of circulation in periphery
Decreased venous return
Decrease in blood pressure
Lack of oxygen in tissues
Fluid loss into tissues
Failure of myocardium, vasomotor center and respiratory center resulting in death

Signs and Symptoms

Patient looks and feels seriously ill
Extreme weakness
Difficulty in orientation
Face—anxious, drawn and pinched in appearance
Skin—ashen gray or cyanotic; cold and clammy
Pulse—rapid, weak, irregular and reduced in volume
Blood pressure—lowered gradually
Respiration—rapid, shallow
Temperature—lowered or subnormal
General diminution of all vital functions
Extreme exhaustion, anoxemia, coma and death, if symptoms are untreated

Treatment

Complete rest, both physical and mental, to avoid additional strain on an already weakening cardiovascular system. The patient should be placed in shock position (elevation of foot of bed by shock blocks).

Control of pain. Although its mechanism is not understood completely, pain is known to increase shock definitely and must be eliminated as early as possible.

Control of body temperature, avoiding overheating or overcooling.

Blood and fluid replacement therapy is based entirely

on the knowledge that there is fluid lost with a diminished cardiac output. The ideal in replacement therapy is to give back to the body the exact amount and kind of fluid that has been lost, as rapidly as possible. Plasma, whole blood, saline and the like are administered intravenously.

Oxygen may be supplied if necessary.

Mental and emotional rest, especially to the patient experiencing psychic trauma, is very important. This may be accomplished partially by maintaining quiet surroundings and reassuring the patient concerning his condition.

Vasoconstrictor agents can be used in a limited number of cases, but should be considered supporting rather than curative therapy. (*See discussion of* Drugs to Treat Hypotension in Pharmacology.)

Conditions Most Likely to Cause Shock

Extensive muscle tissue damage
Fractures—compound and multiple
Extensive burns
Hemorrhage
Damage to internal organs
Intestinal obstruction
Peritonitis
Acute pancreatitis
Gangrene of tissue due to embolism or thrombosis
Prolonged anesthesia and operation

PREDISPOSING FACTORS

Extremes of age
Chronic pulmonary or cardiac disease
Anemia
Diminished blood volume

INSOMNIA

There are many factors contributing to inability to sleep. Chief among them are:
Unfamiliar surroundings
Excitement or overstimulation
Worry, anxiety or grief
Pain or discomfort
Hunger
Excessive heat or cold

MEDICAL AND SURGICAL

Excessive fatigue
Not enough fatigue
Dietary indiscretions

Measures to Induce Sleep Without Drugs

Well-ventilated room
Light but warm bedclothing
Comfortable bed
Quiet surroundings
A warm bath before retiring
Warm milk or a light meal before going to bed
Easily digested food
Sufficient exercise to produce mild fatigue
Rubbing the back and smoothing sheets
Reading that is not stimulating or exciting
Physical relaxation
Mental reassurance

Drugs (*See* Pharmacology)

JAUNDICE (ICTERUS)

Jaundice is the yellowish or greenish staining of the skin, the mucous membranes and certain body fluids with bile pigment. Jaundice is a symptom, not a disease.

Cause

Mechanical interference to the outflow of bile, i.e., obstructive jaundice

Gallstones in common bile duct
Carcinoma of the head of pancreas or of the ampulla of Vater
Acute or chronic inflammation of the common duct —cholangitis
Pressure on duct, either internal or external
Obstruction of biliary ducts in liver

Functional or degenerative changes in liver, i.e., hepatogenic jaundice

Homologous serum jaundice
Infectious hepatitis
Cirrhosis of liver
Toxic hepatitis
Acute yellow atrophy
Chemicals and drugs (chloroform, carbon tetrachloride, etc.)

Systemic reactions, such as severe toxemia of pregnancy, anoxia, nutritional deficiencies, etc.

Injuries of unknown origin.

Treatment

Clinical picture varies with cause, and treatment relates to elimination of the cause where possible.

Obstructive jaundice usually is accompanied by:

Bleeding tendency, which is controlled by vitamin K preparation—menadione and a bile salt preparation or subcutaneous injection of the vitamin alone.

Itching is difficult to control. Usually not found with cancer of the head of the pancreas

Use antipruritic agents (*See discussion in* Pharmacology)

Injections of ergotamine tartrate give temporary relief

Use sedatives or hypnotics to ensure sleep

Part 2.   Diagnostic Procedures

ELECTROCARDIOGRAM

The electrocardiograph is a complicated instrument used to study the rhythm of the heart muscle contraction. The contraction of the heart muscle produces a very delicate electric current. This current is obtained by placing electrodes on the arms or the legs of the patient and connecting them with wires to the electrocardiograph. The current is registered as a series of curves on a moving sheet of photographic paper. The curve is called an *electrocardiogram.*

The curve produced by normal heart action is characteristic. The different types of abnormal rhythm produce typical curves. The physician, therefore, is able to determine the exact type of abnormal rhythm by the kind of curve obtained.

Common Types of Abnormal Rhythm

Sinus arrhythmia
Extrasystole
Auricular fibrillation
Auricular flutter
Heart block

I. HEMATOLOGIC EXAMINATIONS

TEST	NORMAL VALUE	PATHOLOGY INDICATED BY DEVIATIONS
Red Blood Count (Erythrocytes)	4.0 to 5.5 million/cu. mm.	Increase in polycythemia, vera or secondary Decrease in anemias (all types), leukemia
Hemoglobin Females Males	12.0 to 15.2 Gm./100 ml. 14 to 17 Gm./100 ml.	Decrease in anemia (all types), leukemia
White Blood Count Leukocytes	4,500 to 9,500/cu. mm.	Decrease (leukopenia) in aplastic anemia, agranulocytosis, pernicious anemia, deficiency states, some infectious diseases, typhoid, certain viruses, etc. Increase (leukocytosis) in infections and inflammations, leukemia, malignancy, polycythemia vera
Lymphocytes	1,250 to 3,500/cu. mm. 25 to 35 per cent	Increase in infectious mononucleosis, German measles, pertussis, undulant fever, chronic lymphatic leukemia
Monocytes	200 to 1,000/cu. mm. 4 to 10 per cent	Increase in tuberculosis, some infections, monocytic leukemia
Neutrophils	2,500 to 6,500/cu. mm. 50 to 65 per cent	Increase in bacterial, infectious and inflammatory conditions, necrosis, neoplastic diseases, leukemias, and polycythemia vera
Eosinophils	25 to 400/cu. mm. 0.5 to 4 per cent	Increase in infection by animal parasites, bronchial asthma, myelogenous leukemia, allergic reactions, many skin diseases
Basophils	0 to 200/cu. mm. 0 to 2 per cent	Increase in myelogenous leukemia, myeloid metaplasia
Platelets	150 to 300 thousand/cu. mm.	Decrease in some acute infections, pernicious anemia, chronic lymphatic leukemia, acute leukemia, purpura hemorrhagica, following radiation and some cancer drugs Increase in chronic myelogenous leukemia, polycythemia vera, following hemorrhage and trauma

Reticulocytes	0.5 to 2.0 per cent red cells	Increase in pernicious anemia after treatment, hemolytic anemias or after treatment of iron deficiency
Hematocrit (vol. % of red cells)	42 to 50 per cent	Decrease in hemorrhage and other anemias. Increase in large blood plasma or serum loss as in shock, extensive burns; polycythemias
Sedimentation Rate Westegren	less than 15 mm. in 1 hr.	A nonspecific response to tissue damage. Increased rate in chronic infections, neoplasm, localized acute inflammation, acute and inflammatory diseases, chronic infection, infarctions
Wintrobe Male	0 to 9 mm. in 1 hr.	
Female	0 to 15 mm. in 1hr.	
Clotting Time, Venous blood	5 to 10 minutes	Increase in time in hemophilliod diseases, circulating anticoagulant, spontaneous or therapeutic, i.e., heparin
Bleeding Time	1 to 5 minutes	Increase in time in thrombocytopenia

II. CHEMICAL CONSTITUENTS—BLOOD

TEST	NORMAL VALUE	PATHOLOGY INDICATED BY DEVIATIONS
Amylase, serum (Myers and Killian)	Less than 50 units	Elevated in renal insufficiency and in diseases of the pancreas
Bilirubin, total serum	0.1 to 0.8/100 ml.	Elevated when jaundice is present. Indicates obstruction in flow of bile into intestinal tract or hepatic injury
Calcium, serum	9 to 11 mg./100 ml.	Low concentration (hypocalcemia) in hypoparathyroidism, steatorrhea, rickets, osteomalacia, chronic renal disease (uremia). High concentration (hypercalcemia) in hyperparathyroidism, metastatic lesions in skeleton, acromegaly

II. CHEMICAL CONSTITUENTS—BLOOD (Cont.)

TEST	NORMAL VALUE	PATHOLOGY INDICATED BY DEVIATIONS
Carbon Dioxide Content (serum)	23 to 28 mEq./L.	Decreased in acidosis from diabetes, uremia Elevated in alkalosis (metabolic)
Chlorides, serum	98 to 106 mEq./L.	Decreased in alkalosis, fever, pneumonia, vomiting Increased in nephritis, eclampsia, and sometimes in malignancy and cardiac disease
Cholesterol Total serum Esters, serum	150 to 260 mg./100 ml. 80 to 180 mg./100 ml.	Decrease in hepatic disease (esters), hyperthyroidism Increase in nephrosis, obstructive jaundice (cholelithiasis), hypo-thyroidism, diabetes, pregnancy
Creatinine, serum	0.6 to 1.3 mg./100 ml.	Increase in urinary obstruction, acute nephritis, terminal stages of chronic nephritis
Glucose (fasting blood)	70 to 110 mg./100 ml.	Decreased (hypoglycemia) in hyperinsulinism, a complication of pancreatic function Elevated (hyperglycemia) in diabetes mellitus, some adrenal dis-orders, hyperthyroidism
Nitrogen, nonprotein (N.P.N.)	15 to 35 mg./100 ml.	Elevated in inadequacy of renal function, uremia, etc.
Phosphatase acid (Bessey-Laurey) alkaline	0.10 to 0.90 units 5 to 14 King-Armstrong units (adult)	Increased in cancer or prostate Increased in osteoblastic disease of bone, such as Paget's disease, rickets, metastatic cancer, hyperparathyroidism, obstructive liver disease
Phosphorus, inor-ganic serum	3 to 4.5 mg./100 ml.	Decrease in rickets in children, hyperparathyroidism Increase in hypoparathyroidism, adults who have severe fractures, chronic renal disease (uremia)

Potassium, serum	3.4 to 5.2 mg./L.	Increase in adrenal cortical insufficiency, Addison's disease, intestinal obstruction, acute fevers
Protein-bound iodine	4 to 8 mcg./100 ml.	Below 4 = hypothyroidism Above 8 = hyperthyroidism
Proteins—serum Total	6.5 to 8.0 Gm./100 ml.	Decrease in malnutrition Elevated in multiple myeloma
Albumin	4.0 to 5.2 Gm./100 ml.	Decrease in inadequate diet, cirrhosis, nephrosis Elevated in dehydration
Globulin	1.5 to 3.0 Gm./100 ml.	Elevated in liver disease, lymphosarcoma, Boeck's sarcoid, multiple myeloma
Prothrombin, plasma (quick method)	13 to 15 seconds	Prolonged in hepatic disease, anticoagulant drug therapy
Sodium, serum	137 to 145 mEq./L.	Decrease in nephritic acidosis, diabetes mellitus
Urea Nitrogen, serum (BUN)	10 to 22 mg./100 ml.	Decrease in last months of pregnancy, acute hepatic insufficiency Increase in impaired excretion in kidney disease, also in severe burns, shock, intestinal obstruction, acute fever, peritonitis
Uric Acid, serum	3 to 6 mg./100 ml.	Increase in acute or chronic nephritis, cardiorenal disease, leukemia, during remissions in pernicious anemia, eclampsia, gout
SGO—T (Transaminase)	10 to 40 units	Increase in myocardial infarction, acute hepatitis, obstructive jaundice

III. SEROLOGIC TESTS

TEST	NORMAL VALUE	PATHOLOGY INDICATED BY DEVIATIONS
BACTERIAL AGGLUTINATION TESTS	(upper limit of normal titer)	
Widal Test	1:80	Typhoid and paratyphoid (enteric) fevers (salmonellosis) O titer high in infections; high H titer may persist after immunization or infection
Brucellosis (Undulant or Malta fever)	1:40 to 1:80	Higher titer or rise significant in brucellosis
Tularemia	1:20 to 1:40	Rise significant in tularemia
Weil—Felix Test	1:80 to 1:160	Higher titer or rise significant in typhus fever (including Brill's disease) and Rocky Mountain spotted fever
TESTS WITH ERYTHROCYTES		
Heterophile Agglutination Test (Paul-Bunnell Test)	1:64 to 1:128	Higher titer or rise significant in infectious mononucleosis
Latex Fixation Test	less than 1:20	Higher titer in rheumatoid arthritis
Cold Agglutination Test	1:16 to 1:32	Higher titer or rise significant in primary atypical pneumonia
Antistreptolysin Titration	less than 250 units ASL per ml. serum	Group A beta hemolytic streptococcal infection

Test	Normal Value	Pathology Indicated by Deviations
STANDARD TESTS FOR SYPHILIS		
VDRL (Venereal Disease Research Laboratories)	negative	Flocculation test—nonspecific test for syphilis used for screening. Similar principle as other flocculation tests (Mazzini, Kahn, Hinton) but more sensitive. Reported as negative (N); weakly positive (WP); positive (P)
Kolmer (Wasserman)	negative	Complement fixation test—done on all patients with a positive VDRL or positive cerebral spinal fluid. Reported as O, 1+, 2+, 3+, 4+. "BFP"—Biologic False Positive—in infectious mononucleosis, malaria, lupus, some neoplasm, and macroglobinemia
T.P.I. (Treponema Pallidum Immobilization Test)	negative	Used to detect true syphilitic infections, especially when VDRL or Kolmer are positive. Reported as either positive or negative

IV. Urine Tests

Test	Normal Value	Pathology Indicated by Deviations
Quantity	1,200 to 1,500 ml. daily	Increased (polyuria) in chronic nephritis, diabetes insipidus, diabetes mellitus, potassium depletion, psychogenic polydypsia. Decreased (oliguria) in dehydration, shock, acute renal insufficiency
Color	yellow—pale to deep	Red or brown smoky color = blood. Dark yellow or brown = bile (yellow foam forms when shaken). Change in color by certain food and drugs
Transparency	clear	Cloudiness due to phosphates, pus, blood, bacteria
Odor	aromatic odor due to volatile oils	Fruit odor = acetone as in diabetes. Ammoniacal in certain bladder infections. Peculiar odors from certain foods, i.e. asparagus

IV. Urine Tests (Continued)

Test	Normal Value	Pathology Indicated by Deviations
Specific Gravity	1.002 to 1.036	Fixed at 1.010 in chronic renal insufficiency Chronically low in diabetes insipidus, hypercalcemia, potassium depletion, psychogenic polydipsia Chronically high in diabetes mellitus, dehydration
Chlorides	depends entirely on intake	May detect excessive retention or excessive loss of salt if intake is known
Phosphates	2.5 to 3.5 Gms./24 hrs.	Excessive loss in hyperparathyroidism
Urea	20 to 35 Gms./24 hrs. (depends entirely on protein intake and metabolism)	Useful rarely in appraising renal function if plasma urea is known
Ammonia	0.7 Gms. in 24 hrs. (depends on diet and acid-base balance)	
ABNORMAL CONSTITUENTS		
Protein	none	Extra renal proteinuria in cystitis, chronic vaginitis Postural proteinuria occasionally occurs in normal subjects on standing True proteinuria in irritation of kidneys (drugs, bacterial toxins as in acute infectious diseases), nephritis, renal tuberculosis, renal neoplasms, congestion in kidneys from heart disease, later stages of pregnancy
Glucose	none	Increase in diabetes mellitus Transitory increase after strong emotions (fear, anger, anxiety) and assimilation of large amounts of sugar. May be confused with other reducing sugars (e.g. lactose in pregnancy)

Test	Normal Value	Pathology Indicated by Deviations
Acetone Bodies (ketones) acetone diacetic acid	none	Found in diabetic acidosis, limited carbohydrate intake as in fever, gastrointestinal disorders; eclampsia, postanesthetic toxemia, severe dehydration
Urobilinogen	less than 4.0 mg./24 hrs.	Increase in excessive destruction of hemoglobin, functional impairment of liver as in acute hepatitis. Absence in complete biliary obstruction
Hemoglobin	none	Found in extensive burns, transfusions of incompatible blood, hemolytic chemical agents, hemolytic anemia, pyelonephritis, renal calculi, renal tuberculosis, carcinoma of kidney, hemorrhagic cystitis, prostatitis

V. Functional Tests

Test	Normal Value	Pathology Indicated by Deviations
Basal Metabolism Rate	minus 10 per cent to plus 10 per cent of mean standard	Above 10 per cent in hyperthyroidism, infection, neoplasm, pregnancy, heart failure, anxiety Below 10 per cent in hypothyroidism, nephrotic syndrome
Radioactive Iodine Test (24 hr. I131 Uptake Test	15 to 45 per cent uptake in 24 hours	Higher uptake in hyperthyroidism Lower uptake in hypothyroidism, thyroiditis Evidence of decrease I131 uptake in localized area as shown by Geiger counter, indicates possible malignancy (Invalid results if patient recently had drugs with iodine, i.e., dyes such as lipiodal, Lugol's solution, cough syrups with iodides. Pregnancy and lactation are also contraindications for test.)
Bromsulfalein (BSP)	0 to 10 per cent retention after 30 minutes	Increase in hepatic disease

V. FUNCTIONAL TESTS (Continued)

TEST	NORMAL VALUE	PATHOLOGY INDICATED BY DEVIATIONS
Cephalin Flocculation	0 to 1+ precipitate	If precipitation, disease of hepatic parenchyma, protein abnormalities
Circulation Time Calcium gluconate Decholin	arm to tongue, 10 to 16 seconds arm to tongue, 10 to 16 seconds	Prolonged time in most types of heart failure Shortened time in hyperthyroidism, anemia, beriberi
Galactose Tolerance	excretion of no more than 3.0 grams galactose in urine in 5 hours after ingestion of 40 grams of galactose	Increase in excretion in intrahepatic jaundice, hepatic insufficiency
Glucose Tolerance	after ingesting glucose 100 Gms./Kg. body weight, blood sugar is not more than 180 mg./100 ml. after 30 minutes normal in 2 hours and none excreted in urine	If blood sugar remains high, indicates possible diabetes mellitus (test not valid if patient has been on very low carbohydrate intake) "Flat" glucose tolerance type curve suggests intestinal malabsorption
Hippuric Acid	excretion of 3.0 to 3.5 grams in urine in 4 hours after ingestion of 6.0 grams sodium benzoate	Low out put in various forms of hepatitis, other lesions in the liver, cirrhosis
Phenolsulfonphthalein (P.S.P.) intramuscular injection	55 to 75 per cent in urine in 2 hours	Below 40 per cent in impaired function of kidneys Elevated in hepatic disease
Thymol Turbidity Test	0 to 1+	Above 1+ precipitation = hepatocellular damage
Urea Clearance	40 ml. or more blood cleared/minute	Low clearance indicates impaired renal function
Venous Pressure, peripheral vein	60 to 120 mm. water	Elevated in congestive heart failure due to myocardial or valvular disease, in constrictive pericarditis, or pericardial effusion, local increase in part of body due to mechanical venous obstruction

Part 3. Infections and Inflammations

APPENDICITIS

Appendicitis is an acute inflammation of the vermiform appendix. Chronic appendicitis is a poorly understood syndrome and a rarely accepted diagnosis.

Signs and Symptoms
Pain.

Frequently comes on suddenly and is paroxysmal in nature.

Location depends on position of appendix; usually starts in epigastrium and localizes in right lower quadrant.

Nausea and vomiting

Local tenderness

Muscle spasm

Fever 100° to 102° F.

Leukocytosis

Treatment
Diagnosis and early surgical removal

If suspected

Give nothing by mouth

Avoid laxatives

See Preoperative and Postoperative Care, Sect. 1, Part 1, pp. 175 to 177.

PERITONITIS

Peritonitis is an inflammation of the membrane lining the peritoneal cavity. It almost always is secondary to the disease either of the abdominal organs or extending from elsewhere in the body by the way of the blood stream.

Etiology
Peritonitis is secondary to

Perforations in

Appendicitis

MEDICAL AND SURGICAL

     Peptic ulcer
     Diverticulitis
     Carcinoma
     Cholecystitis
Tuberculosis
Gonorrhea in the female
Sepsis associated with abortions or puerperal state
Trauma, surgical or otherwise

Signs and Symptoms

Abdominal pain
Tenderness over involved area (rebound tenderness)
Spasm of abdominal wall
Nausea and vomiting
Distention
Elevated pulse rate
Leukocytosis (25,000 or more per ml. is usual)

Treatment

Antibiotic therapy—Aureomycin, Terramycin, streptomycin (*See* Pharmacology)
Correction of primary focus of infection usually by surgical intervention
Supportive therapy
Gastrointestinal decompression by suction
Position in bed—elevate head to encourage drainage toward pelvis to promote localization
Maintenance of fluid and electrolyte balance

See Preoperative and Postoperative Care, pp. 175 to 177.

PEPTIC ULCER

This is a circumscribed mucosal ulceration resulting from the digestive action of acid gastric juice, and is located in the stomach or the duodenum. It is benign in nature.

Location

Duodenum—most frequently
Stomach
Lower end of esophagus

Etiology

Cause not understood, but there is a relationship between the acid secretion and ulcer formation

Most frequent in people age 20 to 50

Occurs 4 times more frequently in males than in females

More in people of a specific constitutional type, i.e., tall, slim, tense

Brought on by emotional situations

Various types of food that damage mucosa

Diagnosis

History of pain, relieved by food or antacid

Gastrointestinal series—roentgenogram shows ulcer

Gastric expression—high hydrochloric acid content

Signs and Symptoms

Pain, periodic—greatest incidence from October to May

Gnawing or aching, burning

Usually epigastric, may radiate through to back

Occurs 1 to 4 hours after meals

Relieved by food or antacids

Loss of weight from continual vomiting or patient's fear of eating

Vomiting, when associated with obstruction or pylorospasm

Constipation

Severe generalized abdominal pain and collapse associated with perforation

Mild to severe gastrointestinal hemorrhage associated with blood vessel erosion

Treatment

Medical

Rest—physical, mental and emotional

Not necessarily in hospital

Mild sedative or tranquilizer (*See* Pharmacology)

Bland type of diet—frequent, regular feedings— (*See* Diet, p. 559.)

Chemical antacids (*See discussion in* Pharmacology)

Antispasmodics (*See discussion in* Pharmacology)

Avoidance of alcohol, cigarettes and condiments

Education of patient to avoid situations of stress

Psychotherapy

Prevention of fecal impactions which may accompany antacid therapy

Surgical therapy (subtotal gastrectomy)

Indications for

Repeated upper gastrointestinal hemorrhage

Severe uncontrolled gastrointestinal hemorrhage

Obstruction to pylorus

Perforation

Intractable pain that is not controlled by conservative regimen

Inability of patient to follow medical regimen

Ruling out of malignancy in cases of gastric ulcer

Special preoperative and postoperative care of patient with gastric surgery

Preoperative

Reduce bacterial flora by antibiotics and mechanical cleansing (gastric lavage and colonic treatments)

Combat anemia by transfusions

Rehydration in face of prolonged obstruction

High caloric, high vitamin diet for nutritional debility

If obstruction, relieve by gastric decompression by nasogastric tube

Prepare patient for future change in eating habits

Postoperative care

General supportive measures to maintain fluid balance, caloric requirements, patient comfort, etc.

Continued gastric decompression to prevent anastomosis breakdown from overdistention

Graduated oral feedings

Systemic antibiotic therapy to control infection in a contaminated surgical field

Specific drug therapy, vitamin B_{12} and liver, in the case of total gastrectomy

See Preoperative and Postoperative Care, pp. 175 to 177.

Complications

Perforation
Hemorrhage
Obstruction
Threat of development of malignancy

CHOLECYSTITIS AND CHOLEDOCHOLITHIASIS

ACUTE CHOLECYSTITIS

Acute cholecystitis is an inflammation of the gallbladder that may or may not be associated with gallstones.

Etiology

The etiology is unknown, but is associated frequently with

Obstruction of ampulla of gallbladder or cystic duct
Infections such as typhoid fever, paratyphoid fever or influenza

Signs and Symptoms

Nausea, vomiting
Loss of appetite
Right upper quadrant pain radiating through to the back and shoulder
Rebound tenderness
Fever
Leukocytosis (15,000 per ml.)
Jaundice, colicky pain or abdominal mass arouse suspicion of an obstruction of the common or the cystic duct

Treatment

Conservative
Bedrest
Antibiotics
Supportive therapy including rehydration and use of analgesics and sedatives
Fat-free diet
Surgical—cholecystectomy or cholecystostomy as indicated

See Preoperative and Postoperative Care of Patient with Biliary Surgery, p. 217.

MEDICAL AND SURGICAL

CHRONIC CHOLECYSTITIS

Usually chronic cholecystitis is associated with cholelithiasis.

Symptoms
Chronic indigestion
Intolerance to fatty foods
Right upper quadrant pain: recurrent
Eructations ("belching")
Postprandial bloating

Treatment
Conservative
    Fat-free diet (*See* Diet, p. 539)
    Analgesics for pain
    Antispasmodics (*See discussion in* Pharmacology)
Surgical
    Cholecystectomy, if common duct is normal
    Cholecystectomy and choledochostomy, if evidence of common-duct obstruction

CHOLEDOCHOLITHIASIS

Choledocholithiasis is the presence of gallstones in the common duct. Its etiology is not understood.

Signs and Symptoms
Usually associated with cholecystitis; therefore, symptoms are the same
If obstructive
    Jaundice
    Clay-colored stools
    Dark urine with high bile content
    Bile-free vomitus

Treatment
Antispasmodics to relieve biliary colic (*See* Pharmacology)
Analgesics for severe pain (*See* Pharmacology)
Low fat, high protein, high carbohydrate diet (*See* Diet, p. 541
Bile salts (*See* Pharmacology)

Choledochostomy (Surgical exploration of the common bile duct).

Preoperative and Postoperative Care of Patient Having Biliary Tract Surgery

See Preoperative and Postoperative Care, Sect. 1, Part 1

SPECIAL PREOPERATIVE CARE

Antibiotic therapy, if infection is present

Vitamin K, if jaundice is a symptom

Determination of prothrombin time

Low fat diet

Nasogastric tube is often inserted before operation

SPECIAL POSTOPERATIVE CARE

Observation of patient for signs of hemorrhage, hepatic insufficiency or renal insufficiency

Care of patient with a T-tube, if choledochostomy is performed

Be sure tube is not kinked and is free from traction

Check and measure drainage

Management of tube may be highly individualized; therefore, specific instructions will come from surgeon concerned

Careful observation and reporting of

Degree of jaundice

Color of stool

Character and amount of drainage

Presence or absence of bile in vomitus

Distention

Care of patient with nasogastric tube (*See discussion in* Technics.)

INFECTIOUS HEPATITIS

Infectious hepatitis is an acute inflammation of the liver cells caused by a virus.

Etiology

Virus excreted by feces from the patient having the disease, infects food or water, thereby infects others.

Incubation period is 20 to 120 days.

MEDICAL AND SURGICAL

Signs and Symptoms

PREICTERIC STAGE (lasts about 6 days)
Anorexia—profound
Fever 100° to 103° F.
General malaise, fatigability
Headache
Chilly sensation
Nausea and vomiting
Pruritus
Dark urine
Light stools
Constipation and diarrhea
Enlarged liver and lymph glands
Tenderness in liver area

ICTERIC STAGE (few days in mild cases, may persist for 6 weeks in patients with severe liver involvement)
Jaundice, abatement of other symptoms
Reappearance of appetite and sense of well being while jaundice is most marked—signal of the beginning of the recovery stage

Treatment

Bedrest until jaundice is lessened markedly and the liver becomes smaller—about 5 weeks
Bland diet, suck hard candies
Vitamins
Abstinence from alcohol for 6 months
Gastrointestinal precautions
Syringe precautions
Care in handling blood
Supportive care

CONVALESCENT PERIOD
Difficult to appraise clinically
Many patients are weak and depressed long after jaundice disappears
Some complaint of flatulence and fat intolerance
Exercise often tolerated poorly during this period

PROPHYLAXIS
Gamma globulin for those recently closely exposed to fresh cases

HOMOLOGOUS SERUM JAUNDICE

Homologous serum jaundice is an acute inflammation of liver cells caused by a virus. It is different from that causing infectious hepatitis.

Etiology

A very minute amount of virus in blood or blood products is needed to spread the virus
Blood and plasma transfusions
Venipuncture
Syringes and needles inadequately sterilized
Incubation period is from 60 to 160 days

Symptoms

These are the same as for infectious hepatitis except that fever often is absent.

Treatment

Similar to infectious hepatitis
Syringe precautions
Gamma globulin, especially in children

CIRRHOSIS (Laennec's)

Cirrhosis is a degeneration or inflammation of liver cells followed by fibrous tissue supplanting normal liver tissue.

Etiology

Most common in men aged 45 to 65 years
May be unknown
Nutritional deficiency
High alcoholic intake
Exposure to carbon tetrachloride, arsenic, etc.
Viral hepatitis

Signs and Symptoms

May be asymptomatic; this usually is found at autopsy
Usually history of chronic alcoholism and malnutrition
Weight loss
Vomiting and nausea

MEDICAL AND SURGICAL

Anorexia
Low-grade fever accompanied by leukocytosis
Jaundice
Esophageal and gastric varices
Vascular "spider" in skin of face and neck
Bleeding tendency, especially epistaxis
Ascites
Mental changes, confusion, euphoria

Treatment

Bedrest
Nutritious high caloric diet (4,000 to 5,000 calories). (*See* Diet, p. 534)
Vitamin B complex
Alcohol prohibited
Meticulous nursing care
Surgery—portal caval shunt to relieve portal hypertension

ACUTE TONSILLITIS AND PHARYNGITIS

These are inflammatory processes of the lymphoid tissue of the pharynx, often caused by a hemolytic streptococcus.

Signs and Symptoms

Usually sudden onset
Sore throat—
  Severe on swallowing
  Unilateral or bilateral
  At sides of neck under angles of jaw
Chills with onset of fever
Rhinorrhea
Anterior pharynx, swollen, engorged, red—whether tonsils are present or not
Swollen anterior cervical lymph nodes
Elevated erythrocyte sedimentation rate
Leukocytosis (may not be as high in seriously ill)

Treatment

Bed rest
Chemotherapy (*See* Pharmacology)

Hot saline irrigations
Maintain fluid balance
Nutritious diet in the form which is tolerated
Disease of short duration with antimicrobial therapy

PNEUMONIA

BRONCHOPNEUMONIA

Bronchopneumonia is an inflammation of the terminal bronchioles.

Predisposing Factors

Most frequently observed in young children and in the aged.

Common sequela of influenza, whooping cough, measles and diphtheria.

In infants and debilitated persons, it may occur as a primary infection.

The aspiration of infectious materials or particles of food.

Etiology

Various bacteria: the pneumococcus of higher types, streptococcus, influenza bacillus and others.

Virus infections are often responsible (Virus or Primary Atypical Pneumonia).

Symptoms

Onset is gradual and both lungs usually are involved. Affected areas frequently are patchy.

Symptoms are often masked by the primary disease —not distinctive.

The temperature is moderately high and very irregular.

Cough and expectorations increase, sputum rusty or bloody.

Respirations and pulse become more rapid.

The patient is less toxic than in lobar pneumonia.

The temperature usually subsides by lysis.

Complications

Same as in lobar pneumonia, except that lung complications are more prevalent.

Treatment

Indications for treatment the same as in acute bacterial pneumonia.

ACUTE BACTERIAL PNEUMONIA

(LOBAR PNEUMONIA)

Acute bacterial pneumonia is an infectious disease, usually caused by the pneumococcus (*Diplococcus pneumoniae*) and is characterized by inflammation of one or more lobes of the lung.

Etiology

Due in a large majority of cases to the pneumococcus, although a small percentage of cases may be caused by other bacteria (e.g., *Streptococcus hemolyticus* or Friedländer's bacillus).

Usually secondary to injury of respiratory mucosa by viral infection.

Pathology

Stage of congestion—air still passes in and out of lung.
Stage of consolidation—exudate in alveolar spaces.
Stage of resolution—crisis—represents the development of an effective immunity. Exudate is absorbed and air again enters lungs.

Symptoms

Abrupt onset with chill
Rapid rise in temperature to 103° to 106° F.
Malaise and headache
Stabbing pain in chest; patient lies on affected side
Flushed face, cyanosis, herpes, accelerated respirations, respiratory grunt
Cough—tenacious, rusty sputum
Pulse, full and bounding
Skin, hot and moist

Vomiting

Dyspnea—due to pleural pain, consolidation of lung and toxic effect on respiratory center

Abdominal distention

Complications

Specific

Spread to another part of lung

Pleurisy—some effusion in all cases

Empyema

Meningitis, endocarditis, pericarditis are rare today

Nonspecific occurring during acute phase

Paralytic ileus

Peripheral vascular collapse (shock)

Congestive heart failure

Treatment

General Nursing Care

Complete rest and quiet

Proper ventilation, with patient kept warm and protected from drafts

Sleep and relaxation

Special mouth care

Liquid diet, nondistending in nature, preferable during the acute stage, with fluids forced to at least 3 liters. Salty broth to replace sodium chloride

Individual precautions (organisms are present in sputum and cough spray)

Symptomatic

Cough—controlled by codeine or morphine

Pain—controlled by analgesics (codeine, morphine), immobilization of chest (chest binder or strapping with adhesive)

Headache—relieved by icecap or cold compresses

Distention—controlled by daily enemata or colon lavages, poultices or stupes to abdomen with a rectal tube, drugs that stimulate peristalsis and expulsion of flatus (Pitressin, Prostigmine)

Cyanosis and dyspnea best treated by oxygen administration

Delirium—paraldehyde as hypnotic

Circulatory failure—treated by stimulants and intravenous fluids

Penicillin (*See discussion in* Pharmacology)

Streptomycin for that caused by Friedländer's bacillus, *Hemophilus influenza*, etc.

Danger Signals

Failing pulse with increasing rate and increasing respirations

Increasing cyanosis

Cold hands and feet

Moist respirations, sagging jaw

Increasing and excessive restlessness

Increasing distention

PRIMARY ATYPICAL (VIRUS) PNEUMONIA

An acute infectious disease of the respiratory tract characterized by widespread pulmonary infiltration.

Symptoms

Incubation period 2 to 3 weeks

Chilliness

Fever ranging anywhere from a low-grade fever to 102° to 104° F.

Severe headache

Painful and exhausting cough with the production of very little sputum at first; then becomes productive of mucopurulent sputum

Substernal pain

Anorexia

Bradycardia in about 50 per cent of cases

Leukocyte count usually within normal limits

Sore throat

Treatment

Symptomatic and supportive similar to that of bacterial pneumonia

Excellent nursing care as in bacterial pneumonia

Terramycin (*See discussion in* Pharmacology)

Bedrest for several days after temperature is normal

BRONCHIECTASIS

Definition

A dilatation of the peripheral bronchi with resultant structural changes in their walls which are predominantly inflammatory, destructive, or reparative, depending on the development and stage of the process.

Etiology

A prevalent condition

Sequel to pulmonary diseases such as bronchopneumonia, lung abscess, tumors, tuberculosis

May be found without definite antecedent or prevalent pulmonary disease

Signs and Symptoms

Chronic productive cough

Constant foul taste in mouth

Paroxysms of cough on rising in the morning and on reclining at night

Hemoptysis

Chest pain, if condition accompanied by pleurisy or empyema

Fatigability

Gradual weight loss

Signs of chronic sinusitis

Clubbing of fingers and toes

Treatment and Nursing Care

Surgical resection of involved lobes or segments of the lungs (*See* Thoracic Surgery and Nursing Care, p. 231)

Medical management in preparation for surgery and aid in preserving health of those unsuitable for operation:

Postural drainage on rising in the morning and before retiring at night (*See* Nursing Technics)

Antimicrobial drugs, penicillin, streptomycin, etc. May be also given by aerosol therapy (*See* Nursing Technics; *See* Pharmacology)

Cough medications, codeine, ammonium chloride

MEDICAL AND SURGICAL

(*See* Pharmacology), only during acute exacerbations—generally, it is undesirable to suppress cough reflex.

Maintenance of general health

Adequate nutrition

Adequate rest

Avoidance of unnecessary exposure to conditions which predispose to pulmonary infection

A warm dry climate may be advantageous

Complications

Pneumonia which frequently occurs during course of disease

Empyema

Brain abscess

CHRONIC EMPHYSEMA
(Diffuse Obstructive Emphysema)

Definition

A condition characterized by abnormal dilatation of the alveoli or other respiratory structures. The smaller air passages, especially the terminal bronchi, are narrowed and even obliterated.

Etiology

Usually associated with long standing chronic bronchitis.

Signs and Symptoms

Onset—gradual and insidious

Dyspnea on exertion

Cough, deep, hard, spasmodic

Asthmatic attacks

Deep breathing reveals prolonged and often wheezing expirations

Changes in chest structure, i.e. "barrel chest"

In final stages, condition may terminate by extreme pulmonary insufficiency

dyspnea, orthopnea

purulent cough

respirations—inspiratory gasp, prolonged wheezing expiration

marked cyanosis

asthmatic attacks
anoxia
bronchopneumonia (*See* Bronchopneumonia, p. 221)
cor pulmonale with right heart failure
liver enlargement
increased venous pressure
peripheral edema
tachycardia
clubbing of fingers and toes
death often sudden when this occurs

Treatment and Nursing Care

Purpose of Treatment

To improve pulmonary ventilatory function
To prevent, or to treat promptly, recurring respiratory infections
Bronchodilating agents (*See* Pharmacology)
    Ephedrine
    Epinephrine 1:100 as a spray
Codeine (*See* Pharmacology) in nonproductive stages
Breathing exercises, emphasizing diaphragmatic function
Well-fitting lower abdominal belt for asthenic subjects with poor abdominal muscle tone
Prompt attention to any upper respiratory infection, i.e. bed rest, antibiotic therapy
Respirator, especially those with intermittent positive pressure (*See* Nursing Technics)
Cortisone, especially if asthmatic attacks occur with moderately advanced disease
If disease is advanced:
    Patient placed in high Gatch bed
    Use of aminophylline or epinephrine (*See* Pharmacology) to help clear air passages
    Elimination of secretions important, may use tracheobronchial suction (*See* Nursing Technics)
    Positive pressure breathing if anoxia (*See* Nursing Technics)
    Mild sedatives only (*See* Pharmacology)
    Supportive care in relation to fluid, nutrition, physical and mental hygiene

TUBERCULOSIS

Tuberculosis is a disease affecting all ages, but most prevalent in the age of greatest usefulness, that from 20 to 40 years. It affects both sexes. Girls show the greater tendency to develop the disease between the ages of 10 to 30, but after that age males exceed the females in the mortality from the disease. Morbidity and mortality rates are increasing among older people, especially men. The tubercle bacillus attacks the lungs, throat, lymph glands, peritoneum, brain (tubercular meningitis), skin, bones and joints and may simulate many diseases.

Modes of Transmission

The organism gains entrance to the body by way of the mouth and the nose and also is transmitted by droplet infection, close contact with a tuberculous person, and fomites. The sputum dries and floats in the air as dust in dark areas where there is no sunlight. The dust, full of organisms, enters the lungs with the air breathed.

The disease, especially in children, also may be spread through the milk of tuberculous cows.

Our main barrier to the disease is a well-nourished, well-balanced, healthy body.

Tuberculosis is communicated slowly and with difficulty; it often can be arrested if it has not progressed too far. In tuberculosis, scars are always left and the disease, though arrested, may not be cured absolutely.

Heredity

Tuberculosis is not handed down from the parent to the child before birth. Tuberculous parents, however, unless scrupulously careful, may, and often do, infect their healthy children a short time after birth. In such families where tuberculosis exists, children should be brought up with special care as to their surroundings and mode of life, to enable them to resist and to guard against possible infection. Such children should be protected by BCG vaccination.

PULMONARY TUBERCULOSIS

Signs and Symptoms

Onset varies with patient and site of primary lesion

Clinical manifestations often appear later than the appearance of the actual lesion.

Onset usually marked by:

Grippal symptoms which last several weeks

Slow loss of weight

Increasing fatigue

Afternoon fever of a low grade

Impaired efficiency

Cough—in morning in the early stage

Expectoration starts later in disease

Hemoptysis may be first subjective symptom

Pleurisy may cause outstanding initial symptom

Hoarseness, dryness of throat may be present

Malaise, lassitude, fatigue are the most common symptoms of tuberculous toxicity

Tachycardia (80-90 per minute), regular rhythm, then rise in later part of disease

Menarche may be delayed or irregular, usually after disease is well established

Anorexia

Night sweats in the febrile stage

Elevated ESR

Leukocytosis

Diagnosis

A careful examination of the chest

A microscopic examination of sputum (not once but several times) and of gastric contents

Minute study of the case, family history, past life and surroundings. Roentgenogram

In children, the physical signs are too variable to be reliable and are lacking in early disease

Diagnosis is made from

Tuberculin test (*See* Immunity and Disease, pp. 246-249)

Roentgenogram

History of contact

MEDICAL AND SURGICAL

Treatment and Nursing Care

Chief aim is to suppress bacterial activity and to halt the progress of the disease

Bed rest until this aim is achieved

Chemotherapy (*See* Pharmacology)

Streptomycin

PAS

Isoniazid

Combinations of these

Patient encouraged to suppress cough when possible and to expectorate by gently clearing throat

Codeine may be given to help patient get rest

Medical aseptic technic (*See* Nursing Technics)

Maintenance of adequate nutrition, supplying supplement as indicated

Recognition of the long-term nature of this disease

Consideration of pleasant, relaxing environment

Diversional activities consistent with stage of illness

Instruction of patient as to what he can do and the basis for selecting his activities

Recognition of the difficulty patient may experience in accepting the illness, especially if he does not feel particularly ill

Maintenance of outside contacts—family, friends

Vocational rehabilitation should start as soon as condition warrants

Teaching patient principles of care to maintain arrest of disease and prevent recurrence

Thoracic surgery may be advocated (*See* Care of Patient After Thoracic Surgery)

If acutely ill, use similiar measures for any acute illness (*See* Nursing the Acutely Ill Patient)

Home Care

Many patients are being cared for in their own homes under the supervision of a doctor and a public health nurse

Need to help patient and family plan a schedule of activities to insure adequate rest

Principles of care remain essentially the same

Family and patient teaching and supervision is essential in relation to
  Activities and rest
  Drug administration
  Nutrition
  Care of discharges

Prevention and Control of Tuberculosis in the Community

Case finding by
  Observation of symptoms
  Physical examination
  Tuberculin testing
  Examination of known contacts
  Mass roentgen screening
Improvement of living standards
Pasteurization of milk and tuberculin testing of cattle
Prompt treatment of people with active disease
Education in personal hygiene
Rehabilitation of patients with arrested disease to prevent relapse
BCG vaccine—degree of immunity still under discussion (*See* Vaccine)

THORACIC SURGERY (LUNG RESECTION)

Conditions Requiring Thoracic Surgery

Neoplasms, including benign and malignant
Infections
  Bronchiectasis
  Tuberculosis
  Lung abscess
  Empyema
Trauma causing penetrating chest wounds

Specific Diagnostic Procedures

Roentgenogram
Fluoroscopy
Bronchoscopy
Thoracentesis
Bronchography

MEDICAL AND SURGICAL

Types of Surgical Procedures

Segmental resection—removal of a portion of a lobe of the lung

Lobectomy—removal of a lobe of the lung

Pneumonectomy—removal of an entire lung

Closed thoracotomy—insertion of tube into pleural cavity

Open drainage of pleural cavity or lung—empyema or walled-off adherent lung abscess

Specific Preoperative Care (varies with suspected diagnosis)

NEOPLASM

General preoperative preparation that includes measures of correcting abnormalities of nutrition, anemia, etc.

Pulmonary function determined in order that an accurate estimation of pulmonary reserve postoperatively can be made

Prophylactic use of antibiotics, particularly when neoplasm is associated with local suppuration

INFECTIONS

General preoperative preparation that includes measures of correcting abnormalities of nutrition, anemia, etc.

Determination of infectious agent by sputum culture and thoracentesis

Bringing the infectious process under maximum control, achieved by

Antibiotic therapy

Postural drainage

Bronchodilators

General supportive measures, bed rest, etc.

TRAUMA

Usually under emergency conditions

Establish and maintain an open airway by best means available, i.e., nasopharyngeal or endotracheal airways, tracheotomy, etc.

Provide adequate oxygen and carbon-dioxide exchange by positive pressure inhalation, mouth-to-mouth breathing, artificial respiration, etc.

Guard against sucking wounds of chest wall, tension pneumothorax, hemothorax

Preoperative explanation to patient regarding importance of turning and coughing, his need for oxygen tent and chest suction

Special Postoperative Care

Encourage turning and deep breathing

Encourage coughing

Assist patient by supporting chest and holding hands over operative site

Position patient in accord with doctor's specific orders

Care of patient with chest suction (*See discussion in* Technics)

Always have clamp near patient's unit in case suctioning apparatus should fail to work

Watch drainage, especially for signs of hemorrhage

Tracheal suction when necessary. Equipment should be near unit (*See discussion in* Technics)

Antibiotics (*See discussion in* Pharmacology)

Analgesics (*See discussion in* Pharmacology)

Use regularly, but awaken patient to cough and to breathe deeply

Care of patient in oxygen tent (*See discussion in* Technics)

ALLERGY

An allergy is an altered tissue reactivity. An antigen which produces antibodies must be present, then a union of antigen with sensitized cell is effected.

Types of Antigens

Pollens of grasses

Food

Drugs

Proteins

Types of Reaction

Localized edema

Productive

Exudative

Hemorrhagic

233

How Determined

Skin is sensitive to a substance
Family history of allergy—susceptible individual

HAY FEVER

A reaction of the nasal mucosa, the conjunctiva and the bronchial mucosa which is regarded as an anaphylactic or allergic condition excited by a specific antigen to which the individual has been sensitized.

SEASONAL

Depending on the type of pollen to which the individual is sensitive

Symptoms

Itchy eyes, congestion
Sneezing, nasal congestion
Copious thin nasal discharge
Congestion of the eyes, the ears, the nose and the throat
About one third of these people develop asthma

Treatment

Avoidance of pollen (filter on bedroom window, etc.)
Desensitization of patient by injections given 3 to 4 months before the hay fever season begins
Drugs (*See discussion in* Pharmacology)

Antihistaminic drugs—Pyribenzamine, Chlor-Trimeton, Neo-Antergan

Ephedrine 25 mg., 3 to 4 times daily P.O.

Ephedrine or Neosynephrine as nosedrops

PERENNIAL

Nonseasonal (not due to a pollen)

Causes

Dust
Dandruff from animals
Food (wheat, eggs, milk, chocolate, etc.)
Drugs (penicillin, morphine, etc.)
Face powders and other cosmetics (orris root)

Treatment

Removal of causative factor

Desensitization injections

Avoidance of contact with substances which produce symptoms

Antihistaminic drugs

BRONCHIAL ASTHMA

A type of wheezing dyspnea due to constriction of the bronchi and to edema of the bronchial mucosa caused by an allergic response of the bronchial tree to specific antigens.

Etiology

Extrinsic asthma is caused by dust, ingested food or drugs

Intrinsic asthma is most often caused by infections of the respiratory tract

Symptoms

Acute onset often occurs at night

Sense of suffocation and of pressure in chest, non-productive of cough

Shortness of breath, dyspnea accompanied by wheezing

Air hunger—breathing with accessory muscles—patient sits upright or leans forward

Termination of attack—productive cough—thick, stringy, mucoid sputum

Characterized by repeated attacks

Treatment

RELIEF OF SYMPTOMS DURING ATTACK

Epinephrine 1:1,000 solution subcutaneously (*See* Pharmacology)

Epinephrine in oil solution 1:500 intramuscularly for prolonged action (*See* Pharmacology)

Aerosol inhalation of epinephrine 1:100 or Isuprel 1:2 units (*See* Pharmacology)

Aminophyllin (*See* Pharmacology)

Potassium iodide, ammonium chloride—expectorants (*See* Pharmacology)

Oxygen, if asthma attack is severe

Sedatives as adjunctive therapy. Mild doses of barbiturates and tranquilizers

Corticotropin, Cortone Acetate and prednisone give temporary relief if acute attack persists in spite of medications listed above

SPECIFIC THERAPY

Control of causative agent, i.e., elimination of household pets, feather pillows, etc.

Desensitization—injections of antigen and then maintenance of dose as determined by reaction of patient

GENERAL MEASURES

Avoidance of extremes of cold and humidity, especially outdoor exertion in cold, damp weather

Avoidance of upper respiratory infections

Smoking avoided or limited in amount

Elimination of emotional stress

Psychotherapy is only occasionally needed

Maintenance of positive healthy mental attitude is necessary

DRUG ALLERGIES

Sensitivity reaction which occurs during or following the administration of a drug.

Symptoms

Resemblance to serum sickness

Fever

Urticaria

Joint pains

Nausea and vomiting

Lymphadenopathy

Symptoms usually occur 6 to 12 days after start of medication and last 2 to 3 days

Immediate anaphylactic-type reactions occur occasionally in patients with extreme degrees of sensitization (*See* Anaphylaxis)

Treatment

Cessation of suspected drug

Control reaction (*See* Treatment *under* Hay fever, *above*)

Warn patient against further use of drug

SERUM SICKNESS

Due to parenteral injection of a foreign serum (usually horse serum)

Serum involved may be tetanus antitoxin, pneumococcus, diphtheria antitoxin, etc.

Symptoms

Depend on amount of serum given and upon the individual's sensitivity to the serum.

Severe urticaria, pruritus

Painful swollen joints

Enlargement of lymph glands

Fever

Edema of glottis

Treatment

Aspirin to relieve aching joints

Adrenalin, ephedrine

Cortisone, ACTH—most effective today

Supportive

ANAPHYLAXIS

An acute, immediate allergic reaction of profound degree after introduction of foreign serum.

Symptoms

Wheezing, profound difficulty in breathing

Urticaria

Collapse

Acute and severe edema of throat and lungs

Blood pressure at shock level

High pulse rate

Occasionally fatal

MEDICAL AND SURGICAL

Treatment

Prevention by skin testing first

Immediate, if it occurs

Maintenance of open airway

Adrenalin I.V. (*See discussion in* Pharmacology)

Oxygen

Antihistamine drugs (*See discussion in* Pharmacology)

ACTH and cortisone (*See discussion in* Pharmacology)

Measures for treating shock if it occurs (*See treatment for* Shock)

ARTHRITIS

Arthritis—any condition which results in inflammation in a joint. Rheumatism is a term which represents any condition affecting joints, tendons, muscles, and other related structures.

Classification of Diseases of Joints

Arthritis due to infection (gonococcal, suppurative, syphilitic, tuberculous)

Arthritis due to rheumatic fever

Rheumatoid arthritis

Degenerative joint diseases (osteoarthritis, degenerative arthritis)

Neurogenic arthropathy (Charcot's joint)

Arthritis due to gout

Traumatic arthritis

New growths of joints

Intermittent hydrarthrosis

Periarticular conditions (myositis, bursitis, neuritis, etc.)

RHEUMATOID ARTHRITIS

This is a chronic constitutional disease involving the joints with a synovial membrane. It is associated with atrophy and loss of calcium from the limbs. Since it affects chiefly the collagen substance of connective tissue, it is considered one of the collagen diseases.

Differential Diagnosis of Rheumatoid Arthritis and Osteoarthritis

	RHEUMATOID ARTHRITIS	OSTEOARTHRITIS
Average age at onset	3rd and 4th decades	5th and 6th decades
Weight	Normal or underweight	Usually overweight
Condition of bones	Osteoporosis	Condensation of articular margins
Joints involved	Any joint in body	Chiefly knees, spine and fingers
Type	Migratory	Not migratory
Appearance of joints	Periarticular swelling	No swelling
Special signs	Fusiform finger joints	Heberden's nodes
Subcutaneous nodules	Present in 10 per cent of cases	Never present
Roentgen ray	Narrowing and clouding of joint space	Lipping of bony margins of joint
Joint fluid	Turbid. Increased cells and protein	Clear. Few cells. Low protein.
"Specific" serologic reactions	Usually present	Never present
Blood count	Secondary anemia and slight leukocytosis	Normal blood count
Sedimentation of R.B.C.	Considerably accelerated	Normal or slightly accelerated
Course	Usually progressive	Staticnary or slightly progressive
Termination	Ankylosis and deformity	No ankylosis; usually no deformity

Cecil, R. L., and Loeb, R. F.: A Textbook of Medicine, vol. 2, p. 1369, Philadelphia, Saunders, 1959.

[239]

MEDICAL AND SURGICAL

Etiology

Unknown, but certain precipitating factors have been identified.

Severe physical or emotional shock
Fatigue
Trauma
Acute infections, especially respiratory
Sudden or repeated exposure to dampness, rain, cold
Heredity

Symptoms

Onset—usually gradual, may be sudden
Prodromal symptoms
Weakness
Fatigue
Loss of weight
Anemia
Vasomotor disturbances, tingling, numbness of the feet and the hands
Pain and stiffness—usually 1 joint in the beginning—lasts weeks or months before other joints are involved
Swelling of joints of fingers, hands, knees
Migratory nature of joint symptoms
Tendency to develop into chronic state
Ankylosis and deformity of joints if disease is not arrested
Subject to spontaneous remissions

Treatment

Complete and prolonged rest
At least several hours rest daily and a long period of night rest if patient is unable to give up work for a long period of time
Drugs (*See* Pharmacology)
Salicylates—acetylsalicylic acid .6 Gm. 3 to 4 times a day
Gold salts (gold sodium thiosulfate, I.V.) myochrozine, Salganal I.V.
Cortisinone, ACTH
Physical therapy (dry heat, diathermy and exercises) —increase circulation in affected joints
Hydrotherapy

Exercises to
  Preserve function of joint
  Maintain muscle tone
  Prevent deformities
Posturing, especially in bed
  Sleep flat in bed with one pillow
  Foot boards to prevent footdrop
Surgical Treatment (advanced arthritis) (*See* Orthopedic nursing)
  Synovectomy (especially for knees and elbows)
  Arthrodesis
  Arthroplasty
  Osteotomy
Psychotherapy (for mental depression often found in patients)
Good nutrition, especially since many patients are undernourished
Iron therapy for anemia (*See* Pharmacology)
See Rehabilitation Nursing

POLIOMYELITIS
(INFANTILE PARALYSIS)

Poliomyelitis is an acute, viral disease that is characterized in a variable proportion of cases by preliminary manifestations of a general systemic infection; then, in most of the cases, by evidences of acute involvement of the central nervous system; and finally, in the characteristic cases, by irregularly distributed paralyses that at times are sufficient to cause death. Any of these stages may terminate in recovery or death.

Etiology

The causative agent is a filtrable virus and is apparently present in the discharges of the nose and throat, in the spinal fluid and in the feces and urine.

Manner of Transmission

  By droplet infection
  Through human carriers

By flies conveying virus from sewage to food

By swimming in contaminated swimming pools, rivers, etc.

Incidence

In cities, by far the greater number of cases are in the age period of 3 to 7 years, although the incidence in young adults is rising. Pregnant women also are very susceptible.

Incubation Period

3 to 10 days—abortive cases

9 to 13 days—paralytic cases

Classification of Clinical Forms

Minor Illness

Inapparent infection (alimentary infection), commonest form, diagnosis by laboratory tests only

Abortive poliomyelitis—disease did not extend beyond "minor illness" but clinical and laboratory evidence warranted diagnosis

Major Illness

Paralytic poliomyelitis—patient has clear demonstrable paralysis—spinal, bulbar or cranial nerve types

Aseptic meningitis

MAJOR ILLNESS

Symptoms

Abrupt onset

Fever, vomiting, headache

Spontaneous pain in extremities

Hyperesthesia

Sometimes paresthesia

Soreness, stiffness of the back, neck and hamstring muscles

Severe back pain which is relieved by motion

Insidious onset (common in adults)

Little or no fever at first

Patients are uncomfortable and restless rather than sick

Listlessness

Anorexia, sometimes vomiting
Pains in extremities
Hyperesthesia, paresthesia
Similar muscle pains
Febrile period (100° to 103° F.)
  May last 3 to 10 days
  Flaccid paralysis occurs as fever subsides
  Acute retention of urine
Muscle (flaccid paralysis) order of frequency:
  Legs, arms, back, thorax, face, intercostal region and diaphragm
Encephalitic symptoms
  Lightheadedness
  Apprehension
  Twitching of limbs
  Irritability followed by lassitude, drowsiness
Bulbar paralysis
  Involvement of cranial nerve
  Weakness of soft palate, pharynx and vocal cords
  Inability to swallow or to talk clearly
Reflexes
  Normal at first, shift to hyperactivity and then become absent
Moderate leukocytosis 10,000 to 16,000 per ml.

Treatment and Nursing Care

Minor Illness
  Bed rest and isolation, especially in time of epidemics
  Observe for advancement of disease
Major Illness
  Paralytic
    Bed rest—use firm bed and foot boards
    Support of weakened limbs in physiologic alignment
    Hot packs—direct application of hot wet wool from which water has been well wrung to affected limbs—to relieve pain
    Change of patient's position with care
    Sedative, analgesics
    Light diet, encourage fluid intake
    Complete precautions (*See* Nursing Technics)
    Emotional support—anticipate depression

Calm, quiet environment

Bulbar

Treatment of respiratory paralysis depends upon cause

Malfunction of respiratory muscle

Disturbance of central respiratory control center

Obstruction of airway (as with difficulty in swallowing)

Pulmonary edema

Tank respirator for severe respiratory muscle weakness (*See* Nursing Technic)

Maintenance of clear airway

Measures listed under Paralytic when and if patient is removed from respirator

Muscle re-education after acute phase of illness (*See* Rehabilitative Nursing)

Prevention

Vaccination (*See* vaccines)

Early recognition and isolation of infected persons (infectious period 10 to 20 days after onset)

Postponement of elective surgery in nose and throat areas and dental extractions during "polio season."

Part 4.   Communicable Diseases

GENERAL CONSIDERATIONS

Current Approach

Two developments, new immunization agents and the antibiotic drugs, have altered the medical and nursing management of many of the communicable diseases.

The major emphasis today is in the prevention and the control of these diseases. This implies the responsibility to educate the public to methods of preventing these diseases and the early diagnosis and treatment of patients with illness so that complications may be avoided and additional contacts eliminated.

The nurse today must be well informed regarding epidemiology, immunology, and principles of sanitary practice in the home and the community; so that she may fulfill her education role. Also, she must be able to make appropriate observations so that she may become an effective case finder and may help to control these diseases by isolating the infected individual.

Terms Indicating Prevalence of Diseases

EPIDEMIC DISEASE is one that affects a large number of people, in any locality, at the same time.

PANDEMIC DISEASE is one that spreads from one country to another, affecting large groups of people in each country.

ENDEMIC DISEASE is one that is always prevalent in a particular locality, as goiter in Switzerland or cholera in parts of India.

SPORADIC DISEASE is one that occurs occasionally or unexpectedly in regions where it is not usually prevalent.

Information Necessary to Understand
Epidemiologic Factors

Conditions which make a disease communicable

Mode of transmission of organism, i.e., droplet, insect, carrier

Portal of entry to human body, i.e., mouth, blood, etc.

Avenue of exit from body, i.e., nasopharyngeal excretions, excreta, etc.

Behavioral characteristics of organism

Barriers appropriate to preventing spread

Length of time between time of exposure and onset of symptoms

Length of time an infected person is communicable

Public health requirements for preventing these diseases

General Principles of Care

Bed rest for the duration of the fever and from 1 to 3 days longer

Isolation of infected individual (*See* Nursing Technic)

Maintenance of adequate elimination and excretion

Protection against secondary infections

MEDICAL AND SURGICAL

Education of patient, family and visitors in maintaining isolation of patient and his belongings

Immunizing contacts, if warranted

Specific care for each disease

See Specific Disease Table, pp. 250-279

See also Specific Diseases, i.e., poliomyelitis, tuberculosis, infectious hepatitis

IMMUNITY AND DISEASE

Definition

Immunity is the freedom from or lack of susceptibility to a disease. It may be "natural" or it may be due to recovery from an attack of the disease in question—either a recognized illness or an attack so mild as to escape recognition. Immunity sometimes is called *active* immunity when it is developed in response to the disease organism or its products—either through vaccination or an attack of the disease in question. Immunity due to the injection of immune blood or serum from immune persons or animals is called *passive* immunity. Passive immunity is brief (days or weeks); but active immunity may persist for years or even for life. Antitoxins or other antibodies, such as agglutinins which clump bacteria and lysins which dissolve them, are present in immune and convalescent blood.

Carriers

Carriers harbor virulent disease organisms capable of producing disease. This condition may extend beyond recovery as in typhoid fever. Healthy individuals with no history of a given disease, e.g., meningitis, may be carriers.

Skin Tests for Immunity

An antigen (organism, toxin or substitute) is injected into the skin for the purpose of determining the presence of circulating antibodies in a patient.

SPECIFIC SKIN TESTS

Shick Test

Susceptibility to diphtheria

A small amount of diphtheria toxoid is injected

Red tender area at sight of injection, persisting for 7 to 10 days indicates lack of antibodies and, therefore, lack of immunity

Dick Test

Susceptibility to scarlet fever

A small amount of streptococcal toxin is injected

Red tender area at sight of injection, persisting for 48 to 72 hours, indicates lack of antibodies and, therefore, lack of immunity

Tuberculin Test (Mantoux)

Injection of purified protein derivative (PPD) of Tuberculin

Positive red tender area at sight of injection indicates patient has been infected with tuberculosis at some time, not necessarily that he has clinical tuberculosis at the time of the test.

PASSIVE IMMUNITY

Immune serums are prepared from the blood of a person or an animal known to be immune to a specific disease. This immunity may result after natural or artificial injection with bacteria and viruses. The antibodies in the serum are injected parenterally into the patient, and either neutralize the toxins of the micro-organisms or inhibit the growth of the infectious agent.

Human Serum

The gamma globulin fraction of the blood contains the greatest concentration of specific antibodies. It is used in scarlet fever, measles, epidemic infectious hepatitis and mumps.

Animal Serum

Usually horses and rabbits are used for artificial production of immune serums. These sera usually contain antitoxins which neutralize the toxins of the bacteria in the patient's body. They are used mostly for diphtheria, tetanus, gas gangrene, botulism and meningitis.

MEDICAL AND SURGICAL

ACTIVE IMMUNITY

Antigens which may be an organism or a toxin are injected into an individual so that the individual may stimulate the production of his own antibodies. Combinations of toxoids and vaccines from different bacteria often are given to minimize the number of injections.

Toxoid

A toxoid is a toxin which has been modified, usually by formaldehyde, to reduce its toxicity yet maintain its antigenic property.

DIPHTHERIA TOXOID, ALUMINUM HYDROXIDE ADSORBED, U.S.P.

0.5 to 1 ml. × 2 subcutaneously, 4 to 6 weeks interval between doses

TETANUS TOXOID, ALUMINUM HYDROXIDE ADSORBED, U.S.P.

0.5 to 1 ml. × 2 subcutaneously, 4 to 6 weeks interval between doses

Vaccine

A vaccine is a suspension of either attenuated or killed micro-organisms. Vaccines are called by the name of the related disease.

INFLUENZA VIRUS VACCINE, MONOVALENT TYPE A (ASIAN STRAIN), N.N.D.

0.1 ml. × 2, 3 to 4 weeks interval

PERTUSSIS VACCINE, ALUM PRECIPITATED, N.N.D.

1.5 ml. divided into not less than 3 injections given from 4 to 6 week intervals. Booster dose of 0.5 ml. given 1 year after last divided dose

POLIOMYELITIS VACCINE (SALK), N.N.D.

1 ml. dose. Initial dose followed 4 to 6 weeks later by a 2nd dose, 3rd injection given in 7 to 12 months. Booster dose of 1 ml. given 1 year after 3rd dose.

RABIES VACCINE (DUCK EMBRYO), N.N.D.

Given during incubation period after exposure to the disease

1 ml. beneath the skin of the abdomen each day for 14 days

TUBERCULOSIS VACCINE (BCG), N.N.D.

Given only to individuals initially nonreactive to tuberculin test

Administered by multiple puncture or by intradermal injection

SMALLPOX VACCINE, U.S.P.

Injection of content of 1 capillary tube into deeper layer of epidermis

"Nontakes" should be revaccinated

Immunity almost completely lost after 10 years

Revaccination necessary to maintain immunity

TYPHOID VACCINE, U.S.P.

Given subcutaneously in 3 doses of 0.5 ml. to 1 ml. (depending upon manufacturer) at intervals of 1 week

May be accompanied by soreness in arm and general symptoms of headache, nausea and fever for 1 or 2 days

Annual booster dose of 0.1 ml. intradermally or 0.5 ml. subcutaneously

Other diseases for which vaccines are available are cholera, dysentery, Rocky Mountain spotted fever, yellow fever, typhus fever, and paratyphoid fever (A & B).

IMMUNIZATION OF CHILDREN

See Pediatrics

DISEASE	ETIOLOGY AND IN-CUBATION PERIOD	TRANSMISSION	PROPHYLAXIS
Amebiasis (Amebic Dysentery)	Endamoeba histolytica 10 to 21 days	Food and water contaminated by: Human excreta used as fertilizer in tropical countries Healthy carriers Flies and other insects	Active treatment of carriers Proper sanitation Periodic examination of food handlers Control of water and food supply Protection of food from flies and insects
Anthrax	Bacillus anthracis 5 to 7 days	Handling hides, fur or wool of infected animals Using brushes made from hair or bristles of infected animals	Disinfection of hides, wool and furs Sterilization of brushes Vaccination of animals Proper disposal of carcasses of infected animals
Asiatic Cholera	Vibrio comma 1 to 3 days	Contaminated food and water Human carriers Flies	Proper sanitation Control of carriers Vaccination Isolation of infected persons
Bacillary Dysentery	Shigella: dysenteriae paradysenteriae of Flexner sonnei 1 to 6 days	Contaminated food and water Healthy carriers Poor personal hygiene Insanitary conditions Flies as vectors	Treatment of carriers Adequate sanitation Proper screening of food Periodic examination of food handlers

DISEASES

DIAGNOSIS	SYMPTOMS	TREATMENT	COMPLICATIONS AND SEQUELAE

Stool examination
Proctoscopy
Roentgenogram
Agglutination tests
	Diarrhea and abdominal cramps
	Fever
	General debility
	Somatic aching
		Bed rest
		Bland diet
		Drugs:
		  Diodoquin
		  Carbarsone
		  Emetine
		  Chloroquine
		  Terramycin
		  Achromycin
			Perforation of bowel
			Liver abscess
			Scarring and strictures
			Pulmonary abscess

Microscopic examination of lesion or sputum
Blood culture
Animal-inoculation
	Cutaneous form:
	  Intense itching
	  Small papules, rapidly becoming vesicular, then black
	  Swelling of area
	Pulmonary form:
	  Tightness in chest
	  Cough
	  Bronchitis
	  Fever, etc.
		Penicillin
		Immune serum
		Protective dressing to area
		Bed rest
		Supportive
			Septicemia
			Meningitis
			High mortality in pulmonary form

Stool examination Agglutination test Known cases in area	Violent diarrhea with mucous shreds Copious vomiting Collapse Oliguria and anuria Fall in blood pressure Rapid pulse Dehydration	Disinfection of excreta Physiological saline IV Alkali Symptomatic Strict isolation	Mortality rate is high in epidemics
Stool examination Agglutination tests Sigmoidoscopy	Mucous or bloody diarrhea Abdominal cramps Tenesmus Fever Prostration Collapse Dehydration	Strict isolation Disinfection of excreta Heat to abdomen Physiological saline IV Antimicrobial therapy	Broncho-pneumonia Perforation of bowel Prolapse of rectum Stenosis of bowel Peripheral neuritis Encephalitis

DISEASE	ETIOLOGY AND IN-CUBATION PERIOD	TRANSMISSION	PROPHYLAXIS
Brucellosis (Un-dulant Fever)	Brucella: melitensis abortus suis 5 to 21 days	Drinking raw milk Eating butter or cheese made from unpasteurized milk of infected goat or cow Direct contact with infected animal Break in skin-contact with in-fected animal or its excreta	Pasteurization of milk Detection and disposal of in-fected animals Use of rubber gloves when handling in-fected animals or live cultures
Chicken Pox (Varicella)	Virus 2 to 3 weeks —variable	Airborne Direct contact Droplet	Avoid contact Convalescent serum
Dengue Fever (Breakbone Fever)	Filtrable virus 5 to 8 days	Bites of Aedes aegypti mosquito	Rigid mosquito control Screening against mosquitoes

DIAGNOSIS	SYMPTOMS	TREATMENT	COMPLICATIONS AND SEQUELAE

History
Isolation of organism from blood, spinal fluid, secretions, excretions and excised tissue
Specific agglutination
	Acute:
	  Headache
	  Malaise
	  Prostration
	  Fever of intermittent type
	  Profuse diaphoresis
	  Weight loss
	  Severe joint pains
	Chronic:
	  Nervous and mental symptoms
	  Low grade fever
	  Arthralgias
	  Chronic fatigue
	  Anorexia
		Rest is essential
		Tetracycline drugs
		Streptomycin
		Psychotherapy may be indicated
		Symptomatic
			Involved joints
			Peripheral neuritis
			Encephalitis— chronic
			Meningitis— chronic
			Bacterial endocarditis
			Pulmonary infiltration and effusions

Characteristic vesicles-on skin	Rash—appears first on back, then on abdomen, face and whole body
	Before eruption—may be
	  Headache
	  Malaise
	  Anorexia
	  Fever 101° to 102° F.
		Excluded from school and contact with susceptibles
		Rest in bed with diversion
		Force fluids
		Light diet
		Frequent baths except at height of the eruption
		Relieve itching with soothing ointments or by sponging with a solution of bicarbonate of soda (1 dram to 1 pint)
		Use arm cuffs or some protection to prevent scratching
		Antibiotics, if secondary infection
			Disfiguring pox marks
			Secondary infection of lesions

Clinical features
Blood changes:
  Leukopenia
  Lymphocytosis
Studies of blood and urine to make differential diagnosis
	Fever for 2 to 3 days, then remission followed by relapse
	Skin rash
	Severe pain in back and joints
	Severe headache and pain in eyes
	Lymphadenopathy
		Symptomatic
		Supportive
		Absolute bed rest
			Malaise and mental depression may persist for months

DISEASE	ETIOLOGY AND IN-CUBATION PERIOD	TRANSMISSION	PROPHYLAXIS
Diphtheria	Corynebacterium diphtheriae 1 to 7 days, usually 2 to 4 days	Direct contact with patients or healthy carriers Fomites-contaminated clothing, toys, etc. By milk infected by carriers	Determining susceptible persons by Schick Test Immunizing with vaccines, such as toxin-antitoxin or toxoid When disease is prevalent, immunizing exposed person without waiting to determine their susceptibility Quarantine of every diphtheria person Isolation and treatment of carriers
Encephalitis Lethargica (Sleeping Sickness)	Virus (possibly) 4 to 15 days	Not known	

DISEASES—(Continued)

DIAGNOSIS	SYMPTOMS	TREATMENT	COMPLICATIONS AND SEQUELAE
Appearance of membrane Previous reaction of the Schick Test Throat culture	Pharyngeal Sudden onset of pain with difficulty in swallowing Fever 101° to 102° F. Malaise—prostration and increase in pulse rate are out of proportion to amount of fever Grayish-white membrane on tonsil and may spread to soft palate Laryngeal—most severe Mild fever Hoarseness Mild dry tight cough Critically ill within 48 hours Dyspnea Cyanosis Dry hacking (croupy) cough	Strict individual precautions Keep patient flat in bed until danger is past Special care to nose, throat and tongue Fluid diet in concentrated form—give slowly Steam inhalations Intubation when marked respiratory obstruction Tracheotomy, if necessary (See Tracheotomy Care in Nursing Technics) Throat irrigations Diphtheria antitoxin Penicillin to inhibit growth of bacilli	Myocarditis Paralysis—muscles used in swallowing or breathing Bronchopneumonia Otitis media Polyneuritis
Difficult in absence of epidemic	Slow and insidious onset Fever for a few days Headache, vertigo, vague joint pains, restlessness, paralysis of ocular muscles, respiratory disturbances Confusion, apathy, drowsiness, mild stupor Persistent insomnia Long-course—changes may occur as specific areas in cortex are involved, i.e., paralysis, changes in personality Psychic disturbances	In acute stage—as with any acute infection Isolation technic Good posturing principles In later stage Rest Fresh air Reeducation	Some patients partially disabled for 6 mo. to 2 years Others—permanently disabled

DISEASE	ETIOLOGY AND IN-CUBATION PERIOD	TRANSMISSION	PROPHYLAXIS
Filariasis	Wuchereria bancrofti or malayi metazoa	Bite of Culex, Mansonia or Anopheles mosquito Bite of mango fly Bite of coffee gnat	Rigid mosquito and insect control Proper screening against insects
Gas gangrene	Clostridium perfringens or novyi 6 hours to 3 days	Wound contaminated by spores carried into it by dirt	Early débridement of wound, making it a clean open wound in which anaerobic organisms cannot grow
German Measles (Rubella)	Filtrable virus(?) 14 to 21 days	Contact especially with nasopharyngeal secretions	Avoid exposure Contagious during prodromal stage and in 1st day of rash Gamma globulin to exposed woman in 1st trimester of pregnancy
Gonorrhea	Gonococcus (Neisseria gonorrhae) 3 to 5 days	Direct contact	Control by case finding Early recognition of cases Treatment of cases Health education Penicillin tablet (250,000 U) taken within 3 to 4 hours after exposure

DIAGNOSIS	SYMPTOMS	TREATMENT	COMPLICATIONS AND SEQUELAE
Blood films Skin biopsy of lesions	Lymphangitis Fever Malaise Severe headache Elephantiasis Subcutaneous tumors (onchocerciasis) Severe pain	Hetrazan Antimonials Surgical removal of tissue Application of tight bandages	Obstruction and dilatation of lymphatic trunks Extensive fibrosis of skin Hypertrophy of lymph nodes Lowered resistance to infection
Clinical picture Cultures of wound Roentgenographic examination	Severe pain Tissues about wound swollen and discolored Crackling of tissue Exudate of brown frothy fluid from wound Profound toxemia	Penicillin Débridement of wound Antitoxin or polyvalent Erythromycin Supportive esp. fluids	Gangrene may necessitate amputation Mortality rate is high
Presence of enlarged occipital and cervical nodes	Malaise, coryza, headache Pale rash on face, spreads to chest, arms and body in 2 to 3 hours. Lasts 2 days Enlarged occipital and posterior cervical nodes Leukopenia	Isolation about 24 hours Supportive care Watch exposed children from the 11th day through the 19th day following exposure Good skin care Gamma globulin to pregnant woman	When occurs in early pregnancy —abnormality of infant Congenital cataract Septal defects of heart Mental retardation Deaf-mutism

Identified in smears of discharges	Men
	  Sudden onset
	  Pain and burning on urination
	  Purulent discharge
	  Epididymitis and orchitis
	Women
	  Mucopurulent discharge
	  Urinary frequency
	  Burning and pain on urination
	  Abscess of Bartholin's glands
	Children
	  Discharge
		One injection of penicillin—600,000 units of procaine penicillin or 1,200,000 U. of benzathine penicillin G
		Strict hygiene
		Isolation
			Rare if treated
			If untreated:
			Sterility
			Arthritis
			Endocervicitis
			Salpingitis

DISEASE	ETIOLOGY AND IN-CUBATION PERIOD	TRANSMISSION	PROPHYLAXIS
Granuloma Inguinale Venereum	Donovan bodies (Proposed name Donovania gran-ulomatis) Variable 8 days to 12 weeks	Probably direct sexual contact, although disease is not highly con-tagious	See Lympho-granuloma venereum
Hookworm Disease (An-cylostomiasis	Uncinaria americana Ancylostoma duodenale 4 to 6 weeks	Ova are discharged with feces on the soil. Larvae enter skin of person who goes barefoot and enter the circula-tion. Later they are coughed up and swallowed, enter-ing duodenum	Proper sanitation Education as to hygienic meas-ures Wearing of shoes at all times
Infectious jaundice (Weil's Disease)	Leptospira icterohaemor-rhagiae 8 to 12 days	Spirochetes pene-trate skin and mu-cous membranes. In wet places which have been polluted with urine of infected rats, and in some cases infected dogs, these organisms abound	Vaccination
Influenza	Virus Influenza A Influenza B Influenza C 1 to 2 days	Droplet infection	Avoid contacts Care of patient's secretions

DIAGNOSIS	SYMPTOMS	TREATMENT	COMPLICATIONS AND SEQUELAE
Demonstration of Donovan bodies in scrapings of lesions	Superficial lesions of the groin and pubic areas	Cleanliness of area Streptomycin Antimonials Roentgenogram Surgery if necessary Aureomycin Terramycin	Areas heal, leaving small white scars
Stool examination Eosinophilia	Itching of skin between toes Maculopapules which became small vesicles Enlarged regional lymph nodes Profound anemia Bronchitis, if larvae in lungs Capricious appetite (pica)	Anthelmintics. (See discussion in Pharmacology) Iron for anemia Highly nutritious diet	Profound anemia with lowered resistance to disease
History and physical examination Serum and blood determinations Liver function tests Leukocytosis Spinal fluid— pleocytosis	Abrupt onset Fever and chills Headaches Photophobia Severe muscular aching Hepatitis (appears 5 to 6 days) Nephritis	Symptomatic Supportive	Liver dysfunctions are noted over a long period of time Grave prognosis if severe liver or kidney involvement
Organisms found in throat secretions Agglutination test Difficult if non-epidemic	Chills Fever (last 3 to 5 days) Headache Backache Mild upper respiratory symptoms Prostration of varying degrees Cough, nonproductive	Isolation Bed rest High fluid intake Icebag Antipyretics Antibiotics (against secondary invaders) Supportive nursing care	In debilitated, undernourished patients—secondary infections, pneumonia

DISEASE	ETIOLOGY AND IN-CUBATION PERIOD	TRANSMISSION	PROPHYLAXIS
Leishmaniasis: Visceral (Kala-azar)	Protozoan Leishmania donovani Incubation Period not known	Bite of sandflies	Treat infected persons and dogs DDT sprays in areas where sandflies abide Clothing Repellent—dimethyl-phthalate
Cutaneous (Oriental Sore)	Leishmania tropica	Possibly contact with infected persons or with dogs	Same as above
Mucocutaneous (Espundia)	Leishmania braziliensis 6 weeks to 4 months		
Leprosy (Hansen's Disease)	Mycobacterium leprae 2 to 5 years	Contact with infectious persons during transient periods of increased susceptibility	Isolation of patients while cultures are positive
Lymphogranuloma venereum	Filtrable virus 7 to 12 days	Direct sexual contact	A medical and social problem. (See Syphilis)

DIAGNOSIS	SYMPTOMS	TREATMENT	COMPLICATIONS AND SEQUELAE
Smears from blood, liver, spleen, and lymph glands, sternum Blood culture Formal-gel test Antimony test	Remittent or intermittent fever Enlarged spleen and liver Anorexia Weight loss Loss of strength Bleeding gums and nose Discoloration of skin Leukopenia	Antimonials Vitamins Liver Iron Aureomycin	Untreated—fatal Course prolonged if not treated Remissions and relapses Bronchitis Pneumonia Scarring of tissues
	Skin lesions without symptoms	Neostiban Local drug therapy (Pentavalent and Antimony)	
	Destruction of mucous membrane of mouth and nose	General treatment as above	

Microscopic examinations of scrapings from the skin
Animal inoculation to differentiate from tuberculosis
	Lesions—cooler surfaces of body —skin, superficial nerves, nose, pharynx, larynx
	Damage to distal portion of eye and to testicle
	Tendency for transitory states of exacerbation or reactivation
	Loss of sensation in extremities
		Sulfonamides are showing promise in form of:
		  Promin
		  Diasone
		Amethiozone if intolerance to sulfones
		Bed rest, aspirin, histamine during lepra reaction stage
		Postural supports to prevent disfigurement of hands, feet
		Education of patient, family and public to eliminate fear and superstition
		Isolation until patient is bacteriologically negative
			Disfigurement and deformity due to skin infiltration and peripheral nerve destruction

Frei test (a skin test)	In male, a swelling of inguinal lymph glands (bubo) In female, the intrapelvic glands are involved, causing suppuration and scar formation	Sulfonamides Dilatation of the rectum Aureomycin Terramycin	Scarring and stricture, especially in females. Stricture of rectum most common

DISEASE	ETIOLOGY AND IN-CUBATION PERIOD	TRANSMISSION	PROPHYLAXIS
Malaria	Plasmodium: vivax (tertian) malariae (quartan) falciparum (malignant) 12 to 15 hours	Bite of Anopheles mosquito (female)	1. Rigid mosquito control 2. Screening against mosquitoes 3. Drugs to suppress gametocytes (infective form of parasite) in patient's blood
Measles (Rubeola)	Virus 11 days	Secretions from eyes and respiratory passages Direct contact Droplet infection	Avoid contact Convalescent serum Gamma globulin for exposed individuals Education

DIAGNOSIS	SYMPTOMS	TREATMENT	COMPLICATIONS AND SEQUELAE

Clinical signs
Organism identified in blood smears
	Shaking chills
	Periodic fever (tertian and quartan)
	Headache and general discomfort
	Skin hot and flushed after chill
	Delirium
	Extreme thirst
	Profuse diaphoresis
	Nervous manifestations and hemorrhagic episodes (falciparum)
		Symptomatic
		Supportive
		Drugs:
		  Chloroquine phosphate and amodiaquin HCl are effective in suppressing malaria and in treating acute attack
		  Primaquine phosphate—vivax malaria
			Tertian and quartan have frequent relapses
			Falciparum may be rapidly fatal, or patient may entirely recover without relapses

Symptoms Identification of virus in nose and throat secretions Antibody determination	Prodromal (after 10 to 11 days) Catarrhal symptoms Photophobia and burning of eyes Koplick spots Fever 100° to 103° After 2 to 5 days Rash—first appears on face, then neck, trunk and limbs Rash—reddish brown and blanches at first—then elevated and nonblanching Cough productive	Isolate patients Rest until after subsidence of fever Shield eyes from light Codeine for cough Antibiotics to prevent secondary complications Special skin care Oral and nasal hygiene Supportive care	Otitis media Bronchopneumonia Conjunctivitis Fatality high in elderly and tuberculous patients

DISEASE	ETIOLOGY AND IN-CUBATION PERIOD	TRANSMISSION	PROPHYLAXIS
Meningococcal Meningitis (Epidemic cerebro-spinal meningitis)	Meningococcus (Neisseria intra-cellularis) 3 to 10 days	Carriers Secretions of the nose and throat	Avoid contact During epidemics, give sulfadia-zine to involved population
Mumps (Epidemic Parotitis)	Virus Variable— 17 to 21 days	Direct contact Droplet infection	Avoid contact Convalescent gamma globulin after exposure

DIAGNOSIS	SYMPTOMS	TREATMENT	COMPLICATIONS AND SEQUELAE
Identification of organism in blood or spinal fluid	General Signs Fever Headache Prostration Pain in back Nausea and vomiting Stupor, coma Herpes, hemorrhagic skin eruption in any area of body Local signs Increased intracranial pressure Nausea and vomiting Headache Choked optic disk Irritation of meninges Spasm of neck muscles Stiff neck Retraction of head Spasm of spinal muscles Retraction of spine Opisthotonus Spasm of hamstring muscles Positive Kernig's sign	Isolate patient Force fluids Tepid sponge baths for fever Symptomatic and supportive care Maintain nutrition Drugs Sulfadiazine Penicillin Cortisone if circulatory collapse Chloral hydrate or paraldehyde as sedatives Quiet surroundings	Poor prognosis if accompanied by Brain abscess Venous sinus thrombosis Pneumonia Endocarditis Intercurrent infection of respiratory tract Bacteremic complication Permanent sequelae Deafness Ocular palsus Blindness Psychosis Changes in mentality
Clinical picture Complement-fixation test	Chilliness Malaise Fever 101° to 103° F. Swelling of one or both parotid glands Pain about the angle of the jaw and difficulty in moving the jaw Orchitis	Rest in bed Salicylates for pain Heat or cold to affected area Convalescent serum and gamma globulin Isolation Nourishing diet, fluids Demerol and scrotal support if orchitis	Orchitis in boys after puberty

DISEASE	ETIOLOGY AND IN-CUBATION PERIOD	TRANSMISSION	PROPHYLAXIS
Plague	Pasteurella pestis 2 to 10 days	Bite of rat flea Possibly by contact with infected rodents Droplet infection (pneumonia type)	Continual warfare to exterminate rats Rat-proofing of buildings Vaccination lasts 6 months Isolation of infected person
Rabies (Hydrophobia)	Filtrable virus 3 to 8 weeks, depending on site of injury. May be only 10 days if injury is around face or head	Virus is present in saliva of rabid animal and reaches man through bite or other abrasion of skin	Vaccination of animals Suppression of stray animals Licensing of dogs only after vaccination Pasteur treatment when bite has occurred Prompt cleansing and treatment of wound
Rocky Mountain Spotted Fever (Tick Fever)	Rickettsia rickettsiae 2 to 5 days—acute stage 3 to 4 days—mild stage	Bite or skin abrasion contaminated with crushed tick or with feces of vectors: Wood tick Dog tick Lone Star tick (Texas)	Vaccination Avoidance of tick-ridden area Protective clothing Inspection of body at intervals Removal of ticks from skin by forceps or piece of paper, not by bare fingers Ridding dogs of ticks DDT to tick-infected areas

DIAGNOSIS	SYMPTOMS	TREATMENT	COMPLICATIONS AND SEQUELAE

Smears from buboes
Smear of sputum in pneumonic type
Blood culture
Agglutination tests
Animal inoculation
	Swelling and break-
	down of lymph glands (buboes)
	Fatal septicemia
	Pneumonic symp-
	toms (almost in-
	variably fatal)
	High fever
	Nausea and vomit-
	ing
	Diarrhea
	Collapse
		Strict quarantine
		Bed rest
		Drugs
		  Sulfadiazine
		  Streptomycin
		  Tetracycline
		Hot wet applications to buboes
			Mortality rate is high

Suspected animal should not be de-
stroyed but should be watched for development of symptoms
If animal has been destroyed, brain should be sent to laboratory:
  Demonstration of Negri bodies in brain
  Brain tissue in-
oculated into mice
	Depression and irritability
	Difficulty in swallowing
	Intense excitement for 2 to 3 days
	Paralysis and death
		Immediate thorough cleansing of wound
		Anitrabies vaccine
		Symptomatic
		Supportive
		Once symptoms have appeared, disease invariably is fatal
			High mortality

Weil-Felix test Complement- fixation test Animal inoculation History of ex- posure to ticks	Chills and fever Generalized aches and pains Severe prostration Pulse—high and of proportion to fever Respiration elevated in proportion to fever Rash on 4th or 5th day, hemorrhagic in appearance, starting on ex- tremities and spreading to trunk Dehydration Restlessness Hyperesthesia	Chloramphenicol and tetracyclines are the most effective drugs Supportive and symp- tomatic	Secondary pneu- monia Circulatory failure Necrosis

DISEASE	ETIOLOGY AND INCUBATION PERIOD	TRANSMISSION	PROPHYLAXIS

Scarlet Fever	Hemolytic streptococcus
	2 to 5 days
		Direct contact
		Indirect contact
		  Fomites
		  Infected milk
		  Carriers
			Avoid contact
			Dick Test to determine susceptible individuals

Smallpox (Variola)	Virus 10 to 14 days	Direct contact Indirect contact; fomites Airborne route	Vaccination

DIAGNOSIS	SYMPTOMS	TREATMENT	COMPLICATIONS AND SEQUELAE
Clinical picture Identification of organism from nasopharynx discharge Schultz-Carlton reaction	Acute onset Fever 103° to 104° F. Sore throat—very red Headache Vomiting Rash—1 to 3 days after onset. First on chest and back then spreads to abdomen and extremities. Fades on pressure Desquamation 1 to 2 weeks later Circumoral pallor Strawberry tongue Cervical adenitis Leukocytosis Rapid pulse	Isolation Bed rest Force fluids Salicylates Hot saline irrigations Ice collar to neck Skin care Antibiotics—penicillin (See discussion in Pharmacology)	Cervical adenitis Otitis media Mastoiditis Nephritis
Complement-fixation test Staining a smear made from cutaneous lesions or fluid from vesicles	Fever Chills Headache Backache Prostration Papular rash on face spreading to body and extremities Rash also on palms and soles and mucous membranes Papules become pustules—very itchy Desquamation—12th to 14th day Toxicity—delirious, stuporous Leukopenia Leukocytosis in pustular stage Anemia	Isolation Bed rest Force fluids Salicylates for headache Good skin care Bathe lesions with hot water or antipruritic lotions Penicillin to prevent secondary infection at pustular stage Good supportive care Do not remove crusts too rapidly as scarring may result	Abscesses Septicemia Nephritis Respiratory infection Scarring Corneal ulcer Mortality rate greatest under 5 years and over 45 years

DISEASE	ETIOLOGY AND IN-CUBATION PERIOD	TRANSMISSION	PROPHYLAXIS
Syphilis	Treponema pallidum spirocheta 3 weeks	Direct contact, mainly sexual contact Occasionally through break in skin Through placenta from syphilitic mother to fetus	Control program Case finding Early recognition of cases Treatment of cases Health education Penicillin to pregnant women to prevent congenital syphilis

DIAGNOSIS	SYMPTOMS	TREATMENT	COMPLICATIONS AND SEQUELAE
In 1st and 2nd stage —dark-field study of smear Complement-fixation test Wassermann Flocculation test: Kahn Kline Mazzini Hinton	Primary stage Chancre at site of inoculation Painless May ulcerate Enlarged regional lymph nodes— not tender Secondary stage— 4 to 8 weeks later Fever Headache Sore throat Loss of appetite Skin rash—varied in appearance Generalized en-largement of lymph glands Tertiary stage— several months to several years later Granulomatous lesions—known as gummas most common in skin, bone, circulatory and nervous system Charcot joint Aortitis Tabes dor-salis Paresis Congenital— At birth Skin lesions Snuffles Ulcerations of lips Enlargement of liver and spleen Destruction of bone Tertiary at puberty Hutchinson's teeth Interstitial keratitis Deafness Anterior bow-ing of tibial bone	Penicillin (See discussion in Pharmacology) Education of patient and family Early treatment is essential Early—single large dose of long-lasting penicillin Late—procaine penicillin therapy over period of sev-eral weeks	Aneurysm Most fatalities from involve-ment of circu-latory or cen-tral nervous system

DISEASE	ETIOLOGY AND IN-CUBATION PERIOD	TRANSMISSION	PROPHYLAXIS
Tetanus (Lockjaw)	Clostridium tetani 3 days to 4 weeks	Contamination of penetrating wounds with spores carried in soil or other dirty material carried into wound	Active immunization with toxoid Immediate passive immunization with antitoxin Proper surgical care
Trichinosis (Trichiniasis)	Trichinella spiralis A few days	Eating improperly cooked pork from infected animal	Proper cooking of all pork products Avoidance of feeding uncooked garbage to hogs
Trypanosomiasis (African Sleeping Sickness)	Trypanosoma gambiense 10 to 12 days Trypanosoma rhodesiense	Bite of tsetse fly	Screening against tsetse fly, insecticides Chemoprophylaxis (if evidence of outbreak) Pentamidine Subamin sodium
Tularemia (Rabbit Fever)	Pasteurella tularense 1 to 10 days	Bite of infected fleas and ticks Improperly cooked meat of infected rabbits Infection of hands and eyes while dressing infected wild animals	Hunters should avoid animals that appear sluggish and ill Rubber gloves worn while dressing or handling wild animals Proper cooking of meat of wild rabbits Masks for laboratory workers

DIAGNOSIS	SYMPTOMS	TREATMENT	COMPLICATIONS AND SEQUELAE
Clinical picture almost exclusively	Nervousness and irritability Difficulty in chewing and swallowing Stiff neck Rigidity of jaws and facial muscles Risus sardonicus Opisthotonos Convulsions	Quiet, dark environment free from external stimuli Sedation Antitoxin Penicillin Débridement of wound area Tracheotomy in severe cases Maintenance of fluid and electrolyte balance	Disease is highly fatal if short incubation period and rapid progression of symptoms after onset Broncho-pneumonia
History of eating inadequately cooked pork Muscle biopsy Eosinophilia Skin test	Fever Edema around eyes and nose Painful myositis Nervous manifestations	Symptomatic Supportive	Toxemia Myocarditis
Demonstration of parasite in spinal fluid and blood Examination of lymph glands	Irregular fever Increasing debility Generalized aches and pains Drowsiness and lethargy Enlarged lymph nodes Enlarged posterior cervical nodes (Winterbottom's sign) Coma and death	Tryparsamide Suramin-sodium Melarsen Mel B (See Pharmacology)	Mortality rate is high unless treated early
Demonstration of organisms from draining lesions Agglutination tests Culture of sputum Allergic skin tests	Chills and fever Nausea and vomiting Generalized aches and pains Ulceration at site where organism gains entry through skin Lymphadenitis Breakdown of lymph glands	Streptomycin Terramycin Hot moist dressings to local lesions	Peritonitis Ascites Diarrhea Intestinal hemorrhage Meningitis and encephalitis are usually fatal

DISEASE	ETIOLOGY AND IN-CUBATION PERIOD	TRANSMISSION	PROPHYLAXIS
Typhoid Fever	Salmonella typhosa 10 to 12 days	Water and food contaminated by Sewage Carriers among food handlers Flies	Safe water supply Proper sewage disposal Vaccination Periodic examinations of food handlers and known carriers—cholecystectomy for carriers
Typhus Fever (Epidemic Typhus Fever)	Rickettsia prowazeki 10 to 14 days	Bite of body louse Possibly airborne by dried excreta of vector	Vaccination Delousing of population in typhus areas Use of DDT Protective clothing for those attending patient
Vincent's disease	Bacillus fusiformis and Borrelia vincentii (undetermined)	Direct contact Indirect contact	Treatment of inflamed gums and carious teeth Conditions of bad digestion attended to Tonsils chronically infected should be removed

DIAGNOSIS	SYMPTOMS	TREATMENT	COMPLICATIONS AND SEQUELAE
Blood cultures—early Urine and stools—late in disease Blood agglutination	Fever 102° to 103° F. Slow pulse in contrast to high fever Chills Apathy Loss of appetite Headache Drowsiness—coma Skin rash—rose spots—blanch on pressure—principally on trunk few in number Enlarged spleen Bronchitis Constipation or diarrhea Abdominal distention, generalized abdominal tenderness Low white count—2,000 to 3,000	Strict isolation—screen out flies Supportive and symptomatic treatment Maintain fluids High-caloric, high-protein diet Chloramycetin given for 2 to 3 weeks (See discussion in Pharmacology)	Perforation and hemorrhage of intestine Thrombosis Cholecystitis Arthritis
Weil-Felix test Complement-fixation test Typhus rash	High fever Chills Severe headache Severe pains in back and generalized body pains Severe prostration Characteristic maculopapular rash about 5th day, starting on trunk but avoiding hands, feet and face Rash lasts as long as fever Stupor or delirium	Symptomatic Supportive Aureomycin Erythromycin Achromycin	Broncho-pneumonia Involvement of central nervous system Thrombosis Heart failure Otitis media Parotitis Gangrene of skin Renal insufficiency
Clinical picture Smear of ulcer	Sudden onset Marked pain in throat Fever Foul breath Painful superficial ulcer covered with whitish gray membrane Difficulty in swallowing Enlargement of submaxillary lymph nodes	Individual precautions Penicillin (See discussion in Pharmacology) Good oral hygiene Special mouth care after eating	

DISEASE	ETIOLOGY AND IN-CUBATION PERIOD	TRANSMISSION	PROPHYLAXIS
Whooping Cough (Pertussis)	Hemophilus pertussis 7 to 14 days	Direct contact Droplet infection	Vaccine from killed Hemophilus pertussis. Start at 3 to 4 months Expose children to Hyperimmune pertussis serum Hyperimmune pertussis gamma globulin Booster shot to those already immunized
Yaws (Frambesia)	Treponema pertenue A few weeks to 2 months	Direct contact with infected person Possibly through freshly contaminated articles	Protecting all open wounds and abrasions from contamination Isolate infected person until treatment is given

DIAGNOSIS	SYMPTOMS	TREATMENT	COMPLICATIONS AND SEQUELAE
Clinical symptoms Typical cough	Catarrhal stage (1 to 2 weeks) Running nose Sore throat Slight fever Beginning cough Loss of appetite Paroxysmal stage (1 week to 2 months) Cough—spasmodic Paroxysmal Followed by vomiting or expectorating thick mucus More at night and indoors Loss of appetite Vomiting Convalescent stage Cough persists —less spasmodic, less disturbing	Bed rest during catarrhal stage Keep up nutrition Keep child quiet and peaceful to avoid coughing Medication for cough (See discussion in Pharmacology) Antibiotics Hyperimmune pertussis serum or gamma globulin Cough may be frightening to child—reassurance Suction; croup tent with young children if danger of anoxemia Oxygen to patients with increased respiratory rate	Broncho-pneumonia Hemorrhages in conjunctiva or skin Convulsions during paroxysmal stage in infants Otitis media Hernia (umbilical)
Spirochetes seen by dark-field in serum from lesions Wassermann and other tests for syphilis	Primary stage Raised crusted lesions on lower legs Regional lymph nodes enlarged Lesion is granuloma—lasts several months and heals with scar Later stage Widely scattered skin lesions—generalized rash. Lesion is called "frambesia" Pain in head, legs and arms, indicating bone involvement Late lesions—similar to syphilitic gumma—tissue destruction and ulceration Lesions on soles of feet—cause much disability	Penicillin—same as syphilis Surgical treatment for lesions of skin and bones	Essentially a disease of childhood. Destruction of tissue causes great disfigurement and unsightly scarring Secondary infection in lesions

DISEASE	ETIOLOGY AND IN-CUBATION PERIOD	TRANSMISSION	PROPHYLAXIS
Yellow Fever	Filtrable virus 3 to 6 days	Bite of Aedes aegypti mosquito	Rigid mosquito control—DDT Adequate screening against mosquitoes Isolate infected individual for first 4 days of illness Vaccination

DIAGNOSIS	SYMPTOMS	TREATMENT	COMPLICATIONS AND SEQUELAE
Clinical picture Neutralization tests Animal inoculation	Period of Infection Sudden onset Fever Severe headache Backache Pain in legs Prostration Photophobia Faget's sign (slow pulse in relation to temperature) Progressive leukopenia Albuminosis Period of Intoxication Lassitude Depression Jaundice Petechiae Hemorrhage from stomach, in- testine, etc. Vomiting with blood Gums readily bleed Hiccough Coma	Absolute rest is most essential Symptomatic Supportive Isolate patient in mosquito-proof room	Mortality rate is high if hic- cough, copious "black vomi- tus," melena or anuria de- velop

Part 5.   Cardiovascular Diseases

A.   Cardiac Disturbances
NURSING CARE

Rest, Mental and Physical

Freedom from all physical, mental and nervous causes of strain or of anything that throws additional work upon the heart.

Position (in bed) should be that which affords the greatest comfort with the least strain.

When propped up, the support must be firm and nothing should interfere with the respirations. The head, the arms and the knees should be supported and the patient should not be allowed to slip down in bed. When the patient leans forward, there should be proper support.

In giving treatments, in the use of bedpans and in feeding the patient, all exertion and strain should be avoided.

The patient must be free from worry, excitement, irritation or anger.

Sleeping is essential. Sometimes sedatives are necessary.

The Room

In an illness which is apt to be prolonged, the mental attitude has a marked effect on the progress. The room should be bright, cheerful and quiet; the surroundings congenial, free from disorder or confusion. There should be plenty of fresh air and the proper temperature and humidity of the room will lessen the difficulty in breathing and add greatly to the patient's comfort.

Care of the Skin

Daily cleansing baths and frequent massages are

given to refresh the patient, to stimulate the circulation and to keep the skin in good condition. Pressure sores are a real danger.

Diet

The diet has a marked bearing on the patient's comfort and recovery. The circulation in the digestive tract is impaired, so that the appetite and digestion may be poor. Therefore, the food should be tempting and given in fairly small amounts at frequent intervals. The use of salt frequently is restricted. In an acute state the patient may be placed on a full fluid diet. (*See* Diet, pp. 543-546, 567.)

Fluid Intake

The amount given should be measured and charted.

Output

The urine should be measured and charted. The bowels should be regulated for proper elimination.

Exercise as prescribed by the physician.

Rehabilitation of the Cardiac Patient

Aim is to teach the individual to live within the limits of his cardiac capacity.

Nurse must be thoroughly informed about the patient's condition and the limitations which the doctor has indicated for the patient.

Patient's fear of recurrence will be a major problem with which the nurse must deal. A positive approach to teaching the patient and his family how to live with this condition will be helpful in alleviating much of this fear and anxiety.

An equanimity in the patient's life must be the goal, i.e., avoidance of undue emotional and physical strain. Family planning is essential here.

Plans may be made for visits from the public health nurse to assist in health supervision of the patient and his family.

Methods of preventing physical strain may be taught to the patient, i.e., proper method of climbing stairs;

helping homeworker to carry out many activities while sitting—ironing, washing dishes, etc.

Help patient plan for follow-up care, for he must remain under constant medical supervision during the rest of his life.

Stress the importance of avoiding people and situations which predispose to infections, especially upper respiratory.

If the community offers rehabilitative services for the cardiac patient, he should be encouraged to avail himself of their facilities.

If patient returns to work, his employer should fully understand the limitations which the heart condition imposes.

THE CLASSIFICATION OF PATIENTS WITH DISEASES OF THE HEART
(New York Heart Association)

Functional Capacity

CLASS I   Patients with cardiac disease but without resulting limitation of physical activity. Ordinary physical activity does not cause undue fatigue, palpitation, dyspnea or anginal pain.

CLASS II   Patients with cardiac disease resulting in slight limitations of physical activity. They are comfortable at rest. Ordinary physical activity results in fatigue, palpitation, dyspnea or anginal pain.

CLASS III   Patients with cardiac disease resulting in marked limitation of physical activity. They are comfortable at rest. Less than ordinary activity causes fatigue, palpitation, dyspnea or anginal pain.

CLASS IV   Patients with cardiac disease resulting in inability to carry on any physical activity without discomfort. Symptoms of cardiac insufficiency or of the anginal syndrome are present even at rest. If any physical activity is undertaken, discomfort is increased.

Therapeutic Classification

CLASS A   Patients with cardiac disease whose ordinary physical activity need not be restricted.

CLASS B   Patients with cardiac disease whose ordinary physical activity need not be restricted, but who should be advised against severe or competitive physical efforts.

CLASS C   Patients with cardiac disease whose ordinary physical activity should be moderately restricted, and whose more strenuous efforts should be discontinued.

CLASS D   Patients with cardiac disease whose ordinary physical activity should be markedly restricted.

CLASS E   Patients with cardiac disease who should be at complete rest, confined to bed or chair.

No Heart Disease, Predisposing Etiological Factor*

These are patients in whom no cardiac disease is discovered, but whose course should be followed by periodic examinations because of the presence or history of an etiological factor that might cause heart disease. These cases should be recorded as No Heart Disease: Predisposing Etiological Factor and it is essential that the etiological diagnosis also be stated.

Undiagnosed Manifestation*

Patients with symptoms or signs referable to the heart but in whom a diagnosis of cardiac disease is uncertain should be classified tentatively as Undiagnosed Manifestation.

Re-examination after a suitable interval will usually help to establish a definite diagnosis. When there is a reasonable probability that the signs or symptoms are not of cardiac origin, the title Undiagnosed Manifestation should not be used. The diagnosis then should be No Heart Disease.

NOTE: For complete diagnostic criteria, see Nomenclature and Criteria, rev. 1953, prepared by New York Heart Association, distributed by American Heart Association and its affiliates.

* For some patients both diagnoses will apply.

ANGINA PECTORIS

Angina pectoris is a heart condition resulting from partial occlusion of the coronary arteries. The heart cannot meet extraordinary demands made on it, such as unusual muscular or mental effort or emotion.

Symptoms

Sudden severe pain in the heart region. Pain usually radiates to the left shoulder and down the left arm.

A sense of impending death

Dyspnea and a pale, anxious face

The pulse is very variable. Its force is feeble

Attacks last from a few seconds to a minute or two

Prevention of Attacks

Reduce anxiety and sources of irritation

Teach patient to live within his strength and own resources

Avoid "gas-forming" foods

Avoid sudden exertion

Treatment of the Attack

The patient usually is more comfortable in the sitting posture.

Amyl nitrite, nitroglycerine or other vasodilators are effective remedies. (*See discussion in* Pharmacology.)

Morphine may be given by hypodermic.

CARDIAC DECOMPENSATION (INSUFFICIENCY)

Decompensation is a condition in which the heart is unable to maintain an adequate circulation of the blood. It is also called *cardiac insufficiency*. The condition usually occurs in valvular diseases but may also occur in myocarditis, arteriosclerosis, hypertension, etc. The attacks of decompensation may recur and each subsequent attack is apt to be more serious than the previous one.

Causes

Unusual exercise; hard work.

When pneumonia, tonsillitis, typhoid fever, etc., occur in a patient with heart disease.

Results from the absorption of poisons from infected teeth and tonsils.

Symptoms and Signs

Tachycardia

Pain—sticking, precordial or sense of weight

Dyspnea and orthopnea

Cyanosis

Edema

Symptoms of impairment of various systems—nervous, digestive, renal and muscular

PULMONARY EDEMA

Pulmonary edema is an emergency situation in which the lungs become congested and serous fluid is exudated into the alveoli. It occurs most frequently with left ventricular heart failure, but also may be a complication of infections, uremia, bronchial obstruction or may result from the inhalation of irritating fumes.

Symptoms and Signs

Severe dyspnea and orthopnea

Wheezing respirations with loud rales, often heard without the aid of a stethoscope

Cough which is productive of quantities of blood-tinged, watery, frothy sputum

Treatment and Nursing Care

Bed rest—high Fowler's position

Drug therapy (*See* Pharmacology)

Morphine 15 mg. or Demerol 50 to 200 mg.

Digoxin, if heart failure present

Bronchodilators if bronchospasm present

Antibiotic therapy, if condition is pulmonary in origin

Diuretics, if heart failure is present.

Oxygen inhalation by positive pressure. (*See* Nursing Technics)

Venous tourniquets on limbs. (*See* Nursing Technics)

Phlebotomy 250 to 500 ml., if heart failure is present.

Maintenance of cough reflex, if pulmonary in origin.

Maintenance of airways; tracheobronchial suction if necessary. (*See* Nursing Technics)

Continuous nursing care is essential, especially during the acute stage

ACQUIRED DEFECT
(MITRAL STENOSIS)

Definition

This is a scarring and calcification of the mitral valve, usually due to rheumatic fever, that partially prevents ejection of blood from the heart.

Signs and Symptoms

Limited exercise tolerance

Enlargement of left auricle and pulmonary vein

May lead to

Dyspnea, orthopnea

Paroxysmal nocturnal attacks

Pulmonary edema

Hemoptysis

Right-sided failure

Signs of atrial fibrillation, arterial embolism, pulmonary infarction

Treatment

First, medical regimen with limited activity.

Cardiac surgery.

CONGENITAL DEFECT

See Pediatrics for coverage of conditions which àre congenital in origin.

CARE OF THE PATIENT WITH CARDIAC SURGERY

Principles of thoracic surgery (*See* Part 3) and general surgery (*See* Part 1) apply.

Special Preoperative Care

One of the most important considerations is the mental preparation of the patient and his family. This implies careful interpretation of the relationship of surgery to the patient's state of health; so that the patient and his family can make the decision for the operation. Once the decision is made, a general discussion of the expected postoperative period and of the expected results should ensue. All members of the health team must be prepared to answer the patient's many questions and to lend emotional support as the need is evident.

Removal of excess fluid may be accomplished by diuretics (*See* Pharmacology).

Daily weight must be taken.

Patients already digitalized, are continued on their maintenance dose. Those with atrial fibrillation are digitalized so that apical rate is controlled.

Vitamin K (*See* Pharmacology) is often administered as the prothrombin level frequently is low in this condition.

Special Postoperative Care

During early postoperative period patient must be under constant medical and nursing supervision, often in a specialized area.

Main considerations are:

Maintenance of a clear tracheobronchial tract—suction. (*See* Nursing Technics)

Frequent observation of vital signs; especially for evidence of arrhythmias or emboli.

Maintenance of oxygen supply. (*See* Nursing Technics)

Maintenance of fluid balance; careful recording of intake and output. A Foley catheter usually is inserted into the bladder. (*See* Nursing Technics)

Maintenance of dose of digitalis; may be given intravenously during early period.

Maintenance of normal body temperature, often a Therm-o-rite mattress is used.

Observations to detect evidence of complications:

cardiac arrest, hemorrhage, shock, auricular fibrillation, heart block, cardiac decompensation, atelectasis, hemothorax, pneumothorax or emboli.

Maintenance of complete rest; often hygienic care is limited to the basic essentials during the immediate 24 to 48 hours postoperative.

Relief of pain—Demerol. (*See* Pharmacology)

Recognition of and preparation for handling the personality change which many patients undergo shortly after surgery. It usually is an acute depression or anxiety.

Ambulation is started as soon as medical picture warrants it.

Restorative Phase

Assist patient to move from dependent to interdependent stage.

Help patient to gradually increase activity.

Exercises are helpful in restoring full function to left arm.

Diversional therapy is important to help the patient increase his physical and emotional state of well-being.

Referral should be made for a public health nurse to visit the patient and his family for health supervision.

The importance of medical supervision should be stressed and arrangements made for follow-up care. (*See* Rehabilitation of Cardiac Patient)

During the recovery period, some patients experience a febrile illness known as "postcommissurotomy syndrome"—possibly due to a pleuropericardial inflammation secondary to surgical trauma.

SYMPTOMS AND SIGNS:

Pain in chest, neck, and/or shoulders may be due to pleural effusion

High fever

Elevated ESR

Treatment

Bed rest and salicylates.

ACUTE MYOCARDIAL INFARCTION

(Coronary Occlusion, Coronary Thrombosis)

This is an obstruction, generally acute, of a branch of one of the coronary arteries resulting in infarction and death of the myocardium in the area supplied by the occluded vessel.

Symptoms

Severe heart pain, usually beginning without exertion or other obvious reason. It is not relieved by nitrites. Pain is described as sharp, cutting, or as a fullness or heaviness. Pain usually is referred to upper or middle third of sternum. Pain radiates to the left and at times to the right arm, and into the left and the right sides of the neck

Nausea and vomiting frequently occur during or after the onset of pain

In the more severe cases, shock and collapse may occur with the following symptoms: ashen pallor, cold sweat, clammy skin and a rapid, weak pulse

Dyspnea

Very low blood pressure

Apprehension, feeling of dying

Pulse may be imperceptible at wrist, barely perceptible in neck over carotids

Fever, leukocytosis within first 24 hours

Elevated ESR within first 3 to 4 days

Treatment

Absolute physical and mental rest

Bed rest for 3 to 6 weeks; lavatory privileges and sitting in a chair are sometimes allowed

Morphine or Demerol (*See discussion in* Pharmacology) given immediately for relief of pain

Oxygen until pain is relieved and temperature comes down to normal

Anticoagulant drugs (*See discussion in* Pharmacology)

Heparin or others

Dicumarol—for entire period of bed rest

Digitalis, if evidence of congestive failure or atrial fibrillation or flutter

Quinidine sulfate to lessen chance of developing paroxysmal tachycardia or fibrillation (*See discussion in* Pharmacology)

Diet—low calorie, restrictive of salt (*See discussion in* Diet)

Mineral oil to avoid constipation

CARDIAC ARRHYTHMIAS

FIBRILLATION

When the heart muscle becomes excessively irritable, all its bundles of fibers do not beat in harmony; therefore, its rhythm is disturbed. This condition is known as fibrillation and results from the loss of control of the heart muscle by the sinus node.

Atrial fibrillation is a condition in which groups of muscle fibers in the auricles beat by themselves and thus disturb the rhythm of the heart. The condition is recognized when the heart beats are more rapid than the pulse, some of the beats being so weak that they are not transmitted.

Ventricular fibrillation is a condition in which bundles of muscle fibers of the ventricles beat independently, thus disturbing the rhythm of the ventricles. This condition usually is fatal.

Paroxysmal atrial fibrillation is a condition which if evidenced by persistent tachycardia, signs of failure or of discomfort on the part of the patient, should be treated with the following measures:

Bed rest

Digitalis to reduce ventricular rate

Quinidine, if normal rhythm is not returned and there is no sign of failure.

HEART BLOCK

Heart block is a condition resulting from an interference with the conduction of impulses from the sinoatrial node to the ventricle along the atrioventricular bundle. Usually, it is due to arteriosclerosis, rheumatic heart disease, nutritional changes or toxic effects of drugs.

COMPLETE HEART BLOCK

None of the contractions of the atrium reaches the ventricle. The atrium and ventricle beat independently of one another. Usually seen in arteriosclerotic heart disease. Patient complains of syncope and heart rate is around 35.

Treatment

If the heart block is due to digitalis, stop the medication.

Atropine or adrenalin are used sometimes for Adams-Stokes breathing. Pacemaker is used sometimes, especially if cardiac arrest is present.

HEART MURMURS

The contractions of the normal heart produce characteristic sounds resembling "lubb-dupp." Murmurs are abnormal sounds produced when the valves are defective.

Systolic murmurs—sounds which accompany or replace the first sound of the heart.

Diastolic murmurs occur with the second sound of the heart.

Presystolic murmurs usually are rumbling sounds which are heard just before the first sound of the heart.

Importance of Diagnosis

The physician is able to recognize the specific valvular defect by the kind of murmur he hears, and by the region of the heart area where the murmur is heard loudest.

RHEUMATIC FEVER

Definition

This is a febrile disease following an upper respiratory infection caused by Group A hemolytic streptococci. It involves the mesenchymatous tissue of the body. This condition is responsible for the greater part of heart disease in children and young adults. Although the disease is found predominantly in the 5 to 15 year age group, it is by no means limited to this group.

MEDICAL AND SURGICAL

Signs and Symptoms

Variable in manifestations and intensity
Onset may be insidious or acute
Usual symptoms are:
Fever, mostly moderate or low-grade
Pain arising from inflammation of joints
Polyarthritis—migratory in nature
May be vague discomfort in extremities
Joint may be red, swollen, hot, with fluid in the cavity
Large joints of extremities mostly involved
Cardiac involvement—myocarditis, pericarditis
Precordial pain and discomfort
Palpitation
May be signs of failure
Abdominal pain or discomfort
Erythema occurs in some patients
Leukocytosis
Elevated erythrocyte sedimentation rate
Proteinuria

Treatment and Nursing Care

General medical and nursing care to maintain patient in good physiologic balance and comfort
Increase fluid intake
Bed rest is essential
Diversional therapy is necessary to maintain the morale of the patient, especially when bed rest is required after the acute symptoms have disappeared
Drug therapy (*See* Pharmacology)
Penicillin
Salicylates
Cortisone
Adequate nutritious diet
Support of inflamed joints; care in handling them. A foot-cradle may be used to keep covers from touching the joints

Prevention of Recurrences

Prophylactic therapy for all following attack and continued indefinitely if there is any cardiac involvement (*See* Pharmacology)

Sulfadiazine

Oral penicillin (give on an empty stomach before breakfast and at bedtime)

Benzathine penicillin I.M. every 4 weeks

Avoidance of conditions which predispose to upper respiratory infections, i.e., contacts, fatigue, cold, etc.

Prophylactic doses of penicillin before, during and after dental extraction, tonsillectomy or instrumentation of genitourinary tract

BACTERIAL ENDOCARDITIS

This is an inflammation of the endocardium of the heart which includes the valves.

Etiology

Pre-existing valvular abnormality invaded by bacteria, usually *Streptococcus viridans*

Lesions on valves usually result of
Rheumatic endocarditis
Congenital heart abnormality
Syphilitic heart

May follow oral surgery, cystoscopic examination in rheumatic subjects

Invasion of blood stream by bacteria

Diagnosis

Isolation of organism in blood culture

Symptoms

Most common between age of 20 and 40
Insidious onset
Grippal feeling for several weeks
Gradual weakness, fatigability
Anorexia
Fever
Arthralgias
Osler nodes—on pads of fingers or toes—painful, tender, small nodules
Petechiae on mucous membrane and skin
Spleen—palpable
Heart murmurs

Leukocytosis
Albuminuria
Elevated erythrocyte sedimentation rate (ESR)

Treatment

Bed rest in active stage
Penicillin (2 to 5,000,000 units/day for 4 to 6 weeks)
See Pharmacology
Penicillin plus streptomycin (2 Gm. O.D.)
Supportive
Remove foci of infection, such as abscessed teeth

Prevention

Prophylactic therapy of penicillin—several days before and after dental work, tonsillectomy, or instrumentation of genitourinary tract—to all patients with history of rheumatic heart disease.

B. Vascular Disturbances

EMBOLISM

An embolism is defined as a foreign body in the blood stream and, in most cases, is formed by a blood clot which, having become dislodged from its original site, is carried along in the blood. There are many types of emboli—cerebral, pulmonary, etc.

PULMONARY EMBOLISM

The clot is carried to the heart and is forced with the blood into the pulmonary artery where it plugs the main artery or one of its branches. The chief sources of pulmonary embolism are phlebothrombosis and thrombophlebitis of the deep veins of the legs. Other predisposing causes are prolonged bed rest, obesity, postpartum and postoperative states and many cardiac conditions.

Symptoms and Signs

Sudden chest pain
Moderate rise in temperature and pulse rate
Cough, bloody sputum
Mild leukocytosis
Prostration
Nausea
Sweating

Treatment

Bed rest, in sitting position
Narcotic for pain (*See* Pharmacology)
Penicillin (*See* Pharmacology)
Anticoagulant therapy (*See* Pharmacology)
Colon lavage to prevent strain
Oxygen therapy, possibly positive pressure (*See* Nursing Technics)
Drugs to relieve cough (*See* Pharmacology)

THROMBOSIS

A thrombus is a blood clot formed during life within the heart or the blood vessels. Thrombi result from abnormalities in clotting factors, from sluggish circulation, from injury to vessel walls or a combination of these factors. Infection anywhere may injure nearby vessels, especially thin-walled veins. When the intima (the lining layer) of blood vessels is injured, thromboplastin is released. With the aid of calcium prothrombin, and Factor V, thrombin is formed. If the blood current is rapid, any small amount of thrombin would be washed away and neutralized. If the current is sluggish, the thrombin accumulates and, by combination with fibrinogen, fibrin is formed. Thrombi are seen more commonly in veins than in arteries, partly because veins are more subject to infection and partly because of slower circulation. Clotting is especially common when venous flow is obstructed, as in the pelvic veins of pregnant women.

Occasionally, thrombosis of arteries is due directly to inflammation, but usually the thrombus develops over a plaque of thickened and degenerated intima (arteriosclerotic plaque). Thrombi deposited on arteriosclerotic plaques of coronary arteries (blood supply to the heart) may occlude the vessel and give rise to sudden heart failure.

THROMBOPHLEBITIS

Thrombophlebitis is inflammation of the wall of the vein with the formation of a clot. Its cause may be stasis of blood flow in which the blood cells settle out, some abnormality or infection of the lining of the blood vessels, or some abnormality of the clotting mechanism of the blood. It frequently occurs in the lower extremities, and is particularly dangerous because it frequently leads to pulmonary embolism. (*See* Pulmonary Embolism, *above*.)

Occurrence

During periods of prolonged bed rest with associated infection (operations, in puerperium, pneumonia, influenza, etc.)

Trauma to extremity

Extension from focus of infection (osteomyelitis)

Symptoms

Sudden onset

Pelvic veins

Abdominal pain

Nausea or vomiting

Faintness

Superficial vein

Vessel felt as tender cord under skin

Deep popliteal vein

Calf tenderness

Pain on forced dorsiflexion of foot

Fever

Treatment

Bed rest and elevation of foot of bed until clot has had a chance to adhere to the wall of the vessel.

Foot cradle to supply local heat

Anticoagulants to prevent further thrombi from developing (*See discussion in* Pharmacology)

SURGERY: Phlebotomy and thrombectomy for simple, noninflammatory thrombosis of large veins. When temperature is normal, passive and then active exercises to help regain muscle tone and stimulate collateral circulation.

VARICOSE VEINS

Varicose veins are tortuous segmental dilatations of veins that may occur anywhere in the body. (The discussion here is limited to the superficial venous system of the lower extremities, namely, the saphenous system.)

Etiology

Increased postural strain along with defective valves (occupational type)

Obstruction to venous flow as in pregnancy

Signs and Symptoms

Tired, heavy sensation in legs

Cramping of calves at night or in cold water

Swelling of ankle or dorsum of foot

Painful radiation along saphenous nerve

If untreated, condition becomes progressively worse and complications result

Skin becomes atrophied, pigmented and indurated

Ulcers form in pigment areas

Phlebitis in varicose vein

Treatment

Elastic support—must fit snugly; produce tight, even pressure and reach above level of valvular insufficiency

Injection of irritants to produce endophlebitis and thrombosis, either preoperatively or postoperatively

High ligation and stripping of the saphenous vein

If ulcer is present

Rest in bed

Elevation

Warm dressings

Antibiotics applied locally

Surgical excision of ulcer with skin grafting

HEMORRHOIDS

These are varicosities of superficial veins in the anal region, often accompanied by low-grade infection and the development of thrombi. External hemorrhoids are covered by skin. Internal hemorrhoids are covered by mucous membrane.

Etiology
Constipation or straining at stool
Pregnancy or any large abdominal mass
Obesity
Erect posture for long periods of time

Signs and Symptoms (variable)
Bleeding
Pain, if hemorrhoid is thrombosed
Protrusion with evacuation or physical strain
Itching
Backache, if internal hemorrhoids

Treatment
Palliative
Stool kept soft by high residue diet and mild laxatives
Hot packs, sitz baths after defecation
Area kept clean
Anesthetic ointments or suppositories
Nonsurgical
Injection of chemical solution into the hemorrhoids to produce an endophlebitis with resultant thrombosis of the hemorrhoid
For small or moderately large uncomplicated internal hemorrhoids
Surgical—excision of hemorrhoids
Special preoperative care is aimed at providing a sufficiently clean field, i.e., cleansing enemas and purgatives
Special postoperative care
If difficulty in voiding, patient may stand by bed
Analgesics for discomfort
Watch for bleeding

Hot packs and sitz baths
Usually 5 to 7 days will be necessary to establish normal daily stools
Low residue diet (*See* Diet, p. 564)

ANEURYSM

An aneurysm is a localized dilatation of a blood vessel, usually an artery, resulting from a weakness and/or distention of the wall of the vessel.

Etiology

Syphilis (most frequently causes thoracic aneurysm)
Arteriosclerosis (most frequently causes abdominal aneurysm)
Trauma
Congenital

Signs and Symptoms (depend upon location)

Thoracic
Cough, brassy in character
Dyspnea
Dysphagia
Hoarseness
Pain—anginal or constant
May be visible; hear systolic thrill over sac
Abdominal
Excruciating pain when aneurysm erodes into the back
Shock and abdominal rigidity if perforation occurs
Reduction of blood pressure in lower extremities
If untreated, death occurs within 7 to 8 months

Treatment

Symptomatic
Bed rest
Iodides to promote bronchial secretions
Analgesics
Antisyphilitic treatment, if syphilis is the underlying cause
Surgery
Wiring and banding

Resection and wrapping with new type of plastic mesh material

Resection and graft

Mild sedatives

HYPERTENSION

To warrant this term, the increase in pressure must be permanent and 160/100 may be taken as an arbitrary figure for the minimum of hypertension. Hypertension may be found in a variety of conditions. The most important are:

Hypertrophy of the left ventricle

Essential hypertension

With renal disease

With some cases of arteriosclerosis

With endocrine gland disturbance

With increased volume of blood

With increased viscosity of the blood

With obesity

HYPOTENSION

A systolic figure below 110 may be regarded as hypotension. It is significant only in such diseases as Addison's disease or if it is part of a debilitating disease. It is the underlying cause, in this case, not the hypotension that requires treatment.

VASCULAR DISORDERS OF THE BRAIN

CEREBRAL ANOXIA

The brain has no means of storing oxygen or nutrients in tissue, thus cells cannot survive without blood supply for longer than 5 minutes at a normal metabolic rate.

Causes

Hemorrhage

Carbon monoxide inhalation

Cardiac arrest

Vasomotor instability

Respiratory difficulty

Signs and Symptoms

Drowsiness or a more depressed level of consciousness
Lethargy or severe fatigue
Mental confusion
Focal neurologic defects, e.g., hemiparesis, paralysis, ataxia, aphasia, etc.

Treatment

Supportive, in line with cause of anoxia
Hypothermia to decrease metabolic rate, thus decrease need for oxygen and metabolites until more positive treatment can be instituted

CEREBRAL VASCULAR ACCIDENTS

General Principles of Nursing Management

In bed:
Proper positioning in neutral alignment to prevent stretching of weakened muscle
Frequent changes of position to prevent pneumonia, contractures, decreased circulation and skin breakdown
Active range of motion exercises to unaffected limbs to maintain joint motion, decrease spasticity and prevent contractures
Encouragement of patient to do as much for himself as he can—preliminary training to becoming independent and self sufficient
Gradual ambulation—bed to chair, then walking with assistance, to independent ambulation, depending on balance and ability to manage paralyzed side
Early ambulation greatly decreases problems with incontinence of urine and decreased peristalsis
Teach patient to use unaffected limb to assist affected limb in doing exercises with arm, or in getting in and out of bed.
Use of activities of daily living to provide exercises, etc., with minor modification of equipment, as built-up handles on combs, eating utensils, etc.

CEREBRAL INFARCTION

Cerebral infarction occurs when the blood supply to any area of the brain is cut off. This can occur in any blood vessel. Signs and symptoms relate to the area of the brain deprived of blood. The middle meningeal artery is most frequently involved, leading to the typical symptoms of hemiparesis or hemiparalysis

Treatment

Early recognition of impending clot, i.e., transient visual signs, muscle weakness, etc.

Location of thrombus formation by arteriogram—surgical removal, if accessible

Anticoagulant therapy to prevent further formation, depending on age of patient (if under 40, duration of anticoagulation therapy is too long—doctors won't start)

Early ambulation, rehabilitation

CEREBRAL THROMBOSIS

This is an intravascular clot occurring in an abnormal blood vessel. It usually occurs secondary to infection, hypertension, hypotension, defect in the clotting mechanism or arteriosclerotic blood vessels

Signs and Symptoms

Generally sudden onset except in the internal carotid artery in which it is gradual and intermittent

Headache, loss of consciousness, aphasia, convulsions, hemiplegia (more pronounced in arm than in leg), usual visual field defects, facial paralysis, etc.

INTRACEREBRAL HEMORRHAGE

This is bleeding into the brain or the meninges usually as the result of the rupture of an arteriosclerotic blood vessel, although it may result from trauma, aneurysm, blood dyscrasias or other systemic diseases. Usually found in older age groups.

Signs and Symptoms

Sudden onset after physical exertion or emotional stress with headache, loss of consciousness, shock reaction or with evidence of signs of increased intracranial pressure

Focal neurologic signs depend on area of brain involved

Hypertension

Signs of meningeal irritation

Prognosis is poor where coma is present

Treatment

Occasionally, hemorrhage can be surgically removed

Conservative bed rest for prevention of possible repetition of bleeding

Nursing care directed at minimizing exertion of patient to prevent increase of blood pressure and repeated bleeding

Long-term resumption of previous activities at slow rate

Physical rehabilitation measures are dependent on residual abilities of patient

CEREBRAL EMBOLISM

May be single or multiple—these are generally due to cardiac disease, but may occur with thrombophlebitis or fractures of other areas of the body

Signs and symptoms relate to area of the brain and extent of embolization. Treatment symptomatic for the location of emboli and treatment of primary foci

VASCULAR ANOMALIES

ANEURYSM

Aneurysm is a herniation of the wall of a blood vessel with pressure on surrounding brain tissue. The most important complication is leaking or extensive hemorrhage from rupture of aneurysm.

Treatment

Prevent rupture by:

Rest, both physical and emotional

Ligation of accessible vessel feeding aneurysm

ANGIOMA

Angiomas are caused by coiled masses of arteries or

dilated capillary channels. If they are of the surface type, seizures may appear. Treatment is by surgical excision if they are accessible.

MENINGEAL HEMORRHAGE

Subdural

The subdural hemorrhage caused by inflammation, trauma, leaking aneurysm, etc. Treatment is by decompression of the brain by surgery.

Epidural

In the epidural, the dura is pulled from skull during trauma, tearing the middle meningeal artery. The patient is stunned momentarily, but feels well for a few hours. There is sudden loss of consciousness and the pupil on the affected side is dilated. Treatment is by decompression of the brain.

PERIPHERAL VASCULAR DISEASES

ATHEROSCLEROSIS

Atherosclerosis is the leading cause of arterial disease of the extremities of elderly patients. It results from the deposit of patches of lipid-containing material beneath the intimal surfaces of blood vessels, thus narrowing the lumen. Rare before the age of 55 except in cases of diabetes mellitus. Organs most commonly affected are the heart, the brain, and the kidneys.

Signs and Symptoms of Peripheral Atherosclerosis

Mostly in lower extremities
Numbness, tingling, burning sensation in toes
Sense of heaviness and pain
Nocturnal cramps
Intermittent claudication (pain appearing while walking and disappearing after rest)
Foot is colder than normal
Pulse is feeble or absent in posterior tibial and dorsalis pedis arteries
Bilateral, usually confined to lower extremities
Gangrene may result

Treatment

Early recognition
Avoidance of trauma, cold, dampness, infections
Good foot care including proper fitting shoes
Buerger's exercises
Vasodilators (*See discussion in* Pharmacology.)
High carbohydrate, low fat diet (*See* Diet, p. 541)
Treat diabetes, if present
Sympathectomy
Resection and grafting of diseased portion of vessels
Amputation, if gangrene develops

RAYNAUD'S DISEASE

This is a primary form of paroxysmal bilateral cyanosis of the digits with or without local gangrene. Attacks of cyanosis are produced by cold or emotion and are relieved by heat.

Etiology

Cause unknown
Constitutional predisposition—women who are underweight, asthenic, subject to emotional stress

Signs and Symptoms

Usually gradual onset, first attacks usually in winter
Attacks unilateral, soon become bilateral
Fingers become pale, cyanotic and numb
Aching pain, awkwardness in moving digits
Tingling, swelling, throbbing as arterial flow resumes
In 50 per cent of cases, the hands alone are affected
Trophic changes in progressive cases—1 to 4 years after onset

Treatment

Warm clothing
High-caloric diet (*See* Diet, p. 534)
Relaxation and avoidance of mental stress
Avoidance of smoking
Vasodilators (*See discussion in* Pharmacology.)
Regional sympathectomy for progressive type
Psychotherapy may be indicated

MEDICAL AND SURGICAL

BUERGER'S DISEASE

(Thromboangiitis Obliterans)

This is an inflammatory type of obliterative vascular disease affecting the peripheral arteries and veins of men (usually) in early adult life. The course usually runs 6 to 12 years and then advances less rapidly

Etiology

Specific etiology unknown

Suspect infection or activity of some toxic agent

About 50 per cent of the affected patients are Jews

Signs and Symptoms

Persistent coldness of one or both lower extremities

Aching pain in digits, instep, ankles, calf, wrists, or forearm after use of muscles

Color changes in skin

Intermittent claudication

Gangrene may develop

Treatment

Early diagnosis is important

Avoidance of exposure to cold—warm clothing

Avoidance of trauma

Skin care—clean, dry and soft

Avoidance of tobacco (favors extension of disease)

Care if local heat used—danger of blistering

Vasodilators (*See discussion in* Pharmacology)

Absolute bed rest, if pain is present

Heat cradle

Analgesic for pain (with care, danger of addiction)

Change in position of limbs (Buerger's exercise)

Sympathectomy, if gradually advancing disease, and organic occlusion

Amputation of ischemic parts

AMPUTATIONS

An amputation is the removal in whole or in part of an extremity. Consideration is given to obtaining the most useful stump possible, recognizing that the function of the upper extremity is to handle objects and the functions of the lower extremity are to bear weight and to propel the body as in walking.

Indications for Amputation

Reserved in the following instances where all other measures have failed to restore a functional extremity
    Trauma
    Infections
    Tumors
    Gangrene

Specific Preoperative Treatment

Aim is to
    Have the patient in best possible condition
    Minimize possibility of infection with resulting scar formation on stump
    Control any concomitant disorders such as
        Diabetes
        Infection
        Shock accompanying trauma
    Fluids, transfusions, if necessary
    Thorough cleansing and preparation of the skin in the operative area
    Psychological preparation of the patient
    Consultation with a limb maker to establish an ideal stump for future prosthesis

Specific Postoperative Treatment

Posture patients to prevent deformities of the amputated leg stump
    Footboard to maintain dorsal flexion of remaining foot
    Elevate stump to minimize danger of hemorrhage and edema
        Elevate foot of bed
        If pillow, place under entire stump to avoid flexion of knee and allow minimal flexion of hip
    Turn patient, when able, on abdomen several times a day to permit extension of hip

Support stump to avoid outward rotation

Traction may be ordered (*See* Care of Patient in Traction, p. 381)

Posture to prevent deformities of the amputated arm stump

At the shoulder, the arm is maintained in abduction until lessening of pain and tenderness permit exercise

Special observation—hemorrhage

Keep a tourniquet attached to patient's unit until all danger of hemorrhage has passed

Periodic inspection of dressings

Control pain

Analgesics (*See discussion in* Pharmacology)

Phantom pain

Reassuring patient

Diversional therapy

Analgesics given with caution

Prevention of infection in stump

Sterile technic

Antibiotics

Care of stump

Extremely important if patient is to have a satisfactory prosthesis

Patient should be taught stump care

Bandaging—at first to keep dressing in place; later it is used to mold and shrink the stump

Daily observation of stump for signs of abrasions or pressure points

Bathe stump twice daily, being sure it is thoroughly dry

Use powder rather than oil on stump; oil softens tissues and fosters their breakdown

Care of stump sock to be worn inside prosthesis

Fit properly

Change daily, careful washing

Dry thoroughly before wearing

Exercise stump

Emotional support

Rehabilitation

Physical therapy and occupational therapy

Crutch walking (*See discussion in* Technics)

Use of prosthesis

C. Blood Dyscrasias

ANEMIA*

Definition

A term which applies to a condition whereby the peripheral blood falls below the normal range of 12 to 14 Gm. per cent for adult females and 12 to 16 Gm. per cent for adult males. Usually the number of red blood corpuscles also is reduced below the normal range of 4.8 (female) and 5.4 (male) million per cubic ml.

Classification of Anemia

Increased erythrocyte loss or destruction (bone marrow physiologically hyperactive)

Acute erythrocyte loss

Hemorrhage, external

Hemorrhage, internal

Increased erythrocyte destruction

Extrinsic causes

Septicemias

Chemicals

Heat: thermal burns

Natural immunity (transfusion of incompatible blood)

Acquired immunity (Rh factor, pollens, drug)

Intrinsic causes

Abnormal erythrocyte

Abnormal plasma

Secondary hypersplenism (lymphomas, liver cirrhosis)

Decreased erythrocyte production (bone marrow physiologically hypoactive)

Nutritional deficiency

Vitamin B_{12} (macrocytic anemia)

Defective diet

Deficient gastric (intrinsic) factor

Intestinal impermeability (sprue, ileitis)

* Adapted from: Cecil and Loeb: Textbook of Medicine, ed. 10, p. 1117, Philadelphia, Saunders, 1959.

Competitive utilization (tapeworm, intestinal bacteria in diverticuli)

Folic acid (macrocytic anemia)

Defective diet

Intestinal impermeability

Folic and ascorbic acids (macrocytic anemia)

Vitamin B_6 (microcytic anemia)

Iron (hypochromic anemia)

Requirement increase: gradual loss—menstruation, pregnancy.

Decrease in intake—defective diet, diarrhea, gastric anacidity.

Endocrine deficiency (pituitary, thyroid, adrenal)

Toxic

External poisons—benzol insecticides, etc.

Internal toxins—chronic infections, cancer

Physical injury—x-ray, radium, radioactive phosphorus

Mechanical interference

Inadequate marrow capacity—newborn, prematurity

Myelophthisis (leukemia, metastatic cancer)

Idiopathic (aplastic)

Signs and Symptoms

Headache

Poor appetite

Fatigue

Tendency to fainting

Dyspnea on exertion

Rapid pulse

Polyuria, hyposthenuria in chronic anemia

Edema with severe anemia

Other symptoms which may occur (depends on etiology and degree of illness)

Jaundice

Pallor

Enlarged liver and spleen

Paresthesia of toes and fingers

Sore tongue or mouth

Epigastric distress

Treatment (according to etiology) some indicated below

    Hemorrhage
        Control
        Replacement—transfusion with whole blood (*See treatment under* Hemorrhage)
    Extrinsic cause of increased erythrocyte destruction
        Removal of causative agent
        Transfusions of whole blood in red cells
    Decreased erythrocytic production

Nutritional Deficiencies

    Diet to combat deficiency (*See* Diet)
    Drugs (*See* Pharmacology—according to cause)
        Vitamin B_{12} in form of refined liver extract
        Folic acid in folinic acid
        Ascorbic Acid (*See* Pharmacology)
        Vitamin B_6 (pyridoxine)
        Ferrous sulfate or gluconate

Special Considerations in Nursing Care of Patient with Pernicious Anemia (Vitamin B_{12} Deficiency)

Be prepared to help patient in periods of irritability and impatience

Provide for extra warmth

Provide for special mouth care

Help patient to accept fact she will need weekly or biweekly injections

If neurologic symptoms persist, teach patient how to get about safely and easily

BLOOD TRANSFUSION

Blood transfusions are given to treat anemia, and to restore to normal the blood volume depleted by bleeding. Sometimes packed red cells may be used to correct anemia without overexpanding the blood volume if the hemoglobin level is already high. Whole blood must be stored at 5° C. and can be used up to 21 days after collection into a sterile bottle or plastic bag from a blood donor. Other blood products dispensed by a blood bank are pooled liquid plasma, fresh frozen plasma which has antihemophilic globulin activity, dried plasma,

MEDICAL AND SURGICAL

concentrated platelets, albumin solution, fibrinogen, and dextran, an artificial polysaccharide blood volume expander. Pooled products are used with great caution because of the greatly increased chance of including as a donor a carrier of serum homologous jaundice often transmitted by transfusion, and represents the greatest unavoidable risk of blood transfusion.

Blood Grouping

Blood types are important when whole blood is transfused. Tests are made to ensure that the donor's red cells are the same group as that of the intended recipient. Also, a cross-match of patient's cells with donor serum must be done. This is a further check that the donor's cells will not be clumped or agglutinated by the patient's serum when transfused.

Red blood cells contain antigens A or B, A and B, or none. Serum (or plasm) contains antibody alpha or beta, or no antibody.

Blood Group	Cells	Serum	% of Population
O	none	alpha and beta	45
A	A	beta	41
B	B	alpha	10
AB	A and B	none	4

Rh Factor

In 1940, Doctors Karl Landsteiner and Alexander S. Weiner discovered an agglutinogen of great clinical importance which is known as *Rh factor*. They injected the red blood cells of the Rhesus monkey into rabbits and found that these rabbits responded with the production of immune bodies. The serum of these rabbits, when mixed with the red blood cells of humans, caused agglutination or clumping of the red cells in 85 per cent of the cases. These individuals were called *Rh positive*. Since this same serum did not agglutinate the red blood cells of the remaining 15 per cent, these individuals were called *Rh negative*.

The title Rh factor was derived from the first two letters of "Rhesus," the name of the laboratory monkey whose red cells were used for the original experiment.

If Rh-positive blood is injected into the blood stream of an Rh-negative person, the tissues combat the Rh-positive blood by what are called *anti-Rh antibodies*. These antibodies destroy the red blood cells of the Rh-positive blood.

There are two conditions under which these anti-Rh agglutinins can be produced. The first is in connection with repeated blood transfusions. If the patient is Rh-negative and receives transfusions of Rh-positive blood, sensitization may result. The chance that a Rh-negative patient will be sensitized by her first transfusion of Rh-positive blood is 50 per cent and increases greatly with repeated transfusions.

Once sensitization does result and further transfusions of Rh-positive blood are administered, a hemolytic reaction results in which the patient rapidly hemolyzes or destroys the transfused cells. This will be manifest with a rise in temperature, chills, nausea and, perhaps, vomiting, pain in the back, and most important, red urine containing hemoglobin. Several hours later, the patient will show slight or moderate jaundice. An incompatible transfusion may result in sudden death even after as little as 50 ml. A common later result is acute renal shutdown. Every transfusion reaction should be studied thoroughly and, if the Rh factor is found to be the cause, further transfusions may be carried out safely without reaction provided that Rh-negative blood is administered.

The second condition in which the Rh factor plays an important role is in connection with pregnancy. The mechanism here is the same—namely, one of active immunization. The mother may be Rh-negative. If the fetus is Rh-positive, having inherited this factor from the father, and blood of the fetus gets into the mother's circulation she becomes sensitized.

Levine and his co-workers have shown that during pregnancy if the antibodies of a mother who has been sensitized get into the circulation of the fetus, it can so affect the blood of the fetus that stillbirth results, or if the infant is born alive it evidences one or another of the signs of erythroblastosis fetalis. The severity of the disease varies. It may be very mild with slight jaundice lasting a few days. More serious cases require blood transfusion. Rh-negative blood must be administered, however, even though the child is Rh-positive. The child, having received anti-Rh agglutinins from his mother, will hemolyze not only his own blood but also that of any Rh-positive donor. Through the use of so-called "replacement transfusion," blood of the infant is withdrawn so as to remove as much as possible of its own Rh-positive blood containing anti-Rh agglutinins received from the mother. At the same time the Rh-negative blood is transfused into the affected newborn.

Since anti-Rh agglutinins are found also in the breast milk of Rh-negative mothers, this precludes the breast feeding of an infant affected with erythroblastosis.

Importance of Compatible Blood

It is essential that both patient and donor be typed routinely for ABO and for Rh and be shown to be of the same type before a transfusion is given. However, ABO and Rh represent only 2 of the 10 known blood group systems which may cause sensitization of patients with resulting transfusion reactions and erythroblastosis fetalis in exactly the same manner as the above. These are rare but because of the extreme care now practiced with ABO and Rh the Kell, Duffy, Kidd, Lewis, etc., blood systems are assuming increasing importance.

However, most transfusion accidents occur for 1 of 2 reasons: (1) Blood for typing and cross-matching is taken from the wrong patient yet is labeled with the correct name or (2) Blood is given to the wrong patient in the same ward.

LEUKEMIA

This is a state of excessive formation of white blood cells, especially immature forms. It is essentially a malignant disease of the white cells, for they invade all over the body, especially bone marrow, spleen, liver and lymph nodes. The condition arises primarily in the blood-forming organs.

ACUTE LEUKEMIA

Symptoms

Disease of young people, especially children

Fever, shaking chills
Profound anemia
Severe bleeding tendency due to marked decrease in blood platelets
Enlarged lymph nodes and spleen
Spontaneous course of 3 months or less
Abrupt onset
Sudden pallor
Elevated WBC—15,000-30,000 per cubic milliliter

Treatment

Supportive
Transfusions
Drugs (*See* Pharmacology)
Antibiotics, if infection is present
Folic acid antagonists—aminopterin
6-Mercaptopurine
Prednisone, cortisone, ACTH

See Pediatrics for Acute Leukemia in Children, p. 480

CHRONIC LEUKEMIA

Types

Granulocytic—affects persons aged 35 to 45 years
Lymphatic—affects persons aged 45 to 54 years

Signs and Symptoms

Life expectancy from 1 to 20 years, usually 3 to 5 after first symptoms
GRANULOCYTIC
Insidious onset—weakness, pallor, palpitation, dyspnea
Splenic enlargement
Fever—intermittent or remittent
Increased BMR
During acute exacerbations
Tendency to bleed easily (epistaxis, hemorrhage under skin)
Anemia

MEDICAL AND SURGICAL

LYMPHATIC
    Insidious onset
    Painless nontender lymph node—cervical, axillary, inguinal areas
    Pallor
    Loss of weight
    Enlarged spleen
    Anemia
    Elevated BMR

Treatment

Therapeutic agents
    Roentgen ray therapy—treatment of choice
    Radioactive phosphorous (P³²)—granulocytic
    Blood transfusions
    Antibiotics if ulcerations occur
    Myleran (*See* Pharmacology)—granulocytic
    Chlorambucil (*See* Pharmacology)—lymphatic

HEMOPHILIA

This is a hereditary, familial disease occurring only in males, characterized by recurring hemorrhages and prolonged venous clotting time.

Occurrence

Carried as recessive trait by female to male children—50 per cent of cases develop

May skip several generations but family history exists in about one half the cases

Due to a deficiency of blood clotting factor, thromboplastinogen

Symptoms and Signs

Hemorrhage
Hematomas of muscles, joints, kidney
Prolonged bleeding after
    Teeth extraction
    Minor surgery
    Slight injury
Prolonged venous clotting time
Chronic disabling disease

Treatment

Prophylaxis against trauma, surgery, etc.

Many transfusions—should know compatible donor

Injection of Fraction I, which contains antihemophilic factor

Powdered thrombin, oxidized gauze, fibrin foam, etc., placed at site of bleeding if possible

Bed rest, when bleeding occurs

Pain relief—aspirin, codeine, Demerol

IDIOPATHIC THROMBOCYTOPENIC PURPURA

Definition

This is a hemorrhagic condition, resulting from a reduction in blood platelets, which has not been traced to any demonstrable underlying cause.

Signs and Symptoms

More common in women

Petechial hemorrhages and bruises in skin and muscles

Bleeding from nose, mouth, gastrointestinal and urinary tracts

Low platelet count

Increased bleeding time

Bone-marrow tests show increased megakaryocytes, but little platelet formation

Treatment

Splenectomy generally is advised

If surgery is contraindicated:

Blood transfusions

ACTH or adrenal steroids (*See* Pharmacology) effective in controlling hemorrhage

AGRANULOCYTOSIS (AGRANULOCYTIC ANGINA; GRANULOCYTOPENIA)

Agranulocytosis is a condition characterized by a marked diminution in the number of polymorphonuclear leukocytes in the blood, frequently caused by disease, commonly used drugs, radiation, etc.

Frequently, there is an associated inflammation of the gums or throat with swelling and necrosis of these tissues. When lesions are present the disease is called *agranulocytic angina*.

Treatment and Nursing Care

Treat underlying cause

Nursing care is of the utmost importance

Absolute cleanliness of the mouth. Throat irrigations of salt and soda solution (1 tsp. of salt and 1 tsp. of bicarbonate of soda to 1 pt. of water) should be given every hour or whenever necessary

Nutritious diet with an abundance of fluids

Rest in bed

Applications to gums and throat as ordered

Penicillin to control infection

BAL (*See* Pharmacology) when causative agent is gold salt or arsenic

Daily soap suds in saline enema; constipation may lead to perirectal abscess

Medical aseptic technic to prevent contacts from bringing infection to patient

Part 6.   Urologic Disorders

ACUTE NEPHRITIS (GLOMERULONEPHRITIS)

This is an inflammation of the kidneys apparently caused by an allergy to an infection caused by hemolytic streptococcus.

Etiology

History of upper respiratory disease

Primarily a disease of childhood—good prognosis

Signs and Symptoms

History of sore throat

Hematuria

Edema of eyes, face, and dependent parts
Headache
Decrease in urinary output
Elevated blood pressure
Nausea and vomiting
Shortness of breath
Physical findings of cardiac failure
Elevated ESR

Treatment

Bed rest until general manifestations have disappeared

Avoidance of exposure to chilling and to persons with upper respiratory infections

Restriction of sodium chloride in the diet

Penicillin to treat active infection if it persists when glomerulonephritis is first recognized

Symptomatic and supportive care

Remove any potential focus of infection

UREMIA

This is a clinical syndrome associated with advanced kidney disease resulting in retention of urea nitrogen in the blood due to impairment of the filtering function of the kidneys.

Causes

Renal disease

Reduction in renal circulation as in shock, congestive failure, severe dehydration

Obstruction of urinary passage

Increased protein breakdown as in high fever, severe infection

Polycystic disease

Signs and Symptoms

Toxic
    Weakness—anorexia
    Nausea and vomiting
    Headache
    Mental depression, convulsions, restlessness, coma

Stomatitis, inflammation of the bowel
Anemia
Bleeding tendency
Marked pallor
"Uremic frost"—white powdery material clinging to skin—due to crystallized urea from sweat
Chemical Disturbances
Rise of blood nonprotein nitrogen
Dehydration
Loss of sodium chloride through diarrhea, vomiting, and continued renal excretion
Metabolic acidosis due to incompetency of kidneys
Decreased blood calcium causes muscular irritability
Slight hyperkalemia

Treatment

Determination of underlying cause—treatment where possible
Maintenance of body equilibrium as well as possible
Decrease in sodium intake if severe edema, congestive heart failure, malignant hypertension
Intravenous fluids to combat dehydration if indicated
Maintenance of adequate caloric intake; patients should be encouraged to take nourishment in whatever form they desire
Alkali if acidosis, but administration must be guided by chemical and clinical response of patient
Promazine may be helpful in controlling nausea and vomiting
Mild sedation (chloral hydrate). Avoidance of long-acting barbiturates and morphine (only when acute cardiac dyspnea is present)
Calcium P.O. or I.M. for muscular irritability
Symptomatic and supportive nursing care (*See* Care of Acutely Ill Patients, p. 167.)

NURSING CARE OF THE UROLOGIC PATIENT

General

Accurate measurement and recording of all fluid intake and output is essential. The total for the daily fluid intake includes fluid administered by mouth, rectum, hypodermoclysis and intravenous infusion. Fluid output includes urine secreted by voiding, catheterization or drainage tube.

The number of voidings as well as the time and the amount of each should be recorded. The nurse's notes should contain a description of each change of dressing.

Low urinary outputs, catheters that have been removed without an order, and drainage equipment that is not functioning properly should be reported at once.

Odors should be eliminated or reduced to a minimum by frequent change of dressing, careful cleaning of all drainage equipment and good ventilation.

Preoperative

Unless fluids are ordered specifically to be forced or limited, intakes should be maintained between 2,000 and 2,500 ml. The output should be approximately two thirds of the intake. Careful recording is important in determining renal function.

During the preparatory period many patients are provided with retention catheters or drainage tubes to ensure adequate urinary drainage. Drainage through these tubes must be free and uninterrupted at all times. These tubes should be fastened to the draw sheet to prevent pulling upon the tube or catheter. The collecting bottle should be emptied at specified times during the day.

Any change in character or appearance of the urinary drainage should be noted and reported at once. The drainage tubes must be observed closely for patency and free drainage of urine in order that the patient will not experience discomfort from a distended bladder.

Many urologic patients are in the older age group and need special consideration given to initial adjustment to the hospital, mental and personal hygiene, health teaching and accident prevention.

Postoperative

The postoperative care of urologic patients does not differ from that of other surgical patients except in those cases where drainage tubes or catheters are provided to carry off the urine or where urine drains out through the incision.

When the patient returns from the operating room he is made comfortable in bed in the usual manner. It is then necessary to connect the drainage tube with a proper receptacle in which the urine may be collected. This is done by means of a piece of plastic tubing about 5 ft. long which is connected with the drainage tube by means of a glass connecting tube. This tube and connector should be sterilized before using.

Drainage tubing, connections and bottles should be replaced with sterile equipment daily. The drainage bottle provided should have a snug fitting cap with ventilator to provide closed drainage.

Particular attention should be paid to the amount of blood in the drainage or on the dressings and to the color, the blood pressure, the pulse and the respirations of the patient.

During convalescence the principal problem, provided no complications occur, is to keep the patient clean and dry. As a rule, some urine leaks outside of the drainage tube into the dressings at first, but in many cases the leakage stops in a day or two. This leakage of urine can be controlled by the use of special suction drains which remove all urine from within the drainage tube continuously. In the absence of suction drainage, the secret of keeping the patient clean and comfortable is changing dressings very frequently. Use a comparatively small dressing and change this before it becomes completely soaked with urine.

If the urine is not passing through the drainage tube sufficiently, report the fact to the doctor, as a slight adjustment of the tube may be all that is necessary to make it function properly.

Irrigation of the bladder following prostatic and bladder surgery is carried out as the doctor orders.

While urinary wounds may be drained for some time, the drainage tube always is removed eventually in order to allow the wound to heal.

No rectal treatments are given, and temperatures are taken orally after any perineal operation. Many doctors prescribe mineral oil daily to soften the stool.

Cathartics and enemas usually are ordered the 2nd and the 3rd day respectively following operation.

Distention, which occurs frequently following renal and ureteral operations, is treated by poultices, enemas, rectal tubes and prostigmine.

PROSTATE GLAND

The prostate gland is a male accessory sex gland about the size and shape of a horse chestnut. It is trilobed and surrounds the urethra at its origin from the urinary bladder. The prostate produces a thin, opalescent secretion which dilutes the seminal fluid and prolongs the life of spermatozoa.

HYPERTROPHY OF PROSTATE

Occurrence

Usually it occurs in men in the 5th and the 6th decades

Etiology

Its cause is unknown—possibly caused by chronic infection or arteriosclerotic process

Symptoms

Frequency of urination and nocturia
Voiding in small amounts
Painful urination (dysuria)
Burning on urination
Difficulty in starting and stopping the stream
Hesitancy-urgency
Hematuria (occasionally)
High residual urine—acute retention
Pain in lower back, upper legs, perineum and rectum
Dribbling
Overflow incontinence
Urgency incontinence

Diagnostic Treatment

Rectal examination
Cystoscopy—to provide direct visualization of the

bladder and prostatic urethra for stones, tumor, diverticulae, ureteral anomalies, type and degree of intraurethral and intravesical prostatic enlargement.

Blood examinations

Complete blood count—often discloses an elevated white cell count and reduced hemoglobin

Blood urea nitrogen—indicates degree of renal function

Blood sugar—to rule out diabetes mellitus, disease often found in this older age group

Grouping and Rh factor—done preoperatively in event of postoperative hemorrhage

Kline, Kahn or Wassermann tests—positive is a poorer risk and may result in more severe complications

Urine examinations

Routine

Culture

X-ray examination

Roentgenogram of genitourinary tract—to estimate the condition of the kidneys, the ureters and the bladder; to discover the presence of tumors, stones, strictures and metastases.

Roentgenogram of chest—for metastatic lesions, heart size, emphysema

Intravenous pyelogram—to substantiate results of the roentgenogram and to show renal function

Retrograde pyelograms—to demonstrate ureteral strictures or obstruction, calyceal abnormalities; valuable where renal excretory function is poor or when allergy to iodide preparation is known.

Cystogram

Residual urine

Electrocardiogram

Preparation for Operation

This preparation should last from 1 to 4 weeks

Measure intake and output

Indwelling catheter through urethra for drainage

Bladder irrigation only as ordered, usually with

physiological saline, at other times with antiseptic solutions such acriflavine 1:50,000 or antibiotic solutions such as Bacitracin-Neomycin.

Adequate fluid intake: 1,600 to 1,800 ml.

Regular diet, unless sugar is present or there is heart involvement. If these conditions exist, a suitable diet is ordered. In any case, the diet should be interesting and nourishing.

The patient is out of bed each day if there are no complications. This keeps up his morale.

Intestinal regulation, if necessary.

Vas ligation usually done in operating room at the time of the prostatic surgery.

Operation

Prostatectomy—removal of the prostate gland
Suprapubic prostatectomy
Perineal prostatectomy
Retropubic prostatectomy
Transurethral resection

Postoperative Treatment

The retained catheter is connected to drainage, either suction or gravity, upon return from the operating room

Vital signs are watched and recorded every 15 minutes until they are stable

Hypodermoclysis, intravenous infusion or blood transfusion, if necessary

Fluids by mouth as soon as tolerated. Progress to regular diet in 2 or 3 days

Urge fluids to replace blood loss

Measure intake and output

Usually out of bed 1st or 2nd postoperative day

The use of a urethral catheter put in place at the time of surgery, varies with the urologist, but many utilize a large balloon Foley retention catheter (No. 22 or No. 24) to act as a hemostatic agent. Traction also is applied in the first 6 to 8 hours or until bleeding is controlled. The Foley balloon is deflated after bleeding has subsided and the catheter then is taped in place. A smaller size urethral catheter is inserted sometimes after the removal of the suprapubic drain, this lessens the possibility of vesical neck contracture

Distention is controlled by poultices, enemas, early ambulation and a rapidly progressed diet

Ace bandages are used prophylactically postoperatively on all patients with evident peripheral circulatory deficiency

Complications

Shock and hemorrhage
Pneumonia
Bladder spasms
Urinary suppression—an unusual complication
Hiccoughs
Abdominal distention
Wound infections
Thrombophlebitis
Epididymitis
Cardiovascular accident
Myocardial infarction
Bacteremia

Nursing Care

There are special points to be considered in the nursing care of the patient who has had a prostatectomy and who is in the older age group.

PSYCHOLOGICAL ASPECTS

The self concept which affects this patient's adjustment to illness and to future rehabilitation is closely allied to cultural attitudes toward old age; i.e., the tendency to reject the evidences of advancing age, the rejection of the older person in the family and the community. Sudden illness further jeopardizes already diminished self-respect and self-reliance. The patient becomes preoccupied with fears of death and/or permanent disability.

Since the prostate is a secondary sex gland, disease of the prostate or surgery on the prostate have a strong psychosexual component which may affect the patient's mental health. Elderly males often are very concerned about their sexual function and feel threatened with the loss of virility and maleness. In view of the already weakened role which the patient sees himself as playing, this prospect may precipitate depression and helplessness. The patient's fears often are substantiated in that the vas ligation performed with all open surgery on the prostate does result in sterility. However, interference with potency is variable.

The nurse's recognition of the above factors is essential if she is to give intelligent emotional support. Her responsibility for rehabilitation of the patient requires knowledge of community resources which may be utilized in helping the patient to resolve the physical and emotional problems of surgery.

PHYSICAL CARE

See under Nursing Care of the Urologic Patient, p. 320.

TEACHING NEEDS

Careful instructions must be given to each patient concerning

How to get out of bed with gravity drainage setup

How to pin tubing properly when getting back into bed to prevent traction on tubing

Necessity for keeping gravity bottle below the level of the bladder when up and to keep tubing unkinked

Many patients experience difficulty controlling voiding after the removal of their urethral catheter. They have lost some bladder and sphincter tone due to the prolonged catheter drainage, and also notice the absence of the desire to void. The patient is embarrassed to find that he wets when he stands or walks, and can only void in small amounts. In most cases, sensation and control develop quickly. With other patients, it may be a long rehabilitative process requiring muscle training exercises for the perineal and the sphincter muscles. The patient must be encouraged to take the responsibility for this process and, at the same time, be given evidence that the nurse is aware of his feelings about the incontinence and does not find him unacceptable.

Part 7. Cancer

CONCEPTS OF CANCER (CARCINOMA)

Cancer, a major health problem in the United States, causes more than 265,000 deaths per year with about 785,000 under medical care. Fortunately, the outlook for the control of cancer is more promising today than it has been in the past. The medical profession is better equipped to fight it with improved technics in surgery and in the use of radium and x-rays.

The physician and the public are better informed on the need for early diagnosis. That this organized movement to control cancer is producing results daily is evident from the fact that among women especially the cancer death rate has taken a definite downward trend in recent years. An increasing number of people are taking cancer education seriously and are consulting their physicians for the prompt investigation of signs and symptoms that they have learned to suspect as danger signals. Consequently, physicians now have an opportunity to make a contribution of the highest value in preventive medicine by giving such patients the thorough, careful examination which will lead to the detection of early cancer when the chances of cure are best, or to reassurance if cancer is not present.

One of the most recent developments for furthering the early detection of malignant growths is the cytologic test for cancer better known as the Papanicolaou smear test. The smear technic is based on the fact that exfoliated tumor cells may be detected by examination of the secretion of the area in question, as in the case of uterine or vaginal secretion. However, the test should not be considered as a method of final diagnosis. A confirming diagnosis always should be made by biopsy or curettage.

The value of the smear test lies in the fact that it is often possible to make a diagnosis in the incipient stages of disease even before a lesion which can be biopsied is clinically evident.

Danger Signals of Cancer

A painless lump or thickening, especially in the breast, the lip or the tongue

Irregular or unexplained bleeding or discharge from the vagina or breast, especially the nipple

A wound that does not heal, particularly about the tongue, the mouth or the lips

Progressive change in the color or the size of a mole, a wart or a birthmark

Persistent and unexplained indigestion

Any persistent change in normal bowel habits

Blood or bloody mucus in the urine or the stools

Persistent hoarseness, unexplained cough or difficulty in swallowing

Prophylaxis Against Cancer

Careful oral hygiene involving the care of the teeth, repair of cavities, removal of decayed teeth, correction of ill-fitting dentures and other similar measures. Avoidance of undue irritation to the mouth or tongue by excessive use of tobacco or other substances that cause local irritation.

Care of the skin to see that it is kept clean and is not abused by too prolonged or too intense exposure to the direct rays of the sun or to violent changes in temperature or to irritation of the weather. Awareness of abnormal growth of any sort on any part of the body surface.

Tight clothing which compresses or constricts the breast, thus interfering with circulation, must be avoided. Properly supporting brassières should be worn at all times.

All injuries received during childbirth should be repaired at once. The use of metal or other hard pessaries, as well as the persistent use of irritating douches should be avoided.

Food that causes distress or indigestion should be

avoided. Abuse of the gastrointestinal tract may cause abnormal growth of tissue.

Regular bowel habits should be established. The irritating effects of constipation and resulting sluggishness of various related bodily functions can be eliminated.

Since there is some evidence in recent studies that there may be a relationship between tobacco and the incidence of lung cancer, it would seem wise to moderate smoking habits.

Summary

Cancer can be prevented sometimes by correcting possible precancerous conditions early.

Most types of cancer are curable in the early stages. Survival of the patient depends on early diagnosis and prompt treatment by experienced physicians.

Cancer can be detected early, even in many organs that cannot be seen, through modern diagnosis aids.

Cancer must be checked, destroyed or removed through the use of surgery, x-rays and radium, singly or in combination. No drug or ointment will cure cancer.

Successful treatment depends above all upon the patient's presenting himself early, while the cancer is still in such a stage that it can be removed completely.

NURSING CARE OF THE PATIENT WITH CANCER

The general care of the cancer patient is of prime importance. There is much that can be done for the comfort and well-being of the patient besides the removal, the destruction or the retardation of the malignant growth. All hygienic, nutritional and medicinal measures should be adopted that will improve his health and reinforce his powers of resistance.

Following the treatment of the lesion by surgery or irradiation the patient requires medical care, regardless of whether the results have been curative or merely palliative. An attitude of encouragement and hopefulness on the part of the nurse is most important. Sunlight and activity in the open air to the extent of tolerance without fatigue are very beneficial. The diet can be adjusted to meet individual needs for the maintenance of the best possible nutrition with considerable improvements in the patient's general condition. Anemia often can be lessened by appropriate measures directed against its particular cause. Transfusions of blood are desirable in many cases and often give immediate improvement.

The use of drugs for the relief of symptoms is of great importance. Few cancer patients require large doses of narcotics, provided that they receive proper medical and nursing care.

Treatment of complications should be instituted whenever necessary. The proper functioning of heart, lungs, kidneys and other organs is as vital to the cancer patient as to any other.

Much can be done to enhance the sense of well-being and to maintain the morale of the cancer patient by "caring for" the patient.

The care of cancer patients in the home is being recognized as a desirable possibility; not only during the terminal stages of the disease, but also during periods of convalescence or of temporary discharge from the hospital between intervals of treatment. The public health nurse renders a most valuable service in the supervision of the care of these patients.

Since early treatment is essential for recovery, the nurse must assume responsibility for case-finding by,

Encouraging people with evidence of any of the danger signals to seek consultation of physician

Helping the person who has cancer (especially if successfully treated) to recognize the need for continuous medical supervision as well as to know the danger signals indicating need for further treatment.

The nurse must be prepared to be a "good listener" and to evidence empathy as she helps the patient and his family accept the illness, the plan for care and the resultant changes which some therapy causes.

CANCER OF THE SKIN

Cancer of the skin usually occurs on exposed portions of the body, such as the head, the face, the neck or the hands—sites where the skin is subjected most frequently to the effects of chronic irritation, injury, sunlight, chemical agents, etc. These regions of the body are accessible to observation, and thus early diagnosis is possible.

There are many forms of cancer of the skin; but 3 of them are common enough to give here.

The *basal-cell epithelioma* is only slightly malignant. It practically never travels to another part of the body by veins or lymphatics but progresses locally through tissues in its path, even through bone. It is found most commonly on the face in persons beyond the age of 40. It is particularly frequent on the nose and about the eyes and the ears.

In some cases the person may notice a thickened horny area of skin or a wart. Suddenly he becomes aware that this is increasing in extent and thickness. In other cases a scale or scab is noted, which falls off, revealing a minute raw area beneath. Over this a larger scab then forms and thus the raw area extends.

Radium treatment is most successful when the patient is seen at this stage. If no treatment is given and the growth is allowed to continue unchecked, a rodent ulcer forms and spreads to such an extent as to necessitate the removal of an eye or a portion of the nostril or the ear.

In other cases *an old scar may be the base of another type of skin cancer*. The first sign here also is a scaling or scabbing or a warty excrescence. This type is much more serious, as it travels to the lymph nodes early and, unless radical treatment is given, will extend and involve vital organs at a distance.

A third frequent type of cancer of the skin is far more insidious and more malignant, *melanoma*. A bluish-black or dark-brown mole or a hairy mole or a deeply colored wart may be present all one's life on any part of the body. Suddenly, at any age, there may be a change in size or in elevation above the skin, or in color, or there may be the appearance of such a lesion where one never was noted before. This is evidence that activity is going on, and immediate, thorough treatment should be given as the process often is one of rapid metastasis by both lymphatics and blood vessels to vital parts. Operation on these moles or warts does not cause them to spread, as is suggested sometimes. It is wise to find out the advisability of having such dark-colored lesions removed before there is any sign that a malignant change has begun.

CANCER OF THE BREAST

The breast is one of the most common sites of cancer in women.

Signs and Symptoms

Any lump in the breast with or without pain
Alteration in the shape of the breast
Dimpling of the skin of the breast
Retraction of the nipple
Bleeding or discharge from the nipple
Ulceration of the skin of the breast

Treatment

Surgery is required in almost all cases.

Early diagnosis is essential.

Any suspicious breast nodule must be biopsied, before a definitive diagnosis can be made. If the diagnosis is carcinoma, then choice of radical mastectomy, simple mastectomy or radiotherapy must be made in accord with the surgeon's estimate of the extent of the disease. The estimate can be made more accurate by x-ray examination of the lungs and skeletal system and by biopsy of one or more key lymph nodes in the lymphatic drainage system.

The patient should be prepared preoperatively so that if a radical mastectomy (removal of the entire breast, lymph node bearing tissue of axilla and pectoralis major and minor muscles, usually followed by a dermatone skin graft) is undertaken, the extent of the procedure and the necessity for doing so may be understood by the patient.

Specific Care

Recognition of patient's
Fear of cancer itself

Fear of recurrence of cancer

Concern about the disfiguring effects of surgery

Posturing of patient in bed to provide adequate support to shoulder and arm on affected side

Reassure patient if she becomes apprehensive because of difficulty in breathing due to the compression bandage

Teach the patient to use her arm of the affected side in order that a full range of motion can be achieved following the enforced period of inactivity; recognition of the role that many household activities play in providing adequate exercise of arm

Guide patient in the selection of a proper breast prosthesis.

See Preoperative and Postoperative Care, pp. 175-184.

Most important: Teach women the technic of self-examination of breasts at regular monthly intervals to assist with the early diagnosis of cancer of breast.

CANCER OF THE UTERUS

The two cardinal symptoms of cancer of the uterus are persistent vaginal discharge and abnormal bleeding. In cancer of the cervix, the symptoms vary according to the stage of the disease. A discharge or spotting between periods is usually one of the first signs noticed by the patient.

Frequently, there is only a slight watery or yellow-tinged discharge. In other cases with ulceration of the growth, noticeable bleeding may be an early symptom.

The discharge or bleeding at first may be intermittent, frequently occurring after a bowel movement or some form of exertion. Later, it becomes persistent and progressively more severe.

In cancer of the fundus, the same symptoms are present but usually do not appear until about the time of the menopause or later.

Pain commonly does not occur until the disease is well advanced, at which time there are also complaints referable to the bladder and the rectum, as well as fever, weight loss, etc.

Cancer of the uterus can be treated effectively only

by surgery, x-rays, radium or radioactive isotopes, either alone or in combination. The form of treatment selected in any given cancer depends upon the location, the duration, the type, the rapidity of growth of the tumor and the extent of its dissemination.

Early examination by a competent physician is vitally important when any of the danger signals appear.

CANCER OF THE LUNG

Cancer of the lung recently has become the most common primary tumor in men. Metastatic cancer of the lung from a primary tumor elsewhere is a frequent preterminal or terminal event.

Signs and Symptoms

Cough
Chest pain
Hemoptysis
Weakness, weight loss
Hoarseness (upper left lobe)
Pain in shoulder (pulmonary apex)
Pleural effusion
Evidence of plugged bronchus such as
    Atelectasis
    Unresolved pneumonia
    Lung abscess
    Shadow on x-ray picture

Treatment

Removal of lung (pneumonectomy) or a segment of the lung including regional lymphatics

If widespread disease precludes excision, radiotherapy may be of value in palliation

See Care of Patient with Thoracic Surgery, p. 231.

CANCER OF THE LARGE BOWEL

Next to the stomach, the most common site for malignant disease is the gastrointestinal tract.

Signs and Symptoms

These vary widely in different cases.

Blood in the stools
Irregularity of bowel habits
Pain: a later stage
Excessive loss of weight or strength—late in course
of disease
Anemia

Diagnostic Measures

Digital examination
Proctoscopy and biopsy
Barium enema
Stool for guaiac

Treatment

Operations usually are performed to remove tumor and surrounding tissues. The best prognosis occurs when operation is performed before invasion of surrounding tissues and lymphatics by tumor cells.

Specific Preoperative Care

Psychological preparation of patient—particularly where a temporary or a permanent colostomy is anticipated.

Correction of existing anemia

Thorough cleansing of large bowel by colonic irrigations, cleansing enemas and purges

Antibiotics to reduce intestinal flora (*See discussion in* Pharmacology)

Insertion of Foley catheter and ureteral catheters if surgical trauma to urinary systems is likely

Insertion of Miller-Abbott tube prior to surgery if proximal half of colon is to be removed

Specific Postoperative Care

Observation for signs of shock or hemorrhage.

Measurement of intake and output; this is of special importance.

Antibiotic therapy (*See discussion in* Pharmacology)

Colostomy care, if present:

Prevent contamination of abdominal wound from colostomy drainage; usually by sealing with waterproof material.

Open colostomy, usually within first or second day postoperative.

Irrigate colostomy daily after colostomy has been opened.

Teach patient the management of his colostomy.

Offer considerable reassurance and support in helping patient to accept his colostomy.

Perineal wound care, if abdominoperineal resection has been performed

Frequent inspection in early postoperative period to detect abnormal bleeding.

Watch for late hemorrhage after perineal packing is removed.

Sitz baths or perineal irrigations to keep perineal wound clean after packing has been removed.

Care of patient with gastric suction, if present (*See discussion in* Technics).

Care of patient with Foley catheter, if present (*See discussion in* Technics).

See Preoperative and Postoperative Care, pp. 175-184.

CANCER OF THE STOMACH

The most common site of malignancy in the gastrointestinal tract is the stomach. Men are affected 3 times as often as women. The majority of persons affected are between the ages of 40 and 60 years.

Signs and Symptoms

These are variable and often indefinite.

Pain, usually present, may have highly variable pattern

Feeling of fullness or discomfort after eating

Vomiting, usually indicates obstruction

Bleeding, gross or occult, in gastrointestinal tract

Loss of appetite and weight, frequently associated with advanced disease

Mass, infrequently felt in early stages, in upper part of abdomen

Presence of anemia

Diminution of gastric acidity

MEDICAL AND SURGICAL

Diagnosis
Patient's history
Gastrointestinal series
Gastric analysis
Gastroscopy

Treatment
Curative surgery—where there is no gross evidence of the disease beyond the stomach, the lymph nodes and the adjacent resectable organs

Gastrectomy (total or subtotal) and removal of lymphatic drainage areas where possible

Palliative surgery—where there is gross evidence of widely disseminated disease

The tumor is removed for relief of distressing symptoms of obstruction, bleeding, etc.

See Preoperative and Postoperative Care of Patient with Gastric Surgery, *under discussion of* Peptic Ulcer, p. 212.

CANCER OF THE LARYNX

CARE OF PATIENT WITH A LARYNGECTOMY

Laryngectomy is the surgical removal of the larynx, usually done for cancer of the larynx.

Specific Preoperative Nursing Care
Be sure that the patient understands about the operation.

Tell patient that he will go to the recovery room (if the hospital has one).

Arrange for a speech therapist to see the patient before the operation.

If possible, have the patient see an "old laryngectomy" patient who has done well and has learned to speak.

Specific Postoperative Nursing Care
Place patient in a semisitting position
Do not leave patient alone during acute period
Diet—nothing by mouth for about 5 to 7 days. Patient

is fed either by a nasogastric tube or by intravenous route. After 5 to 7 days, the diet progresses from clear fluids to regular food.

Antibiotic therapy (*See discussion in* Pharmacology)

Keep mouth clean (*See discussion in* Technics)

Suction p.r.n.

Clean inner tube p.r.n.

Moist saline compresses over opening p.r.n.

Be sure that tape is threaded through tube and tied securely in a square knot at back of neck so that tube cannot be coughed out.

As soon as possible, teach patient to suction himself and to clean inner tube.

Teach patient how to clean tube, sterilize it, thread with tape and (after doctor has shown patient) supervise him in changing tube.

See that patient has appointment for speech therapy.

Special Equipment Necessary for Care of Patient

Suction machine at bedside with No. 16 whistle-tip catheter

Tray containing solution cup with 5 per cent Sodium Bicarbonate Solution, gauze wipes and thumb forceps at bedside for cleaning tube

Paper and pencil for patient to use in communicating with others

Duplicate sterile laryngectomy tube should be readily available at all times

Part 8. Ophthalmic Disorders

CONDITIONS OF THE LIDS

HORDEOLUM (STYE)

A stye is an inflammation in the small glands of the lid, caused by infection with *Staphylococcus aureus* resulting in an abscess formation.

Treatment

Hot compresses; antibiotic ointment; incision when pointing.

CHALAZION

A noninflammatory, painless swelling due to a chronic infection of one of the meibomian glands. The granuloma which forms is small, round, tensely elastic and grows over a period of weeks or months.

Treatment

Incision and curettage.

BLEPHARITIS

Blepharitis is an infection of the lid margins, usually caused by a staphylococcal organism.

Treatment

Silver nitrate ½ per cent applied to lid margins with swab and irrigated off; antibiotic ointment; Staphylococcus toxoid given subcutaneously in small doses.

ECTROPION

Ectropion is a rolling out of the lower lid—lids fail to close completely. It appears in old age or after injury.

Treatment

Cautery, surgery.

ENTROPION

Entropion is a rolling in of the lower lid. The cilia irritate the eye.

Treatment

Cautery, surgery.

PTOSIS

Ptosis is a drooping of the upper lid. Usually it is due to a failure of the levator muscle but sometimes is due to scar tissue, tumor, myogenic factors (muscular dystrophy, myasthenia gravis), or neurogenic factors (paralytic). It may be congenital or acquired.

Treatment

Surgery or medication for disease process, e.g., neostigmine for myasthenia gravis.

CONDITION OF THE LACRIMAL APPARATUS

DACRYOCYSTITIS

Dacryocystitis is infection in the lacrimal sac and secondary to obstruction of the nasolacrimal duct.

Treatment

Warm compresses, systemic antibiotic therapy; probing and irrigation of duct; surgery to create new passage (dacryocystectomy, dacryocystorhinostomy).

CONDITIONS OF THE ORBIT

CELLULITIS

Cellulitis is usually caused by pneumococci, streptococci or staphylococci, entering the orbit directly or extending from sinuses, styes, or other sources of infection. It may localize and subside spontaneously or it may extend posteriorly causing cavernous sinus thrombosis, meningitis or brain abscess.

Treatment

Hospitalization; hot compresses; chemotherapy; antibiotic ointment locally.

EXOPHTHALMOS

Exophthalmos (proptosis) is a protrusion of the eyeball forward out of the socket. Results may be drying of the cornea, corneal ulcers, and double vision. May be unilateral or bilateral. Causes: (unilateral) inflammation, tumor, trauma, cyts; (bilateral) endocrine diseases, Grave's disease, high myopia.

Treatment

Protect eyeball from drying; attempt to remove the cause; surgery.

CONDITIONS OF THE CONJUNCTIVA

CONJUNCTIVITIS ("Pink Eye")

Conjunctivitis (infection of the conjunctiva) can be due to many causes—pneumococcus, influenza bacillus, staphylococcus, gonococcus, virus, simple allergy, mechanical irritations, vitamin deficiencies, fungus infection, chemical injury.

Symptoms

Redness; discharge; photophobia; lacrimation; and edema.

Treatment

It is important to take cultures, smears and scrapings to determine the organism. This will influence the decision regarding treatment. Treatment: antibiotic drops and ointment—sulfonamides, cortisone and other steroids; saline irrigations to conjunctival sac; cold compresses; prevention of spread of infection.

OPHTHALMIA NEONATORUM

Ophthalmia neonatorum, conjunctivitis of the newborn, is caused by gonococcus or other organisms. The aim should be to prevent the disease by the use of silver nitrate or penicillin drops prophylactically in the eyes of the newborn child.

Treatment

Prompt hospital treatment with chemotherapy; frequent irrigations; protect unaffected eye.

TRACHOMA

Trachoma is an acute or chronic infectious disease of the eyes, that, when untreated or treated poorly, often leads to blindness. It is caused by a virus that usually responds to sulfonamide therapy.

PHLYCTENULAR KERATOCONJUNCTIVITIS

Phlyctenular keratoconjunctivitis is found among people with poor living conditions, malnutrition, tuberculosis or both.

Treatment

Hydrocortisone, diet and underlying disease therapy.

PTERYGIUM

Pterygium is an abnormal conjunctival growth at the inner canthus which grows across the cornea and can compromise vision if it continues across the pupil. The cause is unknown, but it is thought to be an irritative reaction to dust or wind.

Treatment

Surgical excision.

SUBCONJUNCTIVAL HEMORRHAGE

Subconjunctival hemorrhage is recognized by the diffuse, brilliant red color under the conjunctiva. It is terrifying in appearance and has no symptoms. It is caused by injury or occurs as a result of spontaneous rupture of capillary.

Treatment

None. It will absorb in 1 to 2 weeks; avoid heat.

FOREIGN BODIES

For removal of foreign bodies on the conjunctiva, *See discussion in* Technics.

CONDITIONS OF THE CORNEA

FOREIGN BODIES ON THE CORNEA

The nurse may attempt to remove a foreign body from the cornea by gentle irrigation with normal saline solution. If the foreign body is not removed readily in this manner, the patient should be referred to an ophthalmologist. When the foreign body is embedded in the cornea, the doctor uses a local anesthetic, a staining agent such as sterile fluorescein, and a sharp metal instrument (spud) to lift the object off the cornea. An antibiotic ointment is instilled into the conjunctival sac, and a firm patch is applied for 24 hours to allow the cornea to heal.

ULCER

This is a break in the surface of the cornea and, when untreated, may cover the entire surface of the cornea, causing blindness, or may penetrate into the anterior chamber causing endophthalmitis or panophthalmitis with loss of the eye. Ulcers may be caused by bacteria, viruses, fungi, allergy, exposure, 5th-nerve lesions, or vitamin deficiency.

Treatment

Local chemotherapy applied in the form of ointments or drops. Hot compresses. Atropine (0.5% to 1%) to keep the pupil dilated and reduce the pain in the eye. A firm patch is applied to prevent the friction of the lid against the cornea. Corneal grafting is the surgical therapy.

KERATITIS

Keratitis is an inflammation of the structures of the cornea. It may be caused by corneal ulcer, syphilis or tuberculosis.

Treatment

Atropine drops to dilate the pupil and rest eye; cortisone and hot compresses to relieve discomfort.

SYMBLEPHARON

Symblepharon are adhesions of the lids to the cornea or the conjunctiva following severe burns.

KERATOCONUS

Keratoconus is a progressive bulging forward of the

central part of the cornea, occurring often in late 'teens and the early twenties. It is treated by contact lenses or corneal transplant.

CONDITIONS OF THE UVEAL TRACT

UVEITIS

Uveitis is an inflammation of any part of the uveal tract, the vascular coat of the eye.

Iritis—iris
Cyclitis—ciliary body
Choroiditis—choroid

Symptoms

Pain, photophobia, lacrimation, blurred vision, eye injected, cornea cloudy, pupil small and fixed, vitreous cloudy

Etiology

Trauma, known infection, unknown infection (probable systemic infection)

Treatment

Complete medical investigation, hot compresses, dilatation of pupil, chemotherapy, fever therapy, treatment of underlying disease.

Complications

Secondary glaucoma, an increased tension in the eye, cataract.

SYMPATHETIC OPHTHALMIA

Sympathetic ophthalmia is a bilateral inflammation of the entire uveal tract almost invariably caused by a perforating wound that involves uveal tissue. The disease is insidious and usually progresses to blindness, unless the injured eye, which is called the *exciting eye,* is removed before the disease gets well under way in the other eye, which is called the *sympathizing* eye. Usually, it can be prevented by enucleation of exciting eye within 2 weeks after injury.

MEDICAL AND SURGICAL

TUMORS

Benign tumors may occur in almost any eye tissue. The 2 most common malignant tumors are malignant melanoma of the choroid in adults, and retinoblastoma in children, which is hereditary.

Treatment

Benign tumor—careful observation

Malignant melanoma—immediate enucleation of the affected eye, if choroid

Retinoblastoma—immediate enucleation of the affected eye. If both eyes are affected, immediate enucleation of the one in which the tumor is more advanced and radiotherapy to the remaining eye. The systemic use of nitrogen mustards has been successful also.

CONDITIONS OF THE RETINA

RETINITIS

The causes of retinitis may be diabetic, hypertensive, arteriosclerotic, renal.

Treatment

Treatment is directed toward clearing up the medical conditions.

RETINITIS PIGMENTOSA

Retinitis pigmentosa is an extensive bilateral, genetically determined degenerative process. Usually, it leads to complete blindness by middle age from retinal degeneration, migration of pigment into retina, sclerosis of vessels and atrophy of optic nerve.

DETACHMENT OF RETINA

Detachment of retina most frequently is due to trauma. Other reasons are retinal cysts, neoplasm and infection, with about 10 per cent showing no demonstrable cause. High myopia is a predisposing factor. Symptoms: "black spots," and "lightning flashes," blurred vision, loss of part of visual field.

Treatment

Cautery with electric diathermy; scleral resection; vitreous implant; silicone implant, photocoagulation therapy.

RETROLENTAL FIBROPLASIA

Bilateral retinal disease of premature infants which can lead to total blindness. Caused by excessive oxygen use in incubators, stimulating uncontrolled growth of retinal tissue and leading to vascular dilatation and retinal detachment.

Treatment

Preventive, in control of oxygen content in incubators. If recognized rapidly, it may be arrested by discontinuation of oxygen.

RETINOBLASTOMA

For discussion of retinoblastoma, see under Tumors, p. 346.

CONDITIONS OF THE OPTIC NERVE
OPTIC NEURITIS

Optic neuritis denotes inflammation, degeneration or demyelinization of the optic nerve. The cardinal symptom is loss of vision, usually marked. There may be pain in eye region. A variety of diseases can cause this: sinusitis, meningitis, diabetes, viral or bacterial infections, multiple sclerosis, chemical poisoning, etc.

Treatment

Treat the underlying cause, if possible. Systemic cortisone may be helpful for many causes.

OPTIC ATROPHY

Optic atrophy is caused by the death of the nerve fibers. It may be a result of severe neuritis caused by syphilis, wood alcohol or glaucoma.

PAPILLEDEMA

Papilledema is a choked disk, caused by increased intracranial pressure.

CATARACT

Cataract is an opacification of the lens of the eye. The only treatment is the removal of the lens.

Classification on the Basis of Etiology

Senile
Due to diseases such as diabetes, uveitis or glaucoma
Due to trauma, either an intra-ocular foreign body or contusion
Due to radiation—x-rays, radium, ultraviolet, etc.
Due to heat
Congenital

Symptoms

Diminished vision in one or both eyes
Diminished vision in some quadrants
White pupil, due to opacity

Operations for Cataract

Extracapsular extraction—lens nucleus removed with as much cortex as possible
Intracapsular extraction—lens removed in its capsule
Discission (needling)—for congenital cataract, where lens material is more fluid and may be absorbed after being disturbed by knife or needle.

APHAKIA

Aphakia is the state of the eye after the lens has been removed.

The Patient with Aphakia

Strong lenses are necessary for normal vision.
Although vision may be 20/20, the appearance of objects is not the same as with the normal eye. There is need of re-education.

GLAUCOMA

In this insidious disease there is a rise in intra-ocular tension in the eyeball. There is a gradual loss of peripheral vision until total blindness is reached, if untreated. Normal tension is 15 to 24 mm. Hg as measured by the Schiøtz tonometer.

Glaucoma is one of the most frequent causes of blindness.

Symptoms

The symptoms vary from almost none to the following in various combinations: insidious visual loss with "tunnel vision" (central vision intact, peripheral vision lost), halos around lights, increased intra-ocular pressure, redness of eye (ciliary injection), severe eye pain, nausea and vomiting, fixed, moderately dilated pupil.

Treatment

MEDICAL

The instillation of miotics to contract the pupil and to improve the flow of aqueous solution into the Canal of Schlemm. Miotics used are pilocarpine (1 to 4%), eserine (physostigmine) (0.2 to 0.5%), D.F.P. (diisopropyl fluorophosphate).

Sedatives, morphine and antiemetics may be necessary. Diamox (acetazolamide) has been used in conjunction with miotics to control and decrease intra-ocular tension by depressing aqueous production.

SURGICAL

A number of surgical procedures are used for this disease to increase the filtering process of aqueous from the eye and to reduce intra-ocular pressure (iridectomy, iridencleisis, trephine and cyclodialysis).

CONDITIONS OF THE EXTRAOCULAR MUSCLES

STRABISMUS

Strabismus (squint) is a deviation of the eyes from their normal position.

Phoria is a tendency to deviate.

MEDICAL AND SURGICAL

Tropia is an actual deviation.

Convergent strabismus—esophoria, esotropia

Divergent strabismus—exophoria, exotropia

Vertical strabismus—hyperphoria, hypertropia, hypophoria, hypotropia

Treatment

Glasses, exercises (orthoptics), "patching" (occlusion) of a nondeviating eye to force use of weaker one, surgery. Treatment should begin as soon as strabismus is noted. Children do not "outgrow crossed eyes."

AMBLYOPIA EXANOPSIA

Amblyopia exanopsia is blindness due to nonuse of the eye. This occurs in some cases of untreated strabismus. Therefore, it is important to have the condition treated early.

REFRACTION OF THE EYE

In ophthalmology, the term *refraction* refers to the testing of the optical state of the eyes and the correction of visual defects by means of lenses.

Refraction may be done with cycloplegic drugs or without their use (manifest refraction).

"Accommodation" is the adjustment of the eye for vision at various distances, accomplished by the changing shape of the lens by the action of the ciliary muscle to focus a clear image on the retina. It accompanies the act of convergence.

Emmetropia is the term used for normal sight.

Errors of refraction include.

Hyperopia (hypermetropia, farsightedness). Vision is blurred because parallel rays of light are brought to a focus behind the retina. The eyeball is short. Distant vision is better than near vision. Correct with glasses (convex or "plus" lenses).

Myopia (nearsightedness, shortsightedness). Vision is blurred because light is brought to a focus in front of the retina. Eyeball is long. Near vision is better than distant vision. Correct with glasses (concave or "minus" lenses).

Astigmatism. A condition in which there is a difference in the degree of refraction in different meridians of the cornea. Everything appears to be somewhat distorted. Correct with glasses (cylindrical lenses to restore a spherical effect).

Presbyopia (old sight). This normal change occurs about the 5th decade of life as a result of which the so-called near point recedes beyond the distance at which we ordinarily read (about 14 in.).

This is caused by the loss of elasticity of the lens of the eye, as a result of which the eye cannot accommodate as well as in youth. Corrected with plus lenses.

Aniseikonia. A difference between the size and the shape of the 2 eyes, resulting in headache, nausea, etc. Corrected with special lenses.

INJURIES TO THE EYE

FOREIGN BODIES

Foreign bodies in the globe and the orbit. These may be metal, glass, wood, stone, etc. Conclusive diagnosis is made by the use of a special localizing x-ray apparatus.

Treatment

If the substance is magnetic, it may be removed by use of a magnet. Nonmagnetic materials must be removed surgically. The treatment should be prompt in order to avoid infection.

See also Foreign Bodies on the Conjunctiva, in Technics, *and* Foreign Bodies on the Cornea, above.

PERFORATING WOUNDS OF THE GLOBE

These may involve the cornea, the sclera, the iris or the ciliary body and are treated surgically. If the ciliary body is injured, there is danger of sympathetic ophthalmia. The injured eye must be enucleated promptly or treated conservatively with chemotherapy and watched carefully at regular intervals.

BURNS

These may be caused by hot liquids, steam, tear gas, lime, molten metals or chemicals. Frequently, both the conjunctiva and the cornea are burned.

Treatment

Burns require immediate treatment. The conjunctival sac should be washed out immediately with large quantities of water, in order to dilute and remove quickly the caustic substance. Then, after instillation of a local anesthetic and staining agent such as sterile fluorescein, the solid particles, if any, are removed with spuds or sharp instruments by the doctor. Following removal of the foreign body, antibiotic ointment is instilled frequently, and usually the eye is bandaged to prevent further injury. Mydriatics afford eye rest and help to prevent adhesions. Systemic sedation or pain medication may be necessary.

GENERAL PRINCIPLES OF OPHTHALMOLOGIC NURSING

The nurse must gain the confidence of the patient.

The nurse must understand and practice the correct psychological approach to patients with reduced vision.

All her movements, in caring for the eye, must be deliberate, gentle and deft. Her hands must be well cared for with nails not too long.

The nurse must always make herself known to the patient and keep her voice quiet and cheerful.

A patient with both eyes covered must not be left alone for long periods, as this may result in depression and disorientation.

It is the responsibility of the nurse in caring for the newly blind patient to teach and encourage him to be independent as soon as possible.

Diversional therapy is very important to patients with reduced vision.

SELF-HELP AIDS TO BE TAUGHT TO THE EYE PATIENT AND HIS FAMILY

EATING

Posture

Keep arms off the table.

Sit up straight.

Raise food to the mouth—never lower the mouth to food.

Do not try to hurry through a meal.

Have a large table napkin.

Table Setting

1. Table should be set with utensils in the same place at every meal. In Diagram I, A is the bread-and-butter plate (at 11 o'clock); B is the salad or vegetable plate (at 12 o'clock); C is the beverage (at 1 o'clock).

When first sitting down, inconspicuously check that tray, plate, etc., are all in proper place.

2. In the beginning, food should be placed on plate according to the face of the clock (Diagram II).

A. This may be discontinued later.

B. Briefly describe food on his plate to patient at

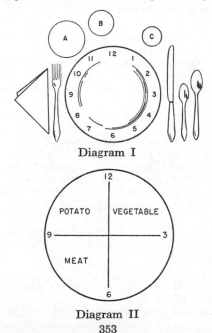

Diagram I

Diagram II

MEDICAL AND SURGICAL

each meal, and in the beginning point out its location (i.e., vegetable is in the 12 to 3 position).

3. At each meal, the patient should be given the same seat at the table, if possible. This helps in orienting the patient to the location of sugar, salt, creamer, etc.

General Hints to Eating

1. A small piece of bread should be used for a pusher.

2. The fork should be used occasionally to push food away from edge of plate toward the center, to prevent its falling off the plate.

3. Continue use of the same utensils as previously; use spoon only when correct.

4. *Never* use fingers to eat foods that should be handled with utensils.

Special Eating Problems

1. Cutting meat
   A. Use Continental method
      a. Knife in right hand, fork in feft
      b. Fork is not transferred to right hand before putting food to mouth
   B. Outline meat by slight tap with fork around edge
   C. Turn prongs of fork down, placing forefinger on back of fork
   D. Place fork near edge of meat
   E. Cut behind prongs
   F. When one large bone is in meat or fish
      a. Locate it by means of light tap of knife
      b. Remove bone by cutting gently around it
      c. Deposit bone on edge of plate

2. Soup
   A. After filling spoon, tilt slightly over bowl
   B. Scrape against opposite rim of bowl and raise to mouth

3. Lettuce
   A. Cut lettuce with salad fork or knife, as with a piece of pie
   B. May ask for salad to be served shredded

4. Fried Chicken

    A. Informal—may pick up bones after big pieces of meat are cut away

    B. Formal—ask for parts of chicken with least bones

5. Potato in Jacket

    A. Use sharp knife to cut, or

    B. Hollow out with fork, placing hand on jacket to hold potato

6. Pie

    A. Flaky—cut with side of fork

    B. Juicy—may be eaten with spoon (Continental style)

7. Preserved Fruits with Pits

    A. Eat juice first

    B. With teaspoon, remove pit or stone before eating fruit

Restaurant Eating

1. Have companion or waiter read menu.

2. Choose easy-to-manage foods, if possible.

3. It is permissible to ask for certain cuts of meat, shredded salads, etc.

FACTORS TO CONSIDER IN HYGIENE OF THE EYES

Health of parents: venereal disease education
Use of prophylactic drops in the eyes at birth
Congenital defects
Muscle anomalies in children
Eye examinations during preschool and school years
Attention to reading habits
Proper illumination
Chlorination of swimming pools
Care in handling conjunctivitis
Foreign bodies
Glaucoma
Cataract
Cancer of the eye—in infancy and in adult life

Part 9. Endocrine Disorders

DIABETES MELLITUS

Definition

Diabetes mellitus is a metabolic disease of the pancreas in which there seems to be a deficiency in the production of insulin in the islands of Langerhans cells, although the function of the islands of Langerhans is related closely to the whole endocrine system. There is an increase in the concentration of sugar in the blood (hyperglycemia) with the consequent secretion of excess sugar in the urine (glycosuria). With this disorder of carbohydrate metabolism, disturbances of protein and fat metabolism are associated frequently with a resulting ketosis.

Etiology

The cause of diabetes mellitus is unknown.

Factors

Obesity is one of the most important factors, especially in people over 40 years of age. Overeating and a large carbohydrate intake are predisposing causes.

RACE. Jews are more susceptible to the disease than other people.

SEX. Men are more subject to the disease than women.

EXERCISE. Lack of exercise leads to obesity and, therefore, is a factor.

INFECTIONS. Acute infections often are followed by a temporary or permanent low carbohydrate tolerance.

FAMILIAL TENDENCIES. About 50 per cent of diabetics show a family history of the disease.

EMOTIONAL DISTURBANCES. Overactivity of the suprarenal, the thyroid and the pituitary (anterior lobe) glands, caused by fear and worry, as well as mental fatigue and mechanical trauma of the floor of the fourth ventricle of the brain, produce a glycosuria that usually is temporary.

Physiology

Hormone secreted in the islands of Langerhans cells in the pancreas is called *insulin*. Insulin is secreted by the normal pancreas at a fairly uniform rate and is increased after ingestion of carbohydrate. It oxidizes sugar and is able also to convert sugar into glycogen which is the form to be stored in muscle and liver tissue until needed for heat and energy.

When the supply of insulin is insufficient, part of the sugar available for body tissues cannot be oxidized properly or stored as glycogen; therefore, excess glucose accumulates in the blood stream and is excreted in the urine.

Onset

The onset is so gradual that it may not be noticed for months, although symptoms are present.

Symptoms

Polyuria, polydipsia, polyphagia, loss of weight, weakness and pruritus, accompanied by hyperglycemia and glycosuria, are characteristic of the disease.

Complications

ACIDOSIS. Insulin must not be omitted unless the urine is sugar free. (Usually, it is given in small amounts in frequent doses, the amount depending on the reports of blood sugar and urinalysis every hour.)

See also Acidosis, p. 185.

INFECTIONS. *Cutaneous.* Sugar in the blood stream is an ideal culture medium for bacteria. Furuncles and carbuncles are common in patients who do not keep sugar-free.

Pulmonary. Diabetics are very susceptible to upper respiratory infections as a result of low resistance, probably due to undernourishment.

Pulmonary tuberculosis is about 4 times more prevalent in diabetic patients than it is in the nondiabetic.

MEDICAL AND SURGICAL

ARTERIOSCLEROSIS generally develops in a patient with a long-continued hyperglycemia. It is attributed also to a faulty fat metabolism, the fat being deposited in the form of cholesterol esters in the arteries with subsequent calcification of the blood vessel walls. The arteries of the lower extremities are involved most frequently. Ulcer and gangrene are due to arteriosclerosis, which causes malnutrition of the parts.

RETINITIS and cataract of the eye are common complications.

NERVOUS SYSTEM. Peripheral neuritis, neuralgia, numbness and tingling, especially of the lower extremities, may be associated with poor circulation.

Diagnosis

Clinical symptoms confirmed by laboratory tests of both the urine and the blood are diagnostic.

A glucose tolerance test is another means for diagnosis. (*See* Diagnostic Tests)

Prognosis

At present, diabetes is a chronic incurable disease. There is a tendency for it to progress in intensity with time. The life expectancy following diagnosis has been increased from 4.9 years in preinsulin days to 13 years. The most striking increase is in the very young.

Treatment

People with a predisposition to the disease should restrict starches and sugar.

Reducing of excess weight in people over 40 years of age.

Personal hygiene. A complete bath should be taken every day, and special care given to the feet by soaking them in warm water and massaging with cocoa butter every night.

Eliminate sources of worry.

Systematic exercise and massage.

Teaching of patient in relation to
    Nature of disease
    Principles of diet and methods of regulation
    Urine testing

Insulin administration
Personal hygiene, especially foot care
Signs of complications and their management
Importance of continuous medical supervision

Diet

Individual diets should be prescribed by the physician to maintain body weight.

See Diabetic Diets, p. 547.

Drug Therapy (*See* Pharmacology)

Insulin
Tolbutamide

Hypoglycemia or Overdosage of Insulin

Nervousness and tremor
Cool, clammy skin
Hunger
Faintness
Psychic disturbances
Convulsions and coma, if untreated

Treatment for Hypoglycemia

Mild Attack
    Put patient to bed
    Carbohydrate in form of orange juice or sugar
Severe Reaction
    Put to bed
    Apply external heat
    If unable to swallow, 20 to 40 ml. of 50 per cent glucose may be given intravenously by the doctor.

A diabetic should carry at all times a lump of sugar and an identification card with diagnosis and treatment needed for insulin shock.

HYPERTHYROIDISM (EXOPHTHALMIC GOITER, GRAVES'S DISEASE)

Hyperthyroidism is a condition resulting from an excessive secretion of the hormone of the thyroid gland.

MEDICAL AND SURGICAL

Etiology

Exact reason for overactivity is not known
More common in women 20 to 30 years of age

Signs and Symptoms

Increased activity of all motor functions
Weight loss although increased appetite
Fatigue; may be masked by restless motor activity
Intolerance to heat
Profuse sweating
Palpitation
Tremors of hands
Increased irritability, frequent emotional outbursts
Protruding eyeballs
Anxious expression
Thyroid gland usually increased in size
Elevated basal metabolism rate

Treatment

MEDICAL
Antithyroid drugs such as propylthiouracil, Tapazole (*See discussion in* Pharmacology)
Radioactive iodine
High-caloric, high-vitamin diet
Control of emotional factors and physical activity
SURGERY—partial thyroidectomy
Preoperative
Medical therapy to bring patient under control—antithyroid drugs and iodine
Provide for optimum relaxation and rest
Peaceful environment, remove causes of anxiety
Tolerance of patient's peculiarities
Avoid boredom
Phenobarbital (*See discussion in* Pharmacology)
Help patient to gain weight
High-caloric, high-vitamin diet
Chart calories, weigh twice a week
Specific therapy for complications of the disease, such as for congestive heart failure
Postoperative
Watch for signs of complications

Hemorrhage especially under suture line where it is not detected easily

Symptoms—difficulty in breathing; swelling in neck

Treated by opening wound immediately

Thyroid storm—in first 3 days after surgery

Symptoms—rise in vital signs, patient becomes disoriented

Treated by oxygen, cooling sponges, I.V. glucose, sedation. Also, antithyroid drugs followed in a few hours by full doses of iodides (*see* Pharmacology). Cortisone, prednisone to prevent renal failure (*see* Pharmacology). Digitalize to control ventricular rate of fibrillation or congestive failure

Parathyroid injury—tetanic movements

Nerve injury—hoarseness

Provide adequate support for head

See Preoperative and Postoperative Care, pp. 175-184.

Nontoxic Nodular Goiter

Surgical treatment indicated

May be malignant growth—need to make differential diagnoses

Pressure symptoms on trachea

May grow into chest and cause pressure

Cosmetic appearance

ENDOCRINE SYSTEM IN VERTEBRATES*

ENDOCRINE GLAND AND HORMONE	PRINCIPAL SITE OF ACTION	PRINCIPAL PROCESSES AFFECTED
Pituitary gland (a) Anterior lobe Growth	General	Growth of bones, viscera and muscles; nitrogen retention
Follicle-stimulating (FSH)	Ovaries	Development of follicles; with LH, secretion of estrogen and ovulation
	Testes	Development of seminiferous tubules, spermatogenesis

* Greisheimer, E. M.: Physiology and Anatomy, ed. 7, Philadelphia, Lippincott, 1955.

Endocrine Gland and Hormone	Principal Site of Action	Principal Processes Affected
Luteinizing (LH) or interstitial cell stimulating (ICSH)	Ovaries	Development of corpora lutea and secretion of progesterone (see FSH)
	Testes	Development of interstitial tissue and secretion of testosterone
Thyrotrophic (TTH)	Thyroid	Growth of thyroid and production of thyroxin
Adrenocorticotrophic (ACTH)	Adrenal cortex	Growth of adrenal cortex and secretion of adrenal cortical steroids
Lactogenic or luteotrophic	Mammary glands and ovaries	Secretion of milk by mammary glands and secretion of estrogen and progesterone
Intermedin	Chromatophore cells in skin of amphibia	Expansion of pigment cells and dispersion of pigment granules; function unknown in man
(b) Posterior lobe Pitressin (pressor and ADH)	Arterioles and cells of kidney tubules	Blood pressure Reabsorption of water; water balance
Pitocin	Uterine muscle	Contraction; parturition, possibly
Thyroid gland Thyroxin	General	Metabolic rate; morphogenesis; physical and mental growth; intermediate metabolism
Parathyroid glands Parathormone	General	Metabolism of calcium and phosphorus
Adrenal glands (a) Cortex Cortin (like desoxycorticosterone)	Kidney tubules	Reabsorption of sodium chloride and elimination of potassium
Corticosterone	General	Carbohydrate metabolism; quantity and quality of intercellular substance; lymphatic tissue in response to stress
Adrenosterone and estrogen and progesterone	General	Like testosterone, estrogen and progesterone
(b) Medulla Epinephrine	Heart muscle and smooth muscle	Pulse rate and blood pressure; same effects as stimulation of thoracolumbar division of autonomic nervous system

ENDOCRINE GLAND AND HORMONE	PRINCIPAL SITE OF ACTION	PRINCIPAL PROCESSES AFFECTED
Ovaries		
Estrogen	General	Development of secondary sexual characteristics
	Mammary glands	Development of duct system
	Accessory reproductive organs	Maturation and normal cyclic function
Progesterone	Mammary glands	Development of alveolar tissue
	Uterus	Preparation for implantation; maintenance of pregnancy
Testes		
Testosterone	General	Development of secondary sexual characteristics
	Accessory reproductive organs	Maturation and normal function
Islet cells of pancreas		
Insulin	General	Utilization of carbohydrate
Placenta (chorionic tissue)		
APL (anterior-pituitarylike)	Same as LH	Same as LH
Estrogen	Same as estrogen	Same as estrogen
Progesterone	Same as progesterone	Same as progesterone
Alimentary tract		
Gastrin	Glands in fundus and body of stomach	Production of gastric juice
Secretin	Pancreas, liver and intestine	Production of watery pancreatic juice (rich in $NaHCO_3$), bile and intestinal juice
Pancreozymin	Pancreas	Production of pancreatic juice rich in enzymes
Enterogastrone	Stomach	Inhibits secretion and motility
Cholecystokinin	Gallbladder	Contraction and emptying
Enterocrinin	Small intestine	Stimulates production of intestinal juice

Part 10. General Principles of Care of the Dermatologic Patient

The following suggestions are not intended in any way to encompass the measures employed by specialists in diseases of the skin. Many of these—notably x-ray therapy—require special knowledge and training. X-ray irradiation has many indications in dermatology that will not be included here,

PART I

Treatment in Acute and Subacute Dermatoses

In this group of diseases belong all the acute cases of contact dermatitis, allergic dermatitis, many of the drug rashes, and toxic erythemas. These diseases constitute the bulk of dermatologic entities requiring good nursing care. The alterations of the skin manifest themselves in various degrees of inflammation, ranging from simple erythema to pronounced edema with vesiculation and oozing, denudation of the epidermis, scaling, crusting, etc. The subjective sensations are itching, burning, soreness and pain; they may be severe.

Treatment is based first on cause and secondly on symptoms. In the former the aim is to eliminate all offending agents (contact allergens, drugs, etc.) which may be brought to light by the patient's history, or by investigations for hypersensitivity (e.g., patch tests). Where it is difficult to determine the cause of the eruption, or where this requires prolonged studies, we may have to depend on symptomatic treatment.

LOCALIZED ACUTE DERMATOSES

Localized dermatoses involve only a portion of the integument. Therapeutic measures will depend on the changes in the skin. In weeping eruptions, wet dressings will prove to be most useful; in fact, salves and pastes are contraindicated. The most commonly used preparations are the following:

Burow's Solution (aluminum subacetate solution 1:20 to 1:40)

Saturated solution of boric acid

Potassium permanganate solution 1:8,000 to 1:12,000, freshly prepared

Physiologic or slightly hypertonic saline solution

Magnesium sulfate (½ to 1 oz. to a quart of water)

Briefly, the actions of wet dressings are as follows:
Cleansing the skin
Removal of crusts and accumulated debris
Soothing action, relieving superficial inflammation
Antipruritic and analgesic action
Maintaining drainage
Astringent and drying action
A tendency to open blisters

The prolonged use of wet dressings will macerate the skin surface and effect keratolytic action

In acute dermatoses without vesiculation and weeping, but with erythema and edema, wet compresses may be used, but for shorter durations. Here the agents of choice will be either shake lotions or powders.

The action of the lotions is superficial, but some absorption may take place. Absorption of topic substances contained in lotions may produce severe systemic symptoms. The action of the lotion ensues after the evaporation of the liquid. The glycerin becomes absorbed by the superficial horny layers of the skin, and the powdery parts adhere, producing a cooling antipruritic and drying effect.

Some patients will not tolerate lotions. They may cause an irritation or an excessive dryness of the skin. They are not well tolerated in the intertriginous areas and cannot be used in hairy parts such as the scalp or the perigenital regions. In such instances, emulsions or liniments will be indicated.

Liniments

Liniments differ from lotions in that the vehicle is an oily liquid. Liniments are less drying because of the oily base.

All active therapeutic agents which can be incorporated in lotions can be included in the liniments. These are convenient preparations for patients confined to bed, since no bandaging is necessary. In their action on the skin, they are similar to the soft ointments.

Powders

Powders will be indicated in some milder forms of dermatitis, especially in the intertriginous areas and

MEDICAL AND SURGICAL

on the feet. They exert a cooling effect on the skin and protect it from irritation. Accordingly, the ingredients are incorporated to produce an antipruritic, astringent or antiparasitic action. The follow-up treatment of the acute dermatoses consists of the application of pastes or salves. Both preparations will be discussed under the treatment of subacute dermatoses.

GENERALIZED ACUTE DERMATOSES

If possible, patients should be hospitalized; if not, a registered nurse should be obtained. These patients may be severely ill with malaise, fever and other symptoms.

The principles of local therapy are similar to those described above. Baths, either cleansing or medicated, may be substituted for the wet compresses. The action of the medicated bath will be:

Soothing
Antipruritic
Anti-inflammatory
Antiseptic
Antiparasitic
Antiseborrheic, according to the medicinal ingredients

From 1 to 3 baths a day, from 20 to 30 minutes in duration, are permissible. Soaps are preferably omitted. At times a soap substitute will be tolerated (Acidolate, pHisoderm, Lowila). In between the baths, lotions, creams, or liniments may be used. The nurse must take all necessary safety precautions when helping patients with medicated baths. This is particularly important when patients have ointments on the skin. It must be remembered that these ointments make the skin very slippery and there is danger of the patient falling.

SUBACUTE DERMATOSES

In subacute dermatoses both the lotions and the liniments may be used during the day. At night, pastes and salves are indicated.

Paste

Paste consists of equal parts of suspended insoluble

366

powders, usually zinc oxide, starch and a fatty substance such as lanolin or petrolatum or their mixtures.

A paste most commonly used, the so-called Lassar's paste, has the following formula:

Zinc oxide	8.0
Starch	8.0
Petrolatum up to	30.0

Pastes tend to absorb secretions and are drying, soothing, protective, antipruritic, etc., according to the medicinal ingredient incorporated. They have a rather superficial action on the skin and as a rule are well tolerated. They are less macerating than ointments. Hairy areas such as the scalp, the armpits, etc., should not be treated with pastes. When pastes are applied to the skin, bandaging usually is indicated. Olive oil or mineral oil may be used for their removal.

Ointments

Ointments are used in subacute dermatoses when the epidermis is intact and thickened, and where deeper pharmacologic action is needed. The base of ointments consists of fat, of either animal or mineral origin. Vegetable fats and oils usually mixed with wax also are used as a base. Petrolatum is a favored preparation, since it is soft, smooth, odorless and does not become rancid. The only disadvantage is that at times it may cause irritation. Both yellow and white petrolatum may be used. Animal fats are lard and lanolin. Lanolin, derived from wool fat, frequently is used since it permits the absorption of equal amounts of water or medicine dissolved in water. Aquaphor (cholesterinized petrolatum) also has the property of mixing with large amounts of water. Many acceptable bases are now available.

The ability of ointments to penetrate the skin is promoted by friction, heat and inunction. Salves act as lubricants and soften the surface of the skin. They will remove scales, crusts and debris from the skin surface. Fat-soluble and oil-soluble medicines incorporated in salves come in close contact with the skin surface and penetrate deeper than when incorporated into paste.

Most of the natural oily ointment bases are immiscible with water. However, the addition of certain surface-active agents leads to the formation of emulsions or dispersion of oil and water. Either the oil is dispersed in the water (oil-in-water emulsions) or the water is dispersed in the oil (water-in-oil emulsions). An example of oil-in-water emulsions base is Hydrophylic Ointment U.S.P. This preparation is penetrating, water washable, not greasy; it may be used in hairy parts. Examples of standard water-in-oil emulsions are hydrous wool fat (lanolin) and Aquaphor (cholesterinized petrolatum). In some skin disorders, these emulsion bases or creams are better tolerated than natural ointment bases. Most drugs mentioned previously can be incorporated in emulsion bases. However, some may be pharmacologically incompatible, e.g., organic acids such as salicylic acid, tannic acid, benzoic acid, etc. (which will break down the emulsion). The proper removal of scales, crusts and other materials from the diseased skin surface is important and often difficult. In acute and subacute dermatoses one should be gentle in order to avoid irritation and bleeding. The preparations used for removal of scales and crusts are the following:

    Olive oil, mineral oil or cottonseed oil
    Boric acid solution 3%
    Potassium permanganate 1:8,000

If these are not available, warm water, or cotton or gauze soaked with warm water may be utilized. In chronic dermatoses these same preparations are helpful, as are benzene, warm water and soap, or the soap substitutes.

PART II

Physical Agents

Radiation Therapy

Superficial roentgen ray, radium, radon, radioactive isotopes and total body irradiation (cathode ray) are employed in the therapy of certain cutaneous malignancies in carefully selected patients. Choice of the modality to be employed depends on many factors (age of patient, type of tumor, location of tumor, etc.) and must be given with vigorously controlled technic. On increasingly rare occasions, small doses of superficial x-rays are given for recalcitrant benign dermatoses. The amount of such x-rays must be much smaller than that which would produce any adverse radiation effects whatsoever.

It is essential that all personnel utilized in radiotherapy be thoroughly trained in its dangers and be aware of protective measures.

Ultraviolet Ray Therapy

Ultraviolet ray therapy is another physical modality that has limited value in certain cutaneous disorders such as acne, psoriasis, etc.

Training in precise technic is essential for both the patient and the technician.

Electrosurgery

Electrosurgery is still another physical method wherein a high-voltage, low-amperage current is used to produce actual desiccation of cellular elements. Remarkably good cosmetic results as well as complete eradication of some of the smaller cutaneous malignancies and certain benign lesions (warts, some moles, etc.) can be predictably achieved if electrodesiccation is combined with thorough curettage, in skilled hands.

Wire Brush Planing (Dermabrasion)

Dermabrasion is now an acceptable method for the therapy of certain disfiguring lesions. The principle is to remove the epidermis with a high-speed rotating wire brush. The method has been highly overexaggerated by the lay press and is only an adjunct to medical and surgical management of selected patients.

Curettage

Curettage is simply the use of a rounded knife for scraping off superficial lesions such as seborrheic keratoses, molluscum contagiosum, etc. It is an excellent method of therapy of such lesions, making excision an infrequent necessity.

Cryotherapy

Cryotherapy consists in the employment of solid carbon dioxide, carbon dioxide snow or liquid nitrogen. At times it is used in the treatment of acne, hypertrophic benign lesions, small keratoses, etc., permitting superficial destruction of lesions with minimal or no scarring.

Chemotherapy

Various highly caustic chemicals (phenol, trichloracetic acid, etc.) are used on rare occasions to destroy superficial benign lesions.

Mohs technic is a method of gradual chemical destruction of tumors with careful histologic control. It is used for the occasional tumor not amenable to other methods.

General Points

It is essential that, whenever possible, the patient be taught to do his own treatments. This enables him to feel some responsibility for his own care and to lessen the sense of dependency on others.

The nature of dermatologic conditions often fosters a feeling of rejection on the part of the patient. The attitude of others toward him is most important; therefore, the nurse must evaluate her own responses to these patients and the sometimes "repulsive appearance" which the dermatologic conditions cause.

PART III

Measures Indicated in Specific Diseases

ACNE VULGARIS

Treatment is general and local.

GENERAL. Well-rounded diet. Exclude all chocolate.

Discourage eating such things as milk shakes, sodas, candy and peanuts between meals. Fruit and milk may be permitted.

Vitamin A and other vitamins may be of help.

Investigate questions of constipation, anemia, low basal metabolism and habits of exercise and rest. Cosmetics with greasy bases must be eliminated. Avoid iodized salt.

Seborrhea nearly always is associated with acne and should be treated.

LOCAL. Thorough cleansing with soap, water and coarse wash cloth, 4 to 6 times a day; mild sulfur lotions; ultraviolet irradiation; express comedones; calamine lotion with phenol as powder base.

Small Comedone Acne with Seborrhea (Oily Skin)

Soap and water; express comedones; local use of sulfur lotions at night; ultraviolet irradiation in doses sufficient to produce peeling; calamine lotion with phenol.

More Severe Forms. Consult physician.

Residual Scarring and Pitting

May be improved by scarification.

ALLERGIC (ATOPIC) DERMATITIS

Determine causative factors if possible—food, foci of infection, bacterial or fungous sensitization.

Use intradermal or scratch test.

LOCAL. *Acute Stages.* Wet dressings; medicated baths; bland ointments and bland oil lotions for soothing effect; hydrocortisone creams are effective.

Chronic Stages. Tar ointments; 10 per cent Naftalan in Lassar's paste; generalized exposures to ultraviolet light; hydrocortisone creams are effective.

ALOPECIA AREATA

Definition

Local temporary baldness.

MEDICAL AND SURGICAL

Treatment

Complete physical examination: search for foci of infection; determine basal metabolic rate; ultraviolet irradiation; vitamins A and B; stimulating salves and lotions; paint areas with phenol once a week (with caution).

CONTACT DERMATITIS

Reactions are essentially the same, whether from plants, chemicals or animal contact. Treatment is essentially the same. Use thorough and alert questioning to find contact agent.

Mild Erythematous Stage

Controlled by wet dressings (preferably cold) of boric acid, Burow's solution, antipruritic lotions or bland creams.

Exudative Vesicular Stage

Wet dressings (continuous) of potassium permanganate, boric acid, magnesium sulfate, Burow's solution; helpful to nick vesicles and let out serum.

If Infected. Medicated baths, such as potassium permanganate, followed by lotions and even employment of systemic antibiotics.

If Very Severe. Systemic corticosteroids are used.

Subsiding Stage

Protective covering with bland ointment or equal parts of plain Lassar's paste and boric ointment; aluminum acetate ointment; plain boric ointment, etc.

When possible in contact dermatitis, prove cause by patch tests. Give thorough instruction in avoiding future contacts.

DERMATITIS MEDICAMENTOSA (DERMATITIS FROM INGESTION OR INJECTION OF DRUGS)

Suspect any rash in a patient receiving medication as due to drugs until proved otherwise. Stop all medication when possible; force fluids; saline catharsis; fluid diet.

LOCAL treatment is essentially the same as for Contact Dermatitis.

Basic treatment is discontinuance of the drug.

In very severe cases, corticosteroids are employed.

DERMATITIS VENENATA (POISON IVY)

Immediately after exposure, if known, or within 24 hours after appearance of rash, cleanse exposed parts, including fingernails, with soap and water, alcohol or other grease solvents. Follow this by lotions.

LOCAL treatment essentially is the same as for Contact Dermatitis.

SPECIFIC. Immunizing agents are employed orally and parenterally, but their exact value is yet to be assessed.

ERYSIPELAS

Definition

An acute severe streptococcal infection

Treatment

Bed rest, penicillin by injection

LOCAL: Wet dressings and penicillin ointment

ERYTHEMA NODOSUM

Definition

Painful pretibial nodules due to drugs, infectious agents and unknown causes

Treatment

Attend to general health. Encourage as much rest as possible, with elevation of the legs. Look for cause in drugs or in foci of infection. Examine the chest, etc., for tuberculosis, coccidioidomycosis.

DISEASES CAUSED BY FILTERABLE VIRUSES

Herpes Simplex

Wet compresses of boric acid, benzoin tincture or 2 per cent ammoniated mercury. Lotio alba and 95 per cent alcohol are excellent remedies.

Recurrent Herpes

Repeated injections of smallpox vaccine, once a week, may help.

Herpes Zoster

LOCAL. Calamine, 2 per cent gentian violet or 2 per cent menthol in collodian.

SPECIFIC. Control of pain essential—many medicaments are used.

DISEASES DUE TO FUNGI

Treatment will depend on the stage of the infection.

IF RAW AND INFLAMED, use wet dressings with liquor aluminum acetate, 1:10 parts of water; or saturated boric acid solution. Apply boric acid or aluminum acetate ointment between wet dressings.

IF SECONDARILY INFECTED, use wet dressings such as 1:10,000 potassium permanganate.

AS INFLAMMATION subsides, use dyes such as 2 to 3 per cent aqueous or alcoholic gentian violet; Ziehl-Neelsen's carbolfuchsin solution, saturated. In chronic cases, undecylenic acid (Desenex), half strength Whitfields' ointment (acidi sal. 1.0, acidi ben. 2.0, pet. alba 30.0), or 6 per cent salicylic acid in alcohol, followed by borated talcum.

SPECIFIC. Griseofulvin 1 Gm. daily P.O. most effective in severe cases.

Tinea Capitis

Examine under Wood's light for extent of involvement. Culture. Treatment with Griseofulvin 1 Gm. daily for an average period of 1 to 2 weeks is curative.

Tinea Corporis

Responds to local fungicides.

Tinea Cruris

The dyes or half-strength Whitfield's ointment at night; calamine lotion during day. Griseofulvin, as above.

Dermatophytosis

Treatment as listed under Fungi above, plus clipping and scraping away dead nails and skin.

Tinea Versicolor

Saturated solution of sodium hyposulfite rubbed in twice daily after bathing with soap and water and using wash cloth. Selenium shampoos applied locally are effective.

FURUNCULOSIS

INCIPIENT STAGE. Local heat; compresses or poultices; appropriate antibiotics

LOCALIZED STAGE. Incision and drainage, culture, antibiotics if indicated

RECURRENT STAGE. Careful evaluation of general health (diabetes mellitus, blood dyscrasias, lymphoma, agammaglobulinemia, foci of infection, intestinal parasites). Strict attention to nasal carrier state

IMPETIGO

Definition

Superficial bacterial infection usually found in children

Treatment

Remove crusts with compresses of warm saline or boric acid. Bacitracin ointment 500 u. per Gm.; Neomycin 5 mg. per Gm.; polymyxin 1,000 u. per Gm. or combination of these are most effective; apply over entire area. Hexachlorophene-containing soaps or detergents are helpful.

INFANTILE ECZEMA

(*See* Allergic Dermatitis, p. 371)

LUPUS ERYTHEMATOSUS

Definition

A local or systemic disease characterized by skin rash,

joint pains, fever, weight loss and involvement of multiple organ systems

Treatment

Avoid exposure to sun, heat or cold.

Adequate diet and rest

Determine whether a local or systemic disease. Antimalarials (*see* Pharmacology) are employed in the discoid type. Corticosteroids often are employed in the systemic type.

PEDICULOSIS

Capitis

Two per cent emulsion DDT applied to the scalp kills the lice and lingers long enough to kill the larvae. One treatment is sufficient. Kwell powder in the hair is an excellent remedy.

Corporis

Boil underwear. Press seams of clothes with hot iron. Dust on DDT powder after soap and water bath; dust also on clothes. Kwell powder is most effective when dusted over the skin.

Pubis

One per cent DDT ointment, Kwell powder, Cuprex; work in the order named. Shave hair. Take frequent baths.

PEMPHIGUS

Definition

A very serious blistering eruption

Treatment

Best treatment is good nursing. Maintain cleanliness. Highly nutritious diet supplemented by vitamins. Corticosteroids, sometimes in very high doses, are needed to control this otherwise fatal disease.

PITYRIASIS ROSEA

Definition

A transient scaly eruption of the trunk, usually not contagious

Treatment

Generalized ultraviolet irradiation to produce mild erythema. (Use bland creams if this causes dryness of skin.) For pruritus, cornstarch baths and antipruritic lotion, such as calamine lotion with phenol, menthol and camphor.

PRICKLY HEAT (MILIARIA RUBRA)

Bathe frequently with cornstarch baths. Dress lightly. Calamine lotion. Powder with talc, cornstarch or zinc stearate. A lotion containing neomycin and hydrocortisone is quite effective.

PRURITUS

Determine cause if possible (may be internal or external).

Senile or dry skins are subject to winter itch. Use fatty soap and bathe daily. Antihistamine drugs may be tried.

LOCAL. Salve or lotion containing phenol or menthol.

PSORIASIS

Definition

A chronic and recurrent scaly eruption. Tends to run in families. Goal of treatment is management.

Treatment

Extreme care must be taken not to overtreat acute psoriasis, as generalized exfoliative dermatitis may result.

ACUTE STAGE. Mild salve, such as 3 per cent ammoniated mercury, can be used. Soothing lotions and baths.

CHRONIC STAGE. Ammoniated mercury and salicylic acid, strong tar salves, anthralin, pyrogallic acid. Object is to peel lesion. Watch for acute irritation.

DIET. Low fat diet. Lecithin in the soybean products is thought to be of value. Vitamins, as vitamin A, or liver may be tried.

Generalized ultraviolet irradiation at night, apply to lesions an ointment of 2 to 4 per cent crude coal tar, 2 per cent zinc oxide and 59 per cent cornstarch in petrolatum. In morning, remove with light mineral oil, *leaving a film of oil,* and then give generalized ultraviolet irradiation; or paint with liquor carbonis detergens, followed by generalized ultraviolet irradiation. Daily or twice daily bathe with soap and water using a wash cloth to remove all scales.

ROSACEA

Definition

A pustular erythematous eruption predominant on the nose.

Treatment

Vasodilators such as coffee, alcohol, condiments and too-hot foods should be avoided. As far as possible, avoid exposure to extreme heat and cold.

Look for foci of infection, especially in teeth, tonsils, sinuses and gallbladder.

Give diluted hydrochloric acid (10%) (10 minums in one half glass of water, t.i.d., a.c.). Lotio alba to be applied at night.

Scarification is of benefit, especially if beginning rhinophyma is present.

SCABIES

Examine and treat contacts. Apply Kwell ointment (hexachlorocyclohexane) following a thorough soap-and-water bath from neck to foot. Change and boil all underwear, sheets and night clothes. Reapply following night. Ten per cent sulfur ointment may be used as above but is followed by dermatitis in many cases. Twenty-five per cent benzyl benzoate emulsion also can be used similarly.

SUNBURN

PREVENT by use of protective cream or lotion. Expose skin to sun in graduated amounts.

LOCAL. Treat as burn. Petrolatum and pressure bandages of extremities; compresses of witch hazel, boric acid or saline solution; albolene, carron or mineral oil; bland creams, dilute vinegar.

URTICARIA (HIVES)

Look for drug (e.g., penicillin) sensitivity; foci of infection; serum reaction; food allergy; sensitivity to external contacts.

AT ONSET. Adrenalin; antihistaminic drugs; saline catharsis; intravenous injections of calcium gluconate; low-protein diet; Corticosteroids.

LOCAL. Antipruritic lotions or bland salves. Oatmeal or cornstarch baths.

VERRUCA PLANTARIS (PLANTAR WART)

Curettage, electrodesiccation, excision, local keratolytic agents, liquid nitrogen and radiotherapy are variously employed. Paint daily with glacial acetic acid and pare off dead skin and wart.

Treatment should be considered carefully, as painful scars can result.

Part II.   Orthopedic Conditions

PRINCIPLES OF PATIENT CARE*

Orthopedic nursing is concerned with the preservation and restoration of the function of the musculoskeletal

* Sections of the material used on pp. 379-382 are quoted directly or paraphrased from Wilde, Delphine: Traction and suspension, Am. J. Nursing 53:1465-1468, 1953.

system. The nurse is always particularly aware of practicing good body mechanics both for the patient and herself. A few of the special knowledges and skills needed are discussed here.

CARE OF THE PATIENT IN A PLASTER CAST

GENERAL CONSIDERATIONS ABOUT CASTS AND SPLINTS

After application of plaster, support contours of cast or splints with pillows or sand bags until dry.

Keep cast uncovered to accelerate drying.

If cast is on an extremity, keep part elevated at first to lessen swelling; watch for signs of circulatory impairment, e.g., color and skin temperature of digits, swelling, inability to move digits; loss of sensation.

Bind all rough edges with adhesive or plaster, padding them first if necessary.

Report any persistent complaints of pressure or burning pain beneath the cast, for the doctor can loosen splints or fenestrate a circular cast to prevent development of a pressure sore.

Keep cast clean by rubbing with damp cloth, when necessary.

Report any weak spots in cast, that would allow motion of the part.

CARE OF PATIENT IN SPICA OR JACKET

Use a bed with a hard mattress and attach a Balkan frame with a trapeze, so that the patient can help in lifting.

Make patient as comfortable as possible by the use of pillows adjacent to cast edges.

Turn patient on abdomen for an hour at least twice a day. For patient in a spica it may be necessary to have a nurse on either side of the bed. The patient is moved to the edge of the bed, on the side of injury. He is instructed to keep arms close to his side. Each nurse puts one hand under the leg and the other hand under the chest, and then turns, the injured leg going uppermost. A large pillow is placed under the abdomen to push cast away from the back; pillow under chest if necessary. At this time, skin care is given to the back, reaching well under the edge of the cast. If there are any reddened areas on the skin, a thermolamp and other prophylactic measures may be used. A powder blower is useful to dust the skin beyond reach of the hand.

If patient is incontinent, bind the edge of the cast around the buttocks with oiled silk and use a thermolamp to dry out any damp areas.

To rub the back of a patient in a jacket, push a piece of flannel through with a long wire.

Provide for proper elimination, especially during first week in plaster, when patient is not yet adapted to position.

Encourage patient to exercise all parts not encased in plaster and to help himself as much as possible.

CARE OF THE PATIENT IN TRACTION AND SUSPENSION

Nursing care of the patient in traction and suspension can be a very satisfying experience, involving not only skills but also a real sense of responsibility for the proper functioning of the apparatus. When the nurse understands what the apparatus is supposed to accomplish, she will be able to note any need for minor adjustments, which often she herself is able to make.

PURPOSES AND METHODS OF TRACTION

Traction is simply the act of pulling upon a part; when it is applied to a patient, the weight of his body acts as the countertraction. The three main purposes of traction are: (1) to obtain and maintain reduction of fractures, (2) to overcome muscle spasm in musculoskeletal conditions, and (3) to lessen or prevent contracture of joints following injury or incident to a disease.

There are various methods of obtaining traction, but some are used more frequently than others. Of course manual traction is used only until a splint is applied or a fracture reduced. Fitted appliances, such as leather anklets for Buck's extension—a simple form of extension without suspension—or head halters for traction on the neck, may be used.

Skin traction usually is accomplished with adhesive tape applied to the part and the ends attached to a spreader on which the pull is exerted by rope and weight.

Skeletal traction exerts the pull on the bone itself by means of a steel pin or a wire drilled through the bone and held taut by a metal yoke. This is the most efficient method, because it produces almost twice as much pull on the bone as other methods and does not cause injury to, or irritation of, the skin.

PURPOSES AND METHODS OF SUSPENSION

Suspension can be defined as the support of a part in some device that overcomes the force of gravity—usually balanced by a sufficient amount of weight to maintain elevation at any desired level. Suspension frequently is used in the treatment of fractures or following orthopedic surgery for one or more of the following purposes: (1) to provide comfortable and evenly distributed support for an extremity, (2) to help maintain alignment of the bone fragments, (3) to provide a form of elevation that is more constantly dependable and higher than pillows, (4) to facilitate moving other parts of the body without causing discomfort in the involved area, and (5) to allow exercise of the involved limb itself, when the apparatus has been mobilized to permit this. Usually, a leg is supported in a Thomas splint with a Pearson attachment, which permits flexion at the knee and also joint motion when this is desired. If a Hodgen splint is used, the fixed angle of flexion does not allow for any motion. An arm is suspended in a flannel or canvas sling attached to spreaders. In fractures of the pubes or ilia, the pelvis may be counterbalanced in a wide canvas sling.

BUCK'S EXTENSION

This is a commonly used simple form of traction. Adhesive or grooved sponge rubber straps are applied to the lower leg with lower ends extending past each malleolus to a spreader; to this in turn is attached a rope going over a pulley and carrying a prescribed weight at the end. The nurse's daily observations in this care are applicable to all forms of skin traction.

The following points should be observed:

Inspection of proximal ends of adhesive for skin irritation. Benzoin tincture may be used to remedy this.

Inspection of Ace or other bandage, which should hold adhesive securely.

Observation of the malleoli for any signs of pressure from the straps.

Noting the position of the foot. Sometimes a foot plate is incorporated in the spreader to give continuous support, but the patient should be encouraged to move the ankle frequently.

Inspection of the traction rope for free movement over the pulley.

Inspection of weights, which should hang freely without chance of resting on the bed or floor.

Continuous observation of the patient's position in bed. If much weight is used, it may be necessary to elevate the foot of the bed in order to obtain adequate countertraction. Turning up the knee gatch will also help. The amount of shoulder elevation permitted is decided by the doctor.

CARE OF PATIENT IN SUSPENSION IN A THOMAS SPLINT

The nurse's daily observation should include the following:

Testing the balance of the splint. It should raise the leg when the patient raises his hips.

Inspection of area under ring of splint. This is apt to cause pressure above the thigh at the groin. Skin areas around the ring should be massaged carefully with alcohol, and any padding that may be used always should be clean.

Inspection of the supporting swathes to see that they are applied evenly, are unwrinkled and are covered by adequate padding. A long piece of felt encased in stockinette makes an excellent "splint mattress."

Inspection of area at knee for any signs of pressure. Should this occur near the fibula head, peroneal nerve damage might result, with inability to dorsiflex the foot.

If the patient has skin traction and suspension, observation points listed for Buck's extension should be carried out.

If the patient has skeletal traction, wire holes should be inspected frequently for signs of irritation.

When suspension is mobilized, the nurse should be sure that weights and pulleys are functioning efficiently. Occasional oiling of pulleys is necessary, and attention to placement of weights may facilitate the patient's exercise routine. The nurse encourages the patient in the prescribed motions that are so important in aftercare, the release of contractures or the later stages of fracture repair.

GENERAL CARE OF THE TRACTION-SUSPENSION PATIENT

The following points, in addition to those above, should be emphasized:

Meticulous back care. The patient usually must spend all of his time in the dorsal recumbent position. Immediate attention to any skin breaks is imperative. A sponge rubber cushion is desirable since the mattress itself should be a very firm one. Powder is a special help in preventing the dampness that may be consequent upon continual contact of the same area with the bedding.

Careful bedmaking. The undersheet always should be changed from the good side and pulled very taut. For top covering, divided linen is desirable so that it can cover the bed below the splint. Small blankets with ties may be used to cover the leg in suspension, which tends to become cold easily because of its elevation and immobilization.

The nurse must know maintenance of position and instruct the patient in keeping the correct alignment of his body and the traction suspension apparatus.

Encouragement of good general hygiene. The patient must be encouraged to help himself in every possible way in preparation for the gradual return to normal function. Conditioning exercises may be used for unaffected extremities and trunk muscles.

Co-operation with the occupational therapist and physical therapist in their part in the total care of the patient.

ADAPTATIONS OF TRACTION

Bryant Traction

This is a form of skin traction used for fractures of the femoral shaft in babies or small children. It is applied to both legs with the pull holding the legs at right angles to the trunk. The weight is sufficient to raise the buttocks slightly off the crib. This helps to maintain good alignment of the fracture when dealing with a young squirmer. Usually, it is necessary to hold the child's body by a restrainer to achieve better countertraction. The nurse strives to maintain the child in this position and observes the adhesive straps frequently because of the tenderness of the baby's skin. Pressure over the heel cord also must be watched for closely; the bandages should be removed and reapplied at least once a day.

Russell Traction

This is used most frequently for older people who have fractures of the femur; even today when internal fixation is the method of choice, it may be used temporarily while the patient's condition is being evaluated for operation. This method uses two traction forces at different angles to give a resultant line of pull in the desired direction. (The principle and mechanics are best explained by the illustration on page 386.)

Careful attention to the position of the patient and the pillows is important because the angle between the thigh and the leg should be 153° and the rope supporting the knee should be at a 90° angle to the pull on the lower leg to produce a resultant force in the long axis of the femur. Unfortunately, an old lady with a fractured hip does not always co-operate in maintaining this position, and the nurse frequently must adjust the pa-

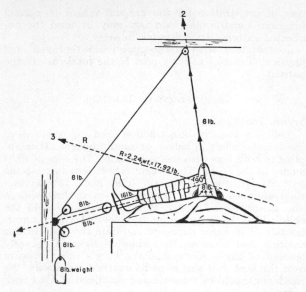

tient's position. The advantage of this type of traction lies in the fact that since less weight is needed, the skin of the older person can tolerate the pull of the apparatus. Protection from pressure under, or at the side of, the knee is obtained by padding the sling with felt or sponge rubber.

Pelvic Sling Suspension

The principle of resultant force is applied also in this apparatus for separated fractures of the pelvis. The hips are supported in a hammock of heavy flannel or canvas, and the sides are pulled inward by the suspending ropes in such a way as to exert pressure on the pelvis. The buttocks clear the bed so that patient's weight acts as one of the forces. This also permits using the bedpan and making the bed without occasioning too much pain. However, the sling must be very well padded, preferably with sponge rubber extending over the edge. Even with this precaution, frequent massage of the sacral area is most essential.

Cervical Traction

The bed should be elevated at the head so that the weight of the patient's body sliding in the other direction acts as countertraction. When a head halter is used, the nurse must see that it fits as well as possible around the chin, to avoid undue pressure. She should check to see that it does not slip down and interfere with the patient's breathing, and she should gently, but frequently, massage the skin under the halter. The traction must be continuous, unless otherwise specified.

Various other forms of traction-suspension are used, but the essentials of care are much the same. The nurse who is diligent in applying these principles will succeed in making life quite tolerable for both the orthopedic patient and herself.

CARE AFTER ARTHROPLASTY OF THE HIP

An arthroplasty is a plastic operation on a joint and is designed to restore motion where there has been limitation and, usually, pain.

After arthroplasty of the hip, the extremity usually is immobilized for about 2 weeks in either cast or suspension and then started on gradual exercise.

The chief responsibility is maintenance of position as ordered by the surgeon—usually moderate abduction and extension of the hip. When the exercise program is started, she encourages the patient in carrying out the prescribed motions.

CARE AFTER SPINE FUSION FOR LOW BACK CONDITIONS

A spine fusion is an operation done to eliminate motion in one or more joints of the spine. The period of bed rest after such surgery varies in different institutions, but the postoperative care usually is as follows:

Preparation of the Bed

Bed board

MEDICAL AND SURGICAL

Firm mattress
Have ready 3 pillows
1 for head
1 to brace back
1 between knees } when lying on either side

Positioning Postoperatively

The patient should be flat on his back for 4 hours. Then he may be rolled to either side like a log, i.e., keeping back in straight line. A turning sheet may be of help in this early period, especially if the patient is heavy. Knees should be moderately flexed with a large pillow between. Change his position every 2 to 3 hours.

Special Points to Check Postoperatively

Evidence of hemorrhage
Vital signs
Ability to move extremities

Elimination

Catheterization often is necessary if the patient does not void in 12 hours. It should be carried out every 8 hours thereafter. If voiding has not become spontaneous by the following day, gravity drainage may be instituted.

ENEMA probably will be necessary on third postoperative day. Prostigmine and rectal tube may have been indicated before this. Mild laxatives may be used.

MEDICATION FOR PAIN should be given fairly freely during first few days, especially if patient tends to be tense, and muscle spasms increase.

Rolling Without Assistance

This may be done in 4 to 7 days, according to patient's ability to splint back and according to amount of discomfort.

Bracing

For men: Knight spinal or similar
For women: Corset with steel reinforcements
Support usually is worn when patient begins getting up. It should be applied by nurse until patient is able to do so without twisting. He is allowed up after 2 to 3 weeks, occasionally sooner.

APPLICATION AND CARE OF BRACES

In assisting with application of the brace, make it as snug as possible. If straps and lacings do not bring the supports in close proximity to contours of the body, the brace needs adjustment.

Under back braces, it is well to wear a high cotton undershirt.

Leather may be kept in good condition with saddle soap.

Locks should be kept free of lint and should be oiled occasionally.

Screws should be checked for tightness.

Part 12. Trauma

BRAIN AND HEAD INJURIES

SKULL FRACTURE

Types

Simple linear

Simple comminuted

Compound. Requires removal of fragments with débridement. May be complicated by increasing intracranial pressure from edema or hemorrhage and by subsequent infection.

Depressed. May require elevation of bone to decompress the brain.

Complications

Brain injury

Hemorrhage

Meningitis

Brain abscess

Osteomyelitis or infected scalp wounds

Cerebrospinal rhinorrhea

BRAIN INJURY

Types

Concussion—shock of the brain resulting from its movement within and against the skull. Its symptoms are momentary loss of consciousness, dizziness, inability to think, headache and emotional instability.

Contusion—usually occurs at temporal and frontal areas. Symptoms are manifested by nervousness, headache and temporary loss of consciousness.

Lacerations of the brain—cerebrospinal fluid is bloody and under increased pressure.

Hemorrhage—arterial bleeding is very dangerous, patient can die very rapidly after loss of consciousness.

Epidural—rupture of middle meningeal artery. Its signs are coma following a head injury, recovery of consciousness (not seen in 50 per cent of cases), lapse into coma with hemiplegia, and signs of increased intracranial pressure.

Subdural—history of head injury may be lacking due to alcoholism. Signs and symptoms may develop immediately or may be delayed for several months. There are possible focal signs, alternating stupor and consciousness, shift of pineal gland seen in skull roentgenogram and signs of expanding intracranial pressure, such as headache, choked disk, nausea and vomiting, etc. Treatment is by evacuation of the clot by suction via trephine holes.

Aerocele—presence of air in the cranial cavity caused by a rent in the dura which opens through the nasal cavities. Treatment is by surgical repair to prevent meningitis.

GENERAL APPROACHES TO HEAD INJURY

Observation for signs of trauma to the brain, spinal cord or vertebra.

Stop bleeding of scalp wound.

Do not use pressure because of danger of forcing bone or blood into the cranial cavity.

Treat for shock and possible tetanus.

Slight elevation of the head.

Establish base line of vital signs every 15 to 30 minutes—particularly the level of consciousness and orientation.

Report bleeding or leakage of colorless fluid from nose, ears, eyes. Do not swab or cover them.

Narcotics and sedatives usually are contraindicated.

Move patient as a log, without flexion of head.

Symptomatic Treatment
  Headache
    Aspirin and caffeine citrate as ordered
    Ice bag as ordered
  Hyperthermia (cerebral)
    Remove woolen blankets
    Aspirin per rectum as ordered
  Hypoxia—respiratory depression, steady rise in pulse
    Caffeine as ordered
    Oxygen
    Keep airway open by
      Tongue held forward
      Patient on side
      Mouth at an angle to the mattress
      Suction whenever necessary
      Nothing by mouth if unconscious or choking on fluids
      Artificial respirations as ordered
  Seizures—*See* Convulsions, p. 188.
  Hemiplegia
    Posture in neutral alignment
    Position changed every 1 to 2 hours
    Passive exercise
    Long-term rehabilitation
  Aphasia
    Establish a method of communication
    Long-term rehabilitation

Postoperative Care

Position as ordered by the surgeon. Usually side of craniotomy is kept uppermost. Gatch level depends on position in which operation has been performed.

Establish base line of vital signs as ordered by the surgeon.

MEDICAL AND SURGICAL

Prevent injury by use of side rails, seizure precautions, wrist restraints and padded side rails whenever necessary.

Prevent wound contamination by covering moist areas with sterile compresses.

Symptomatic treatment as outlined under Symptomatic Treatment, above.

Prevent straining on defecation, retching or coughing, as this may increase intracranial pressure and start hemorrhage.

Deal with problems of personality changes such as negativism, hostility, assaultiveness, emotional lability.

Deal with problems of memory loss and disorientation.

BURNS

CLASSIFICATION

Determine Degree of Severity

FIRST DEGREE. Simple erythema or reddening of the skin accompanied by swelling. The skin remains intact.

SECOND DEGREE. Produces both erythema and destruction of the epidermis with blister formation. Deep layer of skin is destroyed; regeneration of the epithelium is possible.

THIRD DEGREE. Involves destruction of the full thickness of the skin and may also involve deeper structures.

TREATMENT

With all burns the major aim is to keep infection at a minimum. Pressure dressings are no longer the widely used method of treatment. With deep 2nd and 3rd degree burns, except for the hands, the best arrangement is now the "open method." The patient is kept on sterile bed linen, and anyone coming in contact with him wears a sterile gown and gloves and a mask. If the hands are also burned, they are generally bandaged separately in good position and are elevated. Antibiotics may or may not be used. In general, the patients are N.P.O. for the first 48 to 72 hours and fluids are replaced by "cutdown." Often a retention catheter is inserted, and the output should be kept to at least 25 to 50 ml. per hour. When the patient is ready, he is generally placed on a high vitamin, high protein and high carbohydrate diet. There is not complete agreement, but between the 10th and the 17th day, the eschar starts cracking and débridement begins. Once open wounds develop, the new granulation tissue must not be exposed. The best time for grafting depends on the doctor's decision. Some doctors start grafting at the 21st day, some not until the 40th day, and others, very much sooner. If they have not been used before, antibiotics often will be initiated at the time of débridement.

Scale for Determining Percentage of Body Burns

Head—9 per cent
Neck—1 per cent
Upper extremities—9 per cent each
Trunk—36 per cent (18% anterior, 18% posterior)
Lower extremities—18 per cent

First Aid with Burns

Keep the patient warm and quiet.

If clothing adheres, do not remove it. Cover other areas with the cleanest material available.

Get the person under medical supervision.

SHOCK

Most burn deaths in the first 2 to 3 days are due to shock; therefore, prevention of the development of shock by early recognition and appropriate treatment are essential to the patient's welfare.

First Aid

Cut away all burnt clothing. In acid burns, apply weak alkalies after flushing area thoroughly.

In electric burns, remove patient from source of current or shut off electric current.

In hot-water burns or scalds, apply cool compresses, ice, ice bags.

Cover with clean or sterile sheet.

MEDICAL AND SURGICAL

Relief of pain and anxiety—reassurance, sedatives as ordered, etc.

Keep patient warm, but do not overheat. Use light blankets—not in contact with burn.

No hot-water bottles.

Transport to hospital as soon as possible, giving fluids by mouth during journey if possible.

IMPORTANT POINTS

Check patient's temperature, pulse, respiration and blood pressure frequently until stabilized.

Keep accurate fluid balance record.

Maintain strict aseptic technic—to include masks and gowns of all those involved in the patient's care.

Keep patient in quiet, comfortable atmosphere with few visitors.

Turn patient frequently to prevent decubitus.

Encourage deep breathing to prevent hypostatic pneumonia.

Force fluids and diet as prescribed by physician caring for patient.

Keep accurate output records. Foley output measured every hour.

Prevent contracture. Stryker frame helpful.

Section 3

Maternity Nursing

THE CHALLENGE

Childbearing is a natural physiologic process. In itself it has changed little since the beginning of man. However, the revolutionary changes in obstetric care and management have sharply reduced the physical risk to mothers and babies. In addition, socio-economic changes, improved education and the availability of medical care in the United States have greatly influenced the attitudes of people toward childbearing.

Although the tremendous reduction of mortality and morbidity has eliminated a great deal of the fear connected with childbirth, new problems emerge to challenge professional persons concerned with providing and improving maternity care.

Nursing has a vital part to play in identifying and helping to find a solution to these problems. The ability of nursing to accept the challenge of future maternity care lies in the attitudes, knowledge, perception and judgment developed by nurses today.

PREMATERNAL CARE

Prematernal care begins when the female child is developing in the mother's womb and continues throughout infancy, childhood, adolescence, young adulthood, marriage and pregnancy. It is the responsibility, not of professionals alone, but of parents, friends, teachers and clergy as well. It concerns not only physical health, but also attitudes toward family, sex, marriage, childbirth and the host of factors that influence the values of the individual. It is the foundation for prenatal care.

MATERNITY NURSING

MENSTRUAL CYCLE

Menstruation is the periodic discharge of blood, mucous and epithelial cells from the uterus. Normally it occurs from puberty to menopause except during pregnancy and lactation.

ANTEPARTAL CARE

Antepartal care is the medical supervision and support given to prospective mothers during pregnancy.

Objectives

To ensure optimum physical and mental health of mother and baby.

To promote understanding of the process of childbearing and to develop confidence in their parents' ability to meet the demands that will be placed upon them.

Foundations for the baby's organs and systems are laid down before the mother misses her first menstrual period. Hereditary traits of the unborn child are determined at the time of conception. Environment, both in utero and after birth, then becomes the dominant factor. The physical and mental health of the mother and child are achieved through the combined effort of the expectant parents, the obstetrician, the nurse and other members of the health team.

Principles of Antepartal Care

The mother should be under the care of an obstetrician during the entire period of pregnancy. She should report to him as soon as pregnancy is suspected, and then, as a rule, every 4 weeks during the first half of pregnancy and every 2 weeks during the last half, until the last month when the visits may be weekly.

FIRST VISIT

Evaluation of health status—medical and obstetric history and physical examination

Evaluation of adequacy of pelvis

Blood tests—RH and typing, Hgb., test for syphilis

Arrangements for chest x-ray
Urinalysis
Immunization for polio, if necessary

RETURN VISITS
Inquiry into well-being of patient
Observation for signs of complications
Weight
TPR
Blood pressure
Urinalysis
Abdominal examination—height of fundus, position of
baby, fetal heart

PREPARATION FOR CHILDBEARING

The focus and purpose of preparation for childbirth
is to develop the inner resources of parents so that they,
through knowledge and understanding, may actively
participate in the unified effort to provide a positive
and satisfying experience for them throughout the child-
bearing period.

Individual and group conferences or classes are con-
ducted by doctors, nurses and other interested persons
in private offices, hospitals and community health agencies throughout the country. As parents gain knowledge
and understanding of the process of chilbirth and its
resulting responsibilities, their confidence in themselves
and in those to whom they have entrusted their care is
strengthened.

DURATION OF PREGNANCY

Average Duration

280 days, 40 weeks, 9 calendar months, or 10 lunar
months

Expected Date of Labor

Count back 3 months from date of last menstrual
period and add 7 days. Labor may be expected within
2 weeks before or after this date.

WEIGHT GAIN IN PREGNANCY

Suggested Weight Gain

First trimester	— to + 2 pounds
Second trimester	11 pounds
Third trimester	11 pounds
Total	20 to 25 pounds

Distribution of Weight Gain (Approximate)

Baby	7 pounds
Placenta	1 pound
Amniotic fluid	1½ pounds
Breasts	3 pounds
Uterus	2 pounds
Protein storage	4 pounds
Fluids (water)	3 pounds

Excess weight gain needs prompt attention because:
> If due to water retention, can be a sign of pre-eclampsia (*See* Preeclampsia, p. 416)
> If due to fat deposits
>> Adds strain to body
>> Can be a hazard at time of delivery
>> Is a factor in toxemia
>> Is difficult to lose after delivery

SUMMARY OF FETAL AND MATERNAL CHANGES

WEEKS OF GESTATION	GROWTH AND DEVELOPMENT OF EMBRYO-FETUS	PHYSIOLOGIC CHANGES IN MOTHER	SIGNS AND SYMPTOMS
		FIRST TRIMESTER	
Conception	Sperm and ovum unite and immediately begin to divide, until a cluster of cells like a raspberry is formed. It moves down the tube toward the uterus	Progesterone level maintained	Basal body temperature remains elevated
6th to 9th day	Settles into soft velvety uterine lining. Cluster of cells has become a thin-walled sac with a clump of cells on one side. Sends out fingerlike projections to form placenta. Has used up stored food and is living off glycogen from surrounding cells	Mucosa invaded. Glands becoming coiled and enriched by gland secretion. Secretions provide food for baby	Basal body temperature remains elevated
3 weeks	Covered with chorionic villi. Foundations for nervous systems, skin, bone, lungs and G.U. system forming	Production of estrogen and progesterone continues Chorionic activity and change in carbohydrate metabolism	Menstrual period overdue 1 week (amenorrhea) Tingling sensation of breasts Nausea Fatigue
4 weeks	Size—pigeon's egg. Length 1 cm., weight 1 Gm. Rudimentary eyes visible. Buds of arms and legs visible. Sac invaginates to form membranes surrounding amniotic fluid	Chorionic gonadotrophin produced Secretion of estrogen and progesterone continues	Aschheim-Zondek test, white mice —100 hrs. Friedman tests, rabbit—24 hrs. Frog tests: So. Am. clawed toad, 8-16 hrs. Male frog, 2-4 hrs. } 98% accurate Morning sickness (may normally last throughout 1st trimester)

SUMMARY OF FETAL AND MATERNAL CHANGES (Continued)

WEEKS OF GESTATION	GROWTH AND DEVELOPMENT OF EMBRYO-FETUS	PHYSIOLOGIC CHANGES IN MOTHER	SIGNS AND SYMPTOMS
8 weeks	Size—hen's egg. Length 1″, weight 4 Gms. Centers of ossification apparent. Hands and feet disproportionately large due to brain development	Uterus enlarged — size of orange, but ovoid. Blood supply in mucous membrane of vagina and vulva becoming very congested. Cervical glands proliferate, forming a honeycombed network filled with mucous	Frequency of urination. Chadwick's sign—purplish hue to vagina and vulva. Goodell's sign—softened consistency of cervix. Hegar's sign—compressibility of the isthmus of the uterus. Braxton Hicks contractions
12 weeks	Size—goose egg. Length 3½″, weight ½ oz. Fingers and toes evident. Placenta complete. Circulation complete. Rudimentary kidneys secrete a small amount of urine	Uterus at symphysis pubis, size of grapefruit, globular in shape	Uterus palpated at symphysis. Blood sugar rising. Pigmentation of areola. Lethargy and tiredness
		SECOND TRIMESTER	
16 weeks	Length 6″, weight 4 oz. Nasal septum and palate present. Heart beat close. Movements present. Sex can be determined	Uterus rises out of pelvis—3 fingers above symphysis	Frequency disappears. Morning sickness disappears. Secondary areola appear. Colostrum may be noted
20 weeks	Length 10″, weight 8 oz. Lanugo (downy hair) appears. Eyebrows and fingernails present. If born, fetus may make a few efforts to breathe, but invariably succumbs	Uterus half way to umbilicus. Corpus luteum begins to disappear	Mother aware of fetal movements (quickening). *Fetal heart may be heard. *Fetal movements may be felt by examiner. Uterine souffle may be heard. Ballottment may be felt. Umbilicus flush with skin

24 weeks	Length 12″, weight 1½ lb. Skin red and shiny, face wrinkled. Vernix caseosa (fatty cheesy substance) develops on skin	Fundus at umbilicus Increased blood volume	Abdomen slightly distended *Detect fetal skeleton by x-ray Palpate outline of baby Linea nigra appears Chloasma may appear Low Hg. Period of greatest weight gain—4 to 5 lbs./mo.

28 weeks	Length 14″, weight 2½ lbs. Thin and scrawny. Eyelids open. Vernix caseosa abundant. Viable. 2-4% chance of living. Fingerprints set	Fundus midway between umbilicus and xiphoid process. Thyroid and all endocrine glands are more active. Basal metabolism rising (15-25% during latter half of pregnancy) Blood volume at peak (25% increase)	Period of greatest weight gain continues—4 lb./mo. More energetic
32 weeks	Length 16″, weight 3½ lbs. Lanugo disappearing from face. Hair more abundant on head. Amniotic fluid starts to decrease. Old man appearance. Survival rate 40-50%	Fundus ⅔ way to xiphoid process Hormone relaxin affects skeletal articulations of pelvis and thoracic cage	Striae gravidarum more marked Pelvic joints progressively more relaxed Weight gain 3-4 lbs./mo.
36 weeks	Length 18″, weight 5½ lbs. Increased fat, but still very little. Nails reach finger tips. Survival rate 94%	Uterus at xiphoid process. Blood volume begins to fall. Uterus rises to highest level (about 37-38 wk.) then sinks to about level of 34th week	Shortness of breath Umbilicus protrudes Hg. starts to rise Blood pressure rises slightly Lightening Frequency returns
40 weeks	Length 20″, weight 7 lbs. Skin white or pink, not wrinkled. Little lanugo. Bones of skull ossified—nearly together at sutures	Lower uterine segment is relaxed and slightly stretched. Cervix is shortened and soft and the canal is still closed. Basal metabolism still rising (10-25%)	Increased energy

* Positive signs of pregnancy

	OBJECTIVES	SUGGESTIONS
Care of breasts	Support breasts well to prevent sagging and relieve discomfort	Supporting brassiere that lifts breasts upward and toward the opposite shoulder. Attention to wide straps without elastic, a band below the cups, adequate cup size and 2 to 3 fasteners usually meets requirement
		Breasts begin to enlarge by 2nd month of pregnancy and usually reach maximum size by end of 4th month of pregnancy. If interested in breast feeding, nursing brassieres may be purchased and worn during pregnancy as well as during lactation
	Keep nipples clean and dry to prevent soreness and cracking	Wash breasts gently each day, beginning with nipple and working out over breast with a circular motion, removing any dried material. Rinse and pat dry
	Bring out flat or inverted nipples	Grasp flat or inverted nipple between thumb and finger and gently draw out, holding for a few minutes. Repeat 4 or 5 times. This can be done 2 to 3 times a day
Bathing	Stimulate, refresh, relax	Daily baths or showers
	Avoid chilling	Avoid surf bathing, cold sponges and cold shower baths
	Avoid accidents from slipping or falling when stepping into or out of tub	Showers or sponge baths only, during last 2 months of pregnancy
Clothing	Have mother feel comfortable and look attractively groomed	Most women can wear their usual clothing until enlargement of abdomen becomes apparent (4-5 months)
	Be practical, and nonconstricting	Maternity stores have an attractive variety of clothing that hangs from the shoulders to avoid constriction
		Abdominal support is usually unnecessary for those unaccustomed to wearing a girdle, especially in early pregnancy. In the latter months, some are more comfortable in a well-fitted corset (on advice of doctor)
	Wear comfortable, well-fitted low-heeled shoes	Postural changes that occur as abdomen enlarges may be aggravated by high-heeled shoes, with resulting backache and fatigue. Low-heeled shoes should be worn during working hours

	Objectives	Suggestions
	Support stockings from shoulders or waist avoiding downward pressure on abdomen	Garters that encircle the leg should never be worn. Shoulder garters, or ones that come from the waist with front strap below enlarging abdomen are usually satisfactory
Care of teeth	Avoid foci of infection from unsound teeth	Visit dentist early in pregnancy Continue usual good hygiene and good nutrition Consult obstetrician before extensive dental work
Bowel elimination	Avoid constipation	See Constipation (Discomforts of Pregnancy, p. 406)
Marital relations	Continue in moderation until last month of pregnancy Restrict during last month of pregnancy	Usually considered harmless in moderation. Some authorities believe sexual relations in late pregnancy may bring on premature labor, rupture of membranes, bleeding or infection Sexual contact becomes repulsive to some women during pregnancy and in others there may be an increased desire for it. The husband's understanding and support are needed
Rest and Sleep	Prevent fatigue Complete day with energy to spare	Rest is the ability to relax Although 8 hours' sleep is needed by the average person, this must be varied to meet the mother's needs Frequent rest periods do much to prevent fatigue Sit rather than stand, when possible Elevate feet and legs when sitting
Nutrition	Provide for additional needs of mother's body in pregnancy Provide for development of baby	See Nutrition and Diet Therapy, p. 553
Exercise and activity	Promote well-being by steadying the nerves, promoting peace of mind and stimulating the appetite	Woman doing her own housework needs little or no planned exercise from physical standpoint. However, she needs fresh air, sunshine and diversion

MATERNAL GUIDANCE (Continued)

	OBJECTIVES	SUGGESTIONS
	Strengthen some of the muscles used during labor	Walking in the fresh air is undoubtedly best for meeting these objectives Avoid activities that might involve sudden jolts or sudden changes in balance which might result in a fall Specific sports should be discussed with the doctor. The woman accustomed to a certain sport is often permitted to continue it in moderation and at a mild pace Social activities can be continued unless they prove to be fatiguing Avoid long trips. These are especially trying during 1st trimester and last 4 weeks when frequency is a problem. Also it is reassuring to be near accustomed medical supervision
Employment	Avoid work requiring considerable manual labor, long hours, constant standing Avoid fatigue	Should be discussed with doctor. Depends on type of work, physical condition of mother and family responsibilities Some industries do not permit employment after 5th month of pregnancy

DISCOMFORTS OF PREGNANCY

DISCOMFORT	SIGNS AND SYMPTOMS	PRECIPITATING FACTORS	SUGGESTIONS
Morning Sickness	Mild nausea and vomiting. Slight weight loss	Physiologic changes of normal gestation. Possibly emotional factors	Light, sweet meal before arising. Liberal salt, low fat, limited protein, high carbohydrate in small frequent feedings (See Diet)
Heartburn	Burning sensation in lower thorax. Regurgitation of gastric contents into esophagus	Diminished gastric motility. Enlarging uterus displaces stomach upward. Cardiac sphincter of stomach is relaxed in pregnancy. Possible nervous tension and emotional disturbances. Worry, fatigue and improper diet aggravate condition	Aluminum compounds may be prescribed by doctor. Avoid sodium bicarbonate (favors water retention). Frequent small meals, omitting greasy, highly seasoned or undigestible foods
Constipation	Sluggish bowel action. Firm stool	Decreased physical exertion. Relaxation of bowel in association with relaxation of smooth muscle systems all over the body. Late in pregnancy—partial obstruction of lower bowel by presenting part of fetus	Good posture, enabling organs to function with maximum efficiency. Abundant fluids. Roughage in diet. Regular bowel habits. Exercise. Cathartics or suppositories, if ordered by doctor
Flatulence	Gas in digestive tract. Feeling of distention	Bacterial action in intestinal tract. Pressure from enlarging uterus. Lessened motility of gastrointestinal tract	Avoid gas-forming foods. Eat small amounts of food, well masticated. Regular daily elimination
Varicose veins	Enlargement in diameter of a vein with distended areas giving a knotted appearance. Dull, aching pain in legs	Hereditary tendency. Aggravated by advancing age, pregnancy and activities requiring prolonged standing	Avoid standing for long periods of time. Avoid constricting bands, belts or garters

DISCOMFORTS OF PREGNANCY (Continued)

Discomfort	Signs and Symptoms	Precipitating Factors	Suggestions
		Increased venous pressure in lower extremities, pelvic engorgement, increased blood volume, and pressure of enlarged uterus upon veins impede venous flow from extremities Relaxing effect of progesterone on plain muscle may cause lack of tone in walls of veins	Supportive type stockings Sufficient rest Elevate feet when sitting Right-angle position (lie on bed with legs extended upright against wall) several times a day, for 2 to 5 min. each time
Hemorrhoids	Varicosities of veins about lower end of rectum and anus Pain, discomfort Possible bleeding at time of delivery	Like varicosities elsewhere, they are due to pressure interfering with return venous circulation Aggravated by constipation	Relieve constipation Carefully replace into rectum if protruding Ice bag or cold compresses wet with witch hazel or Epsom salt solution Medicated ointments or suppositories may be ordered by doctor
Backache	Aching and discomfort in back	Postural changes to compensate for growing uterus Relaxation of sacro-iliac joints cause backache following excessive exertion Lax abdominal muscles allow uterus to fall forward, throwing center of gravity out of line	Good posture and body mechanics Specific exercises to condition muscles involved A well-fitted corset may be needed Appropriate shoes
Pruritus	Itching of skin	Stretching of skin of abdomen and breasts Hyperactivity of skin glands	Application of baby lotion or hand lotion Soda bicarbonate or starch baths Increased fluids Cleanliness—mild nondrying soap. Rule out glycosuria from diabetes

Discomfort	Signs and Symptoms	Precipitating Factors	Suggestions
Vaginal discharge	Increased vaginal discharge, not necessitating wearing a pad	Increased activity of glands of reproductive tract	Cleanliness
	Profuse yellow discharge Burning and frequency of urination	Possible gonorrhea	*See Gonorrhea*, p. 435
	Profuse frothy discharge Irritation and itching of vulva and vagina	Possible Trichomonas vaginalis	Good hygienic measures Doctor may suggest: Floraquin treatment Douches
	Profuse white, watery, curdy discharge Burning and itching	Possible monilia (yeast infection)	Good hygienic measures Doctor may treat with: Aqueous solution of gentian violet, 1% Babies born of infected mothers frequently develop oral thrush (*See* Thrush, p. 450)
Insomnia	Inability to sleep Wakefulness	Shortness of breath caused by activity of baby and pressure of the enlarging uterus on the diaphragm when mother is lying down	Abdominal breathing and side position following relaxation exercises Warm drink at bedtime Elevate head
Leg cramps	Painful spasmodic muscular contractions	Pressure of enlarging uterus on nerves supplying extremities Fatigue, chilling, tense body posture and insufficient calcium in diet	Quart of milk daily Force toes upward and press on knee to straighten leg Avoid fatigue

MATERNITY NURSING

MULTIPLE PREGNANCY

When two or more embryos develop in the uterus at the same time, the condition is known as multiple pregnancy. Heredity and multiparity are two important factors.

Frequency

Twins—once in 90 births
Triplets—once in 10,000 births
Quadruplets—once in 650,000 births

Development

Identical twins come from a single egg. Fertilization takes place by a single spermatozoon, and early in the ovum's development, it divides into two identical parts. Such twins are always of the same sex and show close physical and mental resemblances. They have one placenta and one chorion, but normally there are two amnions and two umbilical cords.

Nonidentical twins are more common and come from the fertilization of two ova by two spermatozoa. Such twins may be of the same sex or of opposite sexes, and the likelihood of their resembling each other is no greater than that of any brother and sister. Each twin has its own chorion, amnion, cord and placenta.

Twins are likely to be born about 2 weeks earlier than the calculated date of delivery, and the twins usually are about 1 pound lighter than single infants.

Frequent Complications

Toxemia
Postpartal hemorrhage
Uterine inertia
In addition, heaviness of the lower abdomen, back pains and swelling of the feet and the ankles are more commonly experienced in multiple than in single pregnancies.

PREMATURE LABOR

Premature labor occurs after the fetus is viable and before it has reached maturity (between 28 and 38 weeks' gestation). The cause is unknown in 60 per cent of these cases. Premature labor often is signalized by rupture of the membranes at or before its onset.

Contributing Factors

Chronic hypertensive vascular disease
Abruptio placentae
Placenta previa
Untreated syphilis
Toxemias of pregnancy
Congenital abnormalities
Multiple pregnancy
Hydramnios

Treatment

The premature infant should be given every advantage during labor and delivery by avoiding sedatives, analgesics and anesthesia to prevent a drugged infant, and by performing an episiotomy to prevent trauma.

ABORTION

The term *abortion* indicates discharge of the product of conception before the time of viability, 28 weeks.

An early abortion occurs during the first 14 weeks of pregnancy.

A late abortion occurs between the 14th and the 28th week.

An abortion is a miniature labor, and the later it occurs the more nearly it resembles a full-term labor. In late abortion there is the third stage of labor. Abortion is said to occur more frequently about the 14th week, as the attachments of the ovum are still slender and not formed fully. It is most likely to occur at the time of the regular menstrual periods.

Types

THREATENED ABORTION. Is characterized by some bleeding with cramplike pain; the membranes are unruptured, and the cervix is closed or dilated very slightly.

INEVITABLE ABORTION. Same as threatened abortion, except that the cervix is dilated and the membranes may be ruptured.

COMPLETE ABORTION. The ovum is expelled completely, usually early in pregnancy.

INCOMPLETE ABORTION. An emptying of the uterus in which some part of the secundines or embryo has been retained.

CRIMINAL ABORTION. An abortion performed with no legal or legitimate reason.

THERAPEUTIC ABORTION. An abortion performed within the law, or when, if the pregnancy were allowed to continue, the life of the mother would be at stake.

MISSED ABORTION. The fetus is retained in the uterine cavity for weeks, months or years after its death, giving rise to no symptoms, or those varying from mild to marked ones. The fetus may undergo degenerative changes.

HABITUAL ABORTION

Termination of three or more consecutive pregnancies by spontaneous abortion.

Etiology

Malformation of the genital tract; such as infantilism, retroversion
Diseases—chronic or acute
Dietary deficiencies
Severe nervous shock, fright or grief
Trauma—external injury
Defective germ plasm or endometrium
Blood incompatibility

Symptoms

Bleeding due to separation of the ovum from its uterine attachment
Cramplike pains

Treatment

Bed rest
Sedation as needed
Close observation for excessive bleeding
D&C if incomplete

PROPHYLACTIC TREATMENT. This is of the greatest importance. It implies, not merely the treatment of threatened abortion, but, when an abortion has taken place, that the cause should be ascertained and treated in order that a subsequent pregnancy may not be interrupted. Displacement of the uterus must be rectified, endometritis cured, syphilis treated, etc. During the next gestation, particular care should be observed at times corresponding to the suppressed menstrual periods and at the time of the preceding abortion.

ECTOPIC GESTATION

Ectopic gestation refers to a pregnancy in which the fertilized ovum is arrested at some point between the ovary and the uterus and there undergoes some development. The ovum may become implanted in any portion of the tube. The early stages of the development of the placenta are identical in both tubal and uterine pregnancy. The chorionic villi and fetal cells invade the wall of the tube, opening up maternal blood vessels and giving rise to rupture of the tube. In some cases, early rupture is caused by the weakened wall yielding to increased pressure. Rupture usually occurs between the 2nd and 4th months.

The majority, if not all, of abdominal pregnancies are the result of tubal pregnancies. In most instances, the embryo becomes implanted in the peritoneal cavity. Operative intervention usually is considered as soon as the diagnosis is made to save the mother's life from hemorrhage due to detached placenta. If the abdominal pregnancy goes on to term, false labor begins. This may last hours or several days. The fetus may die and become mummified and is termed a *lithopedion*. Occasionally, suppuration may take place.

Causes

Abnormalities of the ovum or of the tube that may favor growth in the tubes

Inflammatory diseases of the tubes

Symptoms

The usual early symptoms of pregnancy

Sudden, intense, knifelike pain on the affected side
Bleeding; slight vaginal or concealed
Symptoms of shock or collapse

Treatment

Keep the patient warm and quiet
Prepare for operation
Prepare for transfusion
Prepare for treatment of shock

Prognosis

Rapid recovery if diagnosed early

HYDATIDIFORM MOLE

A hydatidiform mole is a vesicular degeneration of the chorionic villi. This may develop into chorioepithelioma which is highly malignant.

Etiology

The cause of the mole is unknown.

Signs and Symptoms

Bleeding—at 1 to 3 months after conception. The amount varies and is continuous or comes at intervals.
Uterus is larger than months of gestation indicate.
Passing of cysts.
Pregnancy test shows high titer.
X-ray picture shows no fetal parts.

Treatment

Emptying of the uterus.
Blood transfusion may be indicated.

Follow-up Care

The patient should be followed closely for a year.

PLACENTA PREVIA

Placenta previa is a condition in which the placenta is attached to the lower uterine segment, and its site encroaches upon the internal os.

Types

MARGINAL PLACENTA PREVIA. The placenta is implanted low in the uterus approximating, but not encroaching upon, the internal os.

PARTIAL PLACENTA PREVIA. The placenta partially covers the internal os.

COMPLETE PLACENTA PREVIA. The placenta completely covers the internal os.

Conditions that give rise to a late fixation of the product of conception, permitting the embryo to descend and attach itself low down in the uterus, will cause this condition. This occurs more frequently in multiparous women than in primiparous ones.

Many times the condition is not diagnosed until the bleeding has begun. Bleeding from placenta previa usually occurs after the 7th month and varies greatly in severity. In some cases, the first onset may be so serious as to endanger the patient's life. Often, the first hemorrhage is slight and ceases spontaneously but recurs after several hours or days. The hemorrhage may come on at any time and, in most cases, is not connected with exertion or trauma. The cause of the hemorrhage is the separation of that part of the placenta covering the internal os, when the latter dilates, thus presenting an exposed bleeding surface.

Symptoms

Painless bleeding during the latter part of pregnancy or at the onset of labor.

Treatment and Nursing Care

The treatment includes control of the hemorrhage, promotion of delivery, prevention of infection and treatment for shock.

The most careful antiseptic and aseptic precautions are essential.

The foot of the bed may be elevated and the patient kept absolutely quiet.

These patients should be cared for in a hospital.

Fluids in the form of infusion, transfusion or plasma should be given.

The nurse should remember that bleeding during pregnancy needs prompt diagnosis and treatment. She should do all in her power to carry out her surgical technic in all treatments and should anticipate the needs of the obstetrician.

Check the fetal heart *frequently*.

If bleeding is uncontrolled, immediate delivery may be necessary, either vaginal or abdominal, depending on the placental location.

ABRUPTIO PLACENTA

This is the premature separation of a normally implanted placenta. The separation may be complete, but more often is incomplete, occurring either in the late months of pregnancy or at the beginning of labor. The bleeding may be apparent or concealed.

Etiology

The cause usually is unknown.

Toxemia of pregnancy frequently is present.

Others factors may be
  Maternal vascular disease
  Endocrine imbalance

Symptoms

Local pain and tenderness. The uterus enlarges in size and becomes very firm and boardlike.
  Bleeding
    Evident
    Concealed—suspected by the usual symptoms of hemorrhage; rapid pulse, restlessness, pallor, air hunger, etc.
  Shock
  The fetal parts may be difficult to outline.

Treatment

Preventive—good antepartal care
Treatment for shock
Treatment for control of hemorrhage
Cesarean section or vaginal delivery if cervix is favorable

Prognosis

Fetal mortality is high

Maternal mortality is high in concealed hemorrhage

TOXEMIAS

Classification by the American Committee on Maternal Welfare

Acute toxemia of pregnancy (onset after the 24th week

    Preeclampsia

        Mild

        Severe

    Eclampsia (convulsions or coma, usually both, when associated with hypertension, proteinuria or edema)

Chronic hypertensive (vascular) disease with pregnancy

    Without superimposed acute toxemia (no exacerbation of hypertension or development of proteinuria)

        Hypertension known to have antedated pregnancy

        Hypertension discovered in pregnancy (before 24th week and with postpartum persistence)

    With superimposed acute toxemia

Unclassified toxemia (data insufficient to differentiate the diagnosis)

PREECLAMPSIA

Preeclamptic toxemia may occur in the latter half of pregnancy, during labor or during the puerperium. The diagnosis must be made on the basis of signs and symptoms (albuminuria, hypertension and edema). Convulsions do not occur; it may be mild or severe.

Signs and Symptoms

Headache

Apprehension and depression

Nausea and vomiting

Edema and weight gain

Rise in blood pressure

Albumin in the urine
Visual disturbances
Epigastric pain, rapid pulse and drowsiness
Oliguria

Treatment and Nursing Care

For preventive care, good antepartal care
Proper hygiene, rest, diet, elimination and avoidance of excessive weight gain (over 20 lbs.)
Daily or more frequent check of blood pressure, urine, weight and fetal heart

CURATIVE

The patient should be put to bed
Diet—low in salt
Record the fluid intake and output
Daily administration of barbiturates or other medication to keep patient sedated
Daily administration of diuretics for limited periods of time to reduce edema
If hyperactive reflexes, restlessness, epigastric pain and headache occur, or the blood pressure rises acutely, magnesium sulfate is given intramuscularly or intravenously by single injection or continuous infusion. Morphine sulfate also may be used.
After intensive treatment has been instituted, termination of pregnancy should be considered

ECLAMPSIA

Eclampsia, one of the toxemias of late pregnancy, labor and the puerperium, is marked by convulsions and coma. Signs of an approaching eclampsia nearly always are present, and this condition rarely will occur if the patient has received proper antepartal care. Occasionally, it may be fulminating in character.

Etiology

The cause is unknown. It occurs more frequently in
Primiparous patients
Multiple pregnancies

Its mortality rate is
Maternal 10 to 35 per cent
Fetal 50 per cent

Symptoms

The prodromal signs are those of preeclamptic toxemia. Twitching of facial muscles may immediately precede the generalized convulsions.

Treatment

Prevent patient from injuring herself.

Roll a towel or pad tongue depressors to serve as a mouth gag to prevent biting the tongue.

Keep the patient quiet, as any slight irritation is likely to bring on another convulsion. Morphine and magnesium sulfate are given.

Keep a careful record of convulsions.

Watch closely for signs of beginning labor. Labor in eclamptics often is rapid, and the patient often is in labor when convulsions appear.

Carefully calculated infusions of dextrose.

Oxygen as needed.

Termination of pregnancy after control of convulsions has been achieved.

CHRONIC HYPERTENSIVE DISEASE
(With Pregnancy)

Patients with this condition usually have elevated blood pressure before pregnancy—at least a systolic pressure of 140 mm. Hg and/or a diastolic pressure of 90 or above.

Signs and Symptoms

Eyeground changes
High blood pressure with vascular changes

Treatment

The treatment is similar to that used for preeclampsia.

Prognosis

It is good for both mother and baby if the blood pressure remains below 160 systolic and if albuminuria does not appear. If the blood pressure rises, the prognosis for the fetus is grave.

HYPEREMESIS GRAVIDARUM
(See also Discomforts of Pregnancy)

Mild nausea and vomiting is a common disorder of the 1st trimester. Occasionally this progresses to a stage in which systemic effects such as acetonuria and substantial weight loss are produced. Hospitalization becomes necessary for the regulation of food and fluid. The condition is called hyperemesis gravidarum.

DIABETES MELLITUS

Diabetes affects pregnancy and pregnancy makes diabetes harder to control. Insulin requirement may be increased or decreased.

Frequent Complications

Hypoglycemia (particularly in presence of morning sickness or labor)
Toxemias of pregnancy
Accidents to fetus (spontaneous abortion, premature delivery, congenital malformations)
Large babies

Management

Meticulous supervision (medical and obstetrical)
Maintenance of good nutritional state
Prevention of excess weight gain
Hospitalization for regulation PRN and usually 3 weeks prior to term.

CARDIAC DISEASE

The main cause of heart disease in the child-bearing woman is rheumatic infection. During pregnancy the increased blood volume and body weight put a severe strain on the impaired heart, so that a certain amount of deterioration may be anticipated in the majority of cases. In determining the prognosis of heart disease in pregnancy, the classification of the American Heart Association commonly is employed. The functional capacity of the heart (how it is standing up to the strain of pregnancy) is the criterion by which the efficiency of the heart is assessed. There are four classifications:

Class 1. No limitation of physical activity
Class 2. Slight limitation of physical activity
Class 3. Marked limitation of physical activity
Class 4. Unable to carry on any physical activity without discomfort

Class 1 and 2 patients probably will go through pregnancy safely if sufficient rest can be arranged.

Class 3 and 4 patients must spend most of their pregnancy in the hospital, and, if heart failure develops during the first 12 weeks, therapeutic abortion usually is considered.

NORMAL LABOR

Labor is the process by which the mature products of conception are expelled from the mother's body. Just exactly what initiates labor is not known, but changes in hormonal balance, distention of the uterus from the growing fetus, stretching of the lower uterine segment by the fetal head and pressure on the retrocervical nervous ganglia are thought to be contributing factors.

Signs and Symptoms of True Labor

Regular, rhythmical uterine contractions
Effacement and dilatation of the cervix
Show—blood tinged mucus from vagina

The contraction of the uterus is involuntary and cannot be controlled. During labor the upper part of the uterus (fundus) contracts and retracts (shortening of muscle fiber) exerting pressure on the bag of waters or the presenting part. This in turn exerts pressure on the more relaxed lower segment and the cervix, causing them to dilate and gradually to become a thinned-out muscular tube through which the baby will pass. This process of cervical effacement and dilatation may be visualized if compared with pulling a turtle-neck sweater over the head. The neck (cervix) is taken up and opens up to permit the head to pass through.

419

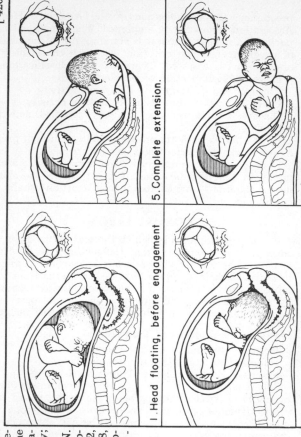

Principal movements in the mechanism of labor and delivery; L.O.A. position. (Eastman, N. J.: Williams Obstetrics, ed. 12, Chap. 15, Fig. 8, New York, Appleton - Century - Croft, 1956.)

1. Head floating, before engagement

2. Engagement; flexion, descent.

5. Complete extension.

6. Restitution, (external rotation).

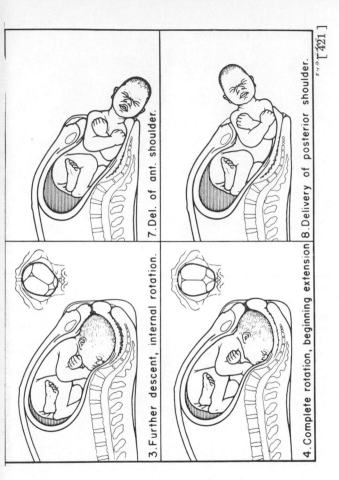

7. Del. of ant. shoulder.

8. Delivery of posterior shoulder.

3. Further descent, internal rotation.

4. Complete rotation, beginning extension

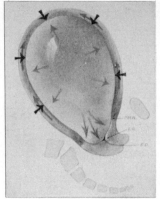
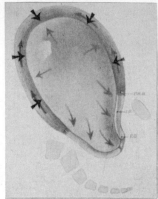

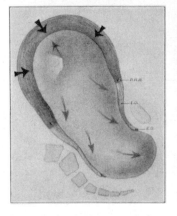

(*Top, left*) Hydrostatic action of bag of waters in effecting cervical effacement and dilatation. In absence of bag of waters, the presenting part acts similarly. Note changing relationships of external os (E.O.), internal os (I.O.), and physiologic retraction ring (P.R.R.). (*Top, right*) Hydrostatic action of bag of waters at completion of effacement. (*Bottom*) Hydrostatic action of bag of waters at full cervical dilatation. (Eastman, N. J.: Williams Obstetrics, ed. 11, Figs. 11-13, New York, Appleton-Century-Croft, 1956)

False Labor

Characterized by irregular, erratic uterine contraction without dilatation of the cervix.

Duration of Labor

This may vary from 1 to 24 hours but averages 14 hours in first labors and 8 hours in multiparous labors. Within normal limits, the length of labor is not as important as *progress* in labor. Whenever *progress* in frequency, intensity and duration of contractions is slowed or the *progress* in the dilatation of the cervix stops or the progress in the descent of the baby through the birth canal is halted, labor ceases to be normal.

The illustration on p. 424 represents a simple method for plotting the course of labor by relating cervical dilatation to hours in labor. The graphs illustrate the average curve for first and multiparous labors.

Stages of Labor

First (dilating) stage. Begins with the first true labor contraction and ends with the complete dilatation of the cervix.

Second stage (stage of expulsion). Begins with the complete dilatation of the cervix and ends with the birth of the baby.

Third (placental) stage. Begins with the birth of the baby and ends with the expulsion of the placenta.

Fourth stage. Sometimes used to describe the period from the expulsion of the placenta to the end of 1 hour postpartum.

Mechanism of Labor (See Fig. 3)

First Stage

Early Labor—Characteristics

Cervix effacing and beginning to dilate

Mild contractions starting in the back and radiating to lower abdomen, usually occurring 10 to 15 minutes apart, lasting about 30 seconds

Blood-tinged mucoid vaginal discharge

Mother may feel excited, relieved, a sense of anticipation mixed with some apprehension

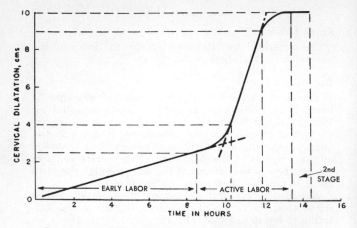

Graphic analysis: (*Top*) Mean primigravid labor pattern; (*bottom*) mean multiparous labor pattern. (Friedman, E. A.: Obstet. Gynec. (NY) 6:567 and 8:691)

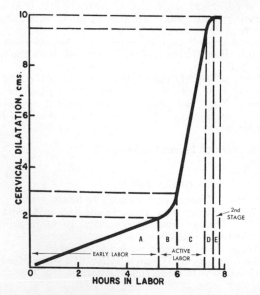

Early Labor—Mother's Needs

Reassurance

Diversion—usually not too uncomfortable. May be ambulatory (if membranes are intact) and carry on with normal activities

Time contractions

Notify doctor and prepare for hospitalization

Active Labor—Characteristics

Cervix dilates from about 3 cm. to 8 cm.

Contractions become stronger—about 3 to 5 minutes apart and lasting 45 to 50 seconds

Mother may feel apprehensive, have greater discomfort and increased pelvic pressure as active phase progresses

Active Labor—Mother's Needs

Continuous support and companionship—*do not leave the mother alone*

Reassurance in regard to condition of mother and baby

Encouragement in using breathing technics during contractions

Instructions to relax pelvic floor during rectal and pelvic examinations

Physical support such as pressure with palm of hand over sacrum during contractions, rubbing back or sponging face

Medication as contractions become stronger

Transitional Phase—Characteristics

Cervix dilating from 8 to 10 cm.—last bit of stretching

May last from 1 to 30 minutes

Contractions strong, every 2 to 3 minutes, lasting 50 to 60 seconds

Apparent amnesia between contractions

Increased bloody show

Increased pelvic pressure, stretching sensation, pain

Increasing restlessness, may have shaking legs

May have perspiration on upper lip and forehead, may feel flushed

May have nausea, hiccoughing, vomiting

May have half-hearted desire to push with contractions

Mother may feel frustrated, irritable, sensitive to palpation or examination, finds it difficult to cope with contractions

May want to be "put to sleep"

Transitional Phase—Mother's Needs

Constant support and observation

If desire to push is present, may be controlled by rapid chest breathing during contractions. Mother should *not push* until cervix is fully dilated

Need for medication to relieve discomfort

SECOND STAGE

Characteristics

May last from 2 to 60 minutes or more

Cervix fully dilated—10 cm.

Strong, expulsive contractions accompanied by an almost uncontrollable urge to push or bear down

Expulsive grunt when exhaling during contraction

Increased bloody show

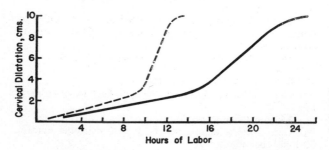

Uterine dysfunction. Composite labor curve denoting prolongation of both the latent and the active phases. Broken line represents the mean curve. (From Friedman) (Eastman, N. J.: Williams Obstetrics, ed. 11, p. 823, New York, Appleton-Century-Croft, 1956.)

Involuntary drawing up and separation of legs

Amnesia between contractions

Increased pelvic pressure and stretching sensation

Rectal bulging, pouching of anus, gradual bulging of perineum, separation of labia and appearance of presenting part at vaginal orifice

See illustration for mechanism of normal L.O.A. presentation

Mother's Needs

Constant support and coaching in using her urge to push with contractions. Instruct mother to take a deep breath (hold knees or, if on delivery table, hold hand grip) and, holding breath with mouth closed, raise head off table and push down with diaphragmatic and abdominal muscles. At the same time, the pelvic floor muscles should be relaxed

Push throughout contraction, rest in between

Stop pushing as presenting part crowns and assist the doctor by panting as he delivers the infant

THIRD STAGE

Characteristics

May last from 1 to 20 minutes or more

Uterine contractions—painless

Mother usually relieved, relaxed, tired

Signs of placental separation:

Uterus contracts, rises in abdomen and assumes globular shape

Cord lengthens

Trickle or gush of blood from the vagina

Mother may be thirsty or hungry, eager to see baby

Mother's Needs

To be assured of baby's condition and identification

To be congratulated on her achievement

To be instructed to push down with uterine contraction to expel the placenta *after* signs of separation have occurred

If physician elects to express the placenta, the mother should be instructed to relax and facilitate the maneuver

MATERNITY NURSING

Characteristics

Uterus is firm with continuous intermittent contractions

Moderate vaginal bleeding—2-3 pads in the first hour

Feeling of exhaustion or, conversely, exhilaration

May have tremors or "nervous chill"

Mother's Needs

Careful observation of vaginal bleeding, consistency of uterus, and temperature, pulse and blood pressure

Rest in a warm, comfortable bed

Fluids, unless contraindicated

NURSING CARE OF THE MOTHER IN LABOR

There are two main objectives of nursing care in labor.

1. Safety—for mother and baby
2. Satisfaction—of the mother's physical, emotional and information needs

To Ensure Safety for Mother and Baby

1. Review record of antepartal course and record all pertinent data pertaining to her care throughout labor
2. Maintain asepsis—perineal shave and enema usually are ordered
3. Maintain hydration by offering fluids unless contraindicated
4. Time contractions—(from beginning of one to beginning of next and from beginning to end of contraction)—record progress
5. Take temperature, pulse and blood pressure every 4 hours
6. Check fetal heart rate every 15 to 30 minutes during first stage, after each contraction during second stage and immediately after rupture of membranes
7. Encourage frequent voiding
8. Avoid fatigue by encouraging rest and relaxation

9. Watch for signs of fetal distress
   a. Absent, irregular, rapid (over 160) or slow (below 120) fetal heart rate
   b. Hyperactivity of fetus
   c. Meconium stained leakage of vagina
10. Watch for maternal danger signs
    a. Vaginal bleeding
    b. Long, painful contractions (over 75 sec.)
    c. Elevation of blood pressure, headache, vomiting
    d. Elevation of temperature, pulse and respirations
    e. Slowing down or cessation of contractions
    f. Exhaustion
    g. Dehydration
    h. Precipitant delivery
11. *Never leave a mother in active labor alone*

Promote Satisfaction by Meeting Mother's Needs*

1. To be sustained by another human being
2. To have relief of pain
3. To be assured of a safe outcome for herself and baby
4. To have her attitude toward and behavior during labor accepted
5. To receive bodily care

INDUCTION OF LABOR

Induction of labor may be used in preeclampsia or other circumstances where initiation of labor is indicated. The procedure consists of artificial rupture of membranes followed by stimulation with highly dilute intravenous Pitocin. Administration of Pitocin should always be under the direct surveillance of the physician.

EPISIOTOMY

Episiotomy is a surgical incision of the perineum employed in the second stage of labor to facilitate delivery. The incision may be:

* Lesser, Marion S., and Keane, Vera R., Nurse-Patient Relationships in a Hospital Maternity Service, p. 100, St. Louis, Mosby, 1956.

Median—directed straight down toward rectum

Medial-lateral—directed down at angle about 1 inch to left or right of rectum

Lateral—directed to side at right angle to the rectum

CESAREAN SECTION

Cesarean section is a surgical operation by which the child is removed from the uterus through an incision in the abdominal and the uterine wall. The most common indications for this procedure are dystocia, toxemia of pregnancy and hemorrhage (placenta previa or abruptio).

COMPLICATIONS OF LABOR
DYSTOCIA (DIFFICULT LABOR)

This is the cessation of *progress* in labor as a result of the mechanisms involved.

Causes of Dystocia

UTERINE DYSFUNCTION OR UTERINE INERTIA. A prolongation of any of the phases of labor as a result of ineffective, weak or in-co-ordinated uterine contractions. Uterine dysfunction may be precipitated by overdistention of the uterus, emotional disturbances or injudicious use of analgesic agents.

ABNORMAL POSITION OR PRESENTATION OF THE FETUS. Aberrations of the normal occiput anterior presentation (such as occiput posterior, breech, face, brow or shoulder presentation) may precipitate an arrest of the passage of the fetus through the pelvis.

CEPHALOPELVIC DISPROPORTION. Any substantial diminution of the capacity of the pelvic canal that makes passage of the fetus difficult or impossible.

ABNORMALITIES OF THE FETUS OR THE GENITAL TRACT. Hydrocephalus, tumors and similar abnormalities may be severe enough to interfere with the normal mechanism of labor.

INJURIES TO THE BIRTH CANAL

Perineal Lacerations

First degree—involving skin and mucous membranes

Second degree—involving perineal muscle but not the sphincter muscles

Third degree—involves perineal and sphincter muscles and may extend through anterior wall of rectum

Lacerations of the cervix, the vaginal sidewalls, the vulva and the tissue surrounding the clitoris and the urethra also may occur in difficult or precipitous labor.

EMERGENCY DELIVERY

What to Do Until Doctor Arrives

Keep your head—don't panic. Thousands of babies come into the world every day with no one to help them.

Mother and baby need immediate help

Baby must breathe.

Mother needs reassurance.

Care for both at same time

Pick baby up gently by the feet, head down, to prevent aspiration of fluid. Encourage mother. After baby cries, place him or her gently on the mother's abdomen where she can see him. This will be reassuring to her, and the weight over the uterus will help it to contract.

Do not touch perineal area—*danger*—infection

Do not pull on cord—*danger*—hemorrhage

If placenta is not delivered

Wait for signs of separation (*see* Third Stage). Nature knows her job. When placenta is delivered, wrap the baby and the placenta in a blanket. Do not cut cord under unsterile conditions.

After placenta is expelled

Feel uterus—must be firm like grapefruit. Danger is hemorrhage. *If* soft and mushy, massage gently until it contracts. Put baby to breast—this may help uterus to contract.

Make mother and baby comfortable and warm.

Give mother fluids.

Encourage mother to move. If she is not in bed or a place where she can lie down, she may move to a more suitable environment.

Instruct mother on care of herself

Need for fluids, food, rest.

Explain the need for uterus to contract, teach her
to feel it periodically and to get help if bleeding
becomes excessive.

Instruct mother in care of baby

Security and warmth—simply by keeping baby
close to her body.

Gentleness in handling.

Nursing—sufficient for baby's nutritional needs.

For choking or cyanosis—hold baby upside down,
clear trachea.

Explain why cord has not been cut.

Emphasize that mother is giving the baby the
essential care it needs.

Summary

Mother needs

Reassurance—someone who knows what to do

Protection against infection—hands off vaginal area

Protection against hemorrhage—hold uterus for
one hour after delivery—massage gently if soft
and flabby—put baby to breast

Nutrition—fluids, food

Baby needs

To breathe—wipe nose and mouth—hold with head
down

Protection against infection—hands off cord—don't
bathe, skin is protected by vernix

Nutrition, warmth, security—all can be supplied by
mother.

Identification—(if in time of disaster) put tag
around baby's wrist with name, date, sex, parents' names, etc.

POSTPARTAL PERIOD
(Puerperium)

The puerperium is the period during which the genital
organs and tract return to their nonpregnant size and
condition following pregnancy and labor and lasts approximately 6 weeks. This is a normal physiologic process but must be watched lest pathologic conditions
develop.

Objectives

Provide medical and nursing care to meet the mother's physical and emotional needs

Give support and encouragement

Explain changes occurring in her body

Give instruction in the care of mother and infant

NURSING CARE DURING THIS PERIOD

Involution

This is the process by which the uterus returns to its nonpregnant state. It is evidenced by:

Firm consistency of the uterus

Steady descent into the pelvis

Normal lochia

Lochia

Rubra: 1 to 3 days, dark red in appearance due to blood from the placental site plus mucus and decidua

Serosa: 6 to 7 days, reddish brown due to serum from healing surfaces

Alba: appears usually by the 10th day, whitish-yellow, disappears around the 14th day

Afterpains

These are caused by contraction and relaxation of uterine muscle. They are more frequent in multiparas, due to poorer tone of the uterine muscle, and also during the nursing period of mothers who are breast feeding, due to action of the parasympathetic nervous system.

Treatment and nursing care:

Administration of analgesics, usually codeine, 30 to 60 mg., and aspirin, 5 to 10 grains

Explanation of cause

Reassurance of patient

Daily Observations

Uterus, for height, consistency and size

Lochia, for amount, color and consistency

Perineum, for normal progress in healing and early detection of infection

PERINEAL CARE. At the present time there is so much variation in perineal care procedures that we do not recommend any one specific technic. The use of sterile water or antiseptic solutions seems of little value since the perineum is considered dirty from an antiseptic point of view, and since solutions would not be in contact long enough to have a germicidal effect. Cleansing the perineum by pouring solutions from a pitcher is outmoded, because this practice may wash organisms from the perineal area into the vaginal canal.

The aims are to make the mother clean and comfortable while preventing infection. Most hospitals use disposable washcloths or cotton balls to accomplish this.

CARE OF THE BLADDER. A distended bladder is one of the causes of postpartal hemorrhage. Catheterization should be avoided if possible, as there is danger of infection due to the presence of lochia and the bladder trauma resulting from labor and delivery. The patient should be encouraged to void 8 to 12 hours following delivery. If the bladder appears distended before this period, it should be emptied by catheterization if the patient is unable to void. The output of urine during the first 2 or 3 days is greater than normal, and retention occurs frequently.

CARE OF THE BOWELS. Constipation often is noted in the postpartal period. After the preliminary cathartic, which is ordered by the physician, the bowels usually can be regulated by fluids, diet and the establishment of a time habit.

Progression and Activity

Any position the patient finds comfortable is permitted. Semi-Fowler's position and activity while in bed should be encouraged. Usually, activities are increased gradually. The patient may be out of bed for 10 minutes on the first day postpartum and may get up progressively the following days as decided by the doctor.

Supportive Care

Since childbearing is a normal physiologic process, the emotional components are as important as the physical ones. A mother's reaction to her newborn baby often is dependent on her acceptance or rejection, in early life, of her parents and family, sex education and marriage, as well as her later reaction toward pregnancy itself.

COMPLICATIONS OF THE POSTPARTAL PERIOD

COMPLICATION	ETIOLOGY	SIGNS AND SYMPTOMS	TREATMENT	NURSING CARE	PROGNOSIS
Mastitis	*Staphylococcus aureus* *Streptococcus pyogenes* *Micrococcus pyogenes*	Pain in one quadrant of the breast Redness Swelling of the affected part Chill Elevation in temperature Malaise	*Prophylactic* Washing hands Prevention of fissured nipples *Symptomatic* Ice bags Supporting breast binder Infant is taken from the breast temporarily *Medication* Antibiotics or chemotherapeutic agents Analgesics	Instruction in good breast hygiene Careful daily inspection of breasts, especially the nipple area Administration of treatment ordered	Favorable Recovery is usually prompt following treatment
Postpartum hemorrhage	Uterine atony Retained secundines Precipitate labor Lacerations along the birth canal Vulvar varicosities Blood dyscrasias	Blood loss of 500 cc. or more Evidence of shock Boggy uterus on palpation	*Prophylactic* Proper management of fundus during the hours immediately following delivery Oxytocic preparations *Symptomatic* Uterine and vaginal packing may be necessary Shock therapy Hysterectomy when bleeding not controlled otherwise Removal of placental fragments by curettage Blood transfusions	Observation of: Fundus, height and consistency Vital signs Bleeding, amount, color and consistency	Favorable if bleeding is controlled
Late postpartum hemorrhage (Same as above, but occurs after first 24 hours following delivery)					

COMPLICATIONS OF THE POSTPARTAL PERIOD (Continued)

COMPLICATION	ETIOLOGY	SIGNS AND SYMPTOMS	TREATMENT	NURSING CARE	PROGNOSIS
Puerperal Infections: Types Endometritis Parametritis Peritonitis or pelvic cellulitis Pelvic thrombophlebitis (see above) Septicemia	Streptococcus Staphylococcus Gonococcus Colon or gas bacillus Any pus-producing organism	Malaise, headache, backache and general discomfort Chilly sensations or a distinct chill Elevation of temp. as high as 105-106° F. Scant, odorless lochia to profuse foul-smelling lochia	*Prophylactic* Asepsis during labor and throughout the puerperium *Symptomatic* Sulfonamide and antibiotic therapy Promotion of drainage by placing the patient in Fowler's position Blood transfusion or plasma	The patient should be kept quiet and as comfortable as possible	Favorable with treatment
Urinary tract involvement	Bladder atony due to overdistention Trauma Presence of bacteria	Inability to void or Urinary frequency Inability to empty bladder Burning on urination Temperature elevation Incontinence	*Prophylactic* Frequent emptying of bladder during labor and immediately postpartum Instruction in good personal hygiene Catheterize every 8 hours or p.r.n. *Symptomatic* Sulfonamides and/or antibiotics Instillation of mild antiseptic irritant Indwelling catheter, if involvement is severe	Observation Aseptic technic	Favorable with treatment
Phlebitis (See Medical-Surgical Section, p. 296)					

Fears and apprehensions may accompany pregnancy for the mother who knows little about the whole process, causing resentment. Even if the child is wanted, she may vacillate between happiness and resentment. The role of the doctor or nurse in teaching the patient about the physical and emotional changes taking place during pregnancy, parturition and the postpartal period is invaluable in alleviating many of her anxieties. Her husband can be equally important in planning with her for enough pleasant diversion and relaxation during pregnancy so that she will avoid both boredom and overexertion.

After the baby is born, the mother is often keyed up and oversensitive. Underlying this may be a feeling of inadequacy to care for her child. This may be overcome to a great extent by mothers' classes and individual teaching and encouragement by the nurse and doctor.

Many mothers go through a period of moderate depression the 3rd or 4th postpartal day. Often this is referred to as the "third-day blues." At this time the climax and excitement of childbirth are over and yet she may have minor discomforts such as engorgement, after-pains and perineal discomfort. She is also getting tired of the hospital routine, and longs for home and familiar surroundings. The full realization that the baby is completely dependent on her may come after the mother leaves the hospital. This causes an overwhelming emotional feeling, particularly if she does not realize the necessity of self-sacrifice as well as the satisfaction and enjoyment involved in being a parent.

THE NORMAL NEWBORN

The relief that comes to parents once the baby is born is followed by their concern over the mental and the physical condition of their baby and their ability to be good parents. It is important for them to know what a newborn looks like and how he behaves before their baby is born.

The nurse, who, with the doctor, functions as teacher for these parents, must have a sound understanding of the physical characteristics and the behavior of the normal newborn infant and must be able to interpret them to the parents.

THE NORMAL NEWBORN

	PHYSICAL APPEARANCE	BEHAVIOR
Weight at birth	Average: 7-7½ lbs. (3,178-3,405 Gm.) Normal: 5½-9½ lbs. (2,500-4,300 Gm.)	10% of birth weight usually lost by end of 3-4 days. This is regained by end of 2 weeks
Length	19"-21" (48-53 cm.)	
Head	¼ total length Circumference 12½"-14" 31-35 cm.) Skull bones not united, leaving two soft spots (anterior fontanel, diamond shaped, closes approx. 1½ years; posterior fontanel, triangle shaped, closes 6-8 weeks) Moulding may or may not be present Hair may or may not be present	Can raise head for a short time when prone and not at all when supine
Face	Nose flat and pudgy Eyes have no expression, may appear crossed due to weak muscle. Blue-gray in color, except for some Negro babies Lower jaw appears to recede Lips—upper lip may have small tubercle resembling blister, due to sucking Tongue does not extend far beyond the margin of the gum, sometimes giving the appearance of being tongue-tied	Eyes closed most of time Reacts to bright lights and large objects Sucking reflex well developed. May suck fingers or entire fist. Lips sensitive and this reflex is stimulated by touch "Rooting" reflex present when cheeks touched
Neck	Short—head appears to be resting directly on shoulders. Muscles weak	Unable to support head because of weak muscles. Falls when not supported
Chest	Round Breast engorgement may be present in either male or female, due to placental transmission of hormones from mother to baby Respirations—irregular	Abdomen—not chest—moves when breathing

Abdomen	Round—protrudes because of size of abdominal organs in relation to rest of body. Poor muscle tone— diastasis of abdominal muscles
Extremities	Arms and legs flexed (fetal position) Legs bowed. Hands semiclosed
Color	Ruddy complexion. Extremities may be cyanotic due to poor circulation Skin may appear mottled with prominent superficial veins
Skin	Thin. Peeling may be present on trunk and extremities Areas of hemangiomatosis may be present on eyelids, nose, upper lips and neck Petechia may be present on face Vernix caseosa—cheeselike material covers body Some areas may be covered with a downy hair (lanugo) In Oriental, Negro and Mediterranean people there may be a triangular area on back of buttocks that is bluish-gray These skin reactions are normal and will disappear as the infant grows older

When awake baby jerks, wiggles and has continuous, purposeless movements of legs and arms arches back. When not eating, the baby will be sleeping; he twitches, stretches, yawns, sneezes and makes peculiar noises during sleep

Nursing Observations

RESPIRATIONS

Rate: The normal respiratory rate for the newborn infant is considered to be 35 to 45 respirations per minute but may vary 20–100 per minute.

Rhythm: Respirations are usually irregular with brief periods of apnea.

Characteristics: Abdominal-diaphragmatic breathing rather than chest breathing is done. Discharges collect in the nasal passage, causing breathing to sound stuffed up.

[439]

BOWEL MOVEMENTS

TYPE	COLOR AND CONSISTENCY	NUMBER	DAY OF LIFE	SIGNIFICANCE
Meconium plug	Thick grayish-white mucous plug 2-5 cm. in length	1	1st or 2nd	Usually precedes first meconium stool
Meconium	Thick, black, sticky, tarry	4-5	1-3	Absence of gastrointestinal obstruction
Transitional	Thin, slimy with some undigested food, brown-green in color	1-6	3-5	Remaining meconium plus the first feedings
Breast fed	Golden, orange-yellow, soft, mealy	1-8	4-5+	
Formula fed	Light, yellow pasty	1-3	4-5+	
Diarrhea	Pale yellow or grass green; watery mucous, pus or blood is rare but may be present	Frequent		Should be reported immediately, and infant should be isolated

URINE

Frequency: Twelve to fifteen times daily
Color: Usually pale yellow, but diaper may be stained pink due to uric acid crystals

OBSERVATIONS DURING MORNING CARE

Observation	Appearance	Significance
Fontanel	Should be flat	Sunken fontanel may mean dehydration; bulging fontanel may mean infection or tumor growth
Position	Head should be in mid-line position and give impression of good balance. No mechanical difficulty in turning it from right to left should be present. Extremities flexed; fists semiclosed	Any habitual flexion of head to one side accompanied by rotation of chin to opposite side is abnormal. Any flaccidity is abnormal
Cry	Lusty	
Reactions	Reaction to sudden noises or abrupt movements should elicit Moro reflex; arms and legs should move freely	Limited movement or failure to move a limb should be reported
Umbilical cord	Should appear to be drying; oozing may be present. Should be kept dry and clean	Bleeding or signs of infection should be reported
Breasts	May be engorged and oozing	Should be left alone. Engorgement is a hormonal reaction and will subside
Sucking	Vigorous	Indicative of infant's ability to swallow
Weight loss	Initial weight loss the first 3-4 days of life should not exceed 10% of birth weight	Marked weight loss on 3rd day with temperature elevation usually means dehydration. It should be reported so that additional fluids can be given

OBSERVATIONS DURING MORNING CARE (Continued)

OBSERVATION	APPEARANCE	SIGNIFICANCE
Color	Jaundice	Within the first 24 hours should be called to physician's attention immediately
	Jaundice on 2nd or 3rd day	Usually considered physiologic and should disappear by the end of the 2nd week
	Acrocyanosis	Usually caused by immaturity of the circulatory system; if extensive should be reported
Genitalia	Girl—Vaginal discharge or bleeding	Hormonal reaction and will subside
	Boy—Circumcision, for bleeding or infection	Excessive bleeding or signs of infection should be reported
Mouth	Pink and moist	White patches on tongue and buccal surfaces may be indicative of thrush (*See* Disorders of the Newborn, p. 449)

INFANT FEEDING

BREAST FEEDING

The most suitable food for the baby is breast milk, because it contains the essential food constituents for the baby in the most digestible form.

Objectives

To promote confidence of the mother in her own ability to breast feed

To promote complete emptying of the breasts by
    Correction of retracted or inverted nipples
    Prevention of extreme or prolonged engorgement
    Putting the infant to breast when hungry
    Making certain that the infant is not filling up on air

To promote adequate relaxation in order to decrease tension

To promote good circulation

Each breast is composed of fifteen to twenty lobes, each of which is composed of lobules. These lobules contain many cells with an epithelium lining in which milk is produced. They are connected by ducts opening into a larger duct, which empties into a collecting sinus, or ampulla, at the base of the nipple.

Successful lactation presupposes adequate glandular tissues, the hypertrophy incident to pregnancy and the liberation of the secretion.

Colostrum, the breast secretion prior to the establishment of the milk flow, is higher in protein and lower in fat than breast milk.

Engorgement

This is a venous and lymphatic stasis of the breasts in preparation for lactation. Usually it occurs on the 3rd and 4th days of the puerperium and lasts for about 48 hours. This condition occurs about 24 hours earlier in the multiparous patient than the primiparous patient. It is manifested by pain, redness and swelling. Such palliative measures as supporting binder, ice bags and sedatives will provide the relief needed. During the engorgement period, the baby should be allowed to nurse for short periods.

Milk Secretion

Breast milk usually begins to flow on the 3rd or the 4th day after the birth of the baby. It is stimulated by the baby's nursing.

Care of the Breasts

The breasts should be washed gently with soap and water daily. The mother should wash her hands thoroughly before nursing the baby. The baby should grasp the entire nipple, and the length and frequency of nursing periods should be limited.

Sore Nipples

A complaint of sore nipples should not be overlooked as this may lead to an abrasion or fissure. Prophylactic measures are: short nursing periods, nursing on alternate breasts at feeding time and the local application of ointments.

Cracked Nipples

If the nipples become cracked, the baby should not nurse for a 24-hour period, to allow time for healing. Various ointments may prove to be helpful. Occasionally, if the condition does not respond to treatment, the baby must be removed from the breasts permanently.

FORMULA FEEDING

The doctor will prescribe the formula. If no pediatrician has been chosen, a standard formula approved by the medical staff and adopted by the hospital, will be used.

The doctor will also advise concerning the feeding schedule. For the normal baby a 3 to 5 hour schedule usually is used, although considerable variation is permitted.

PREPARATION AND COMPOSITION OF FORMULA (*see* Diet, p. 578)

WARMING THE BOTTLE. If using a screw-on cap, loosen cap. Gently shake bottle before warming. Warm the bottle by standing it in a pan of hot water. To test for the right temperature, dry the bottle, remove the cap and drop a few drops of milk on the inside of the wrist.

They should feel warm. If using nipples with a cross cut instead of holes, it will be necessary to shake the bottle to get the drops for testing.

ENLARGING NIPPLE HOLES. The holes in most of the new nipples are too small. There are two ways to enlarge the holes:

Method 1. Using a razor blade, make two small cuts (about $1/4$-$1/8$ in.) through the rubber so that the cuts form a cross. No milk will come through the nipple until the baby sucks. Nipples cut out in this way are available in many drug stores. The cut is called a cross-cut or crucial incision.

Method 2. Stick the eye of a needle into a cork; the cork will form a handle. Hold the needle in a flame until it is red hot and then make one stab in each hole of the nipple. Repeat if necessary. The holes should be large enough to allow the milk to drop quickly from the bottle without pouring in a stream (at about the same rate of speed of a clock ticking).

FEEDING OF FORMULA OR WATER. Hold the baby in an upright position to feed. Be sure the bottle is held up so that the neck of the bottle is always full of milk. After each feeding the baby should be held in the upright position and patted gently on the back to help bring up the air he may have swallowed. This may be necessary several times during a feeding.

The regular water supply of some cities does not require boiling before offering to the infant to drink. If you are in doubt of the water supply, sterilize a bottle of water at the time of formula sterilization. If the infant cries, or it is otherwise indicated, water may be offered halfway between feedings. Water need not be warmer than room temperature.

CARE OF THE NIPPLES AND BOTTLES AFTER USE. Immediately after feeding the baby, rinse the nipples in cold running water. Force the water through the holes in the nipples to remove any milk that might clog the holes. Drain the nipples and allow them to stand exposed to the air.

Throw away any formula left in the bottle. Rinse and then fill the bottles with cold water. Leave to soak until they are washed.

DISORDERS OF THE NEWBORN

Complication	Etiology	Signs and Symptoms	Treatment	Nursing Care	Prognosis
Asphyxia neonatorum	Obstruction of air passages with mucous or amniotic fluid	*Mild asphyxia* The baby presents a congested or livid appearance, marked cyanosis, satisfactory but slow pulse; muscle tone remains good	Observe the principles of resuscitation: Clear the air passages Mouth-to-mouth breathing Keep the baby warm	Carrying out of treatment ordered Observation Reporting of any change in condition	Favorable, responding well to external stimuli
	Interference with placental circulation because of tetanic contraction, prolonged labor, separation of placenta, prolapsed cord	*Severe asphyxia* The baby presents a pale and waxy appearance, lips blue, body limp. The only evidence of life is a slow, weak, or perhaps very rapid heartbeat audible only with a stethoscope	Stimulate respiration by: Certain resuscitative apparatus, such as Flagg or Kreiselman resuscitators Medications: respiratory and heart stimulants		Grave, usually due to cerebral injury
	Narcosis due to drugs such as morphine and the barbiturates				
	Cerebral injury				
	Hemorrhage		Oxygen by catheter, mask or bed		
Atelectasis	Obstruction of the bronchi from aspiration of mucous or amniotic fluid	Respiratory grunt Respirations shallow and rapid Mostly abdominal respirations Pallor and cyanosis	*See* Asphyxia neonatorum, above	*See* Asphyxia neonatorum, above	This is dependent upon the establishment of adequate expansion of the lungs
	Cerebral damage resulting in interference with normal				

	function of the respiratory center, thorax and respiratory muscles / Poorly developed or displaced lung due to an enlarged heart or diaphragmatic hernia				
Caput succedaneum	Birth injury following prolonged labor in which the membranes have ruptured before the cervix is fully dilated	Diffuse compressible and movable swelling on presenting part of head, usually the occipital region	None. The area is absorbed and disappears within a few days	Observation	Favorable
Cephalhematoma	Birth injury causing hemorrhage beneath the periosteum and occurring most often on one or both parietal bones. Occurs frequently after forceps delivery but may occur after a normal delivery	Usually not apparent immediately following birth. Swelling of scalp, quite similar in appearance to caput suc. However, there is a gradual increase in size during first week of life	No specific treatment. Swelling disappears spontaneously in 6-8 weeks	Observation	Favorable
Diarrhea	See Section on Pediatrics.				

DISORDERS OF THE NEWBORN (Continued)

COMPLICATION	ETIOLOGY	SIGNS AND SYMPTOMS	TREATMENT	NURSING CARE	PROGNOSIS
Erb's paralysis (arm)	Caused by stretching and tearing of the brachial plexus during delivery	Entire arm hangs limp and the hand rotates inward Movement of the fingers usually is present	Same as that followed for nerve injuries: Put the part at rest The aim is to keep the muscles relaxed without stretching The doctor may order this position maintained by securing the arm with bandages	Observation Care in handling of infant	Recovery depends on the extent of injury to the 5th and 6th cervical nerves Usually disappears within several weeks but may be permanent
Facial paralysis	Usually caused by pressure of forceps during delivery	Paralysis of the muscles of one side of the face, more noticeable when infant is crying or feeding	Observation	Observation	Usually disappears within several hours or days
Hemorrhage (cord)	Usually due to slipping of cord tie or clamp	Bleeding from cord stump	Application of new ligature or clamp	Observation	Favorable
Hemorrhagic Disease of the Newborn	Internal or external bleeding	Blood characteristics: Increase in bleeding and clotting time	Blood transfusions Vitamin K	Observation	Favorable Infant usually responds quickly to treatment

Platelets may be
  decreased
Marked reduction
  in prothrombin
Digestive tract
  signs:
Blood stained vom-
  itus
Tarry stools
Bleeding from skin
  or cord stump
In severe cases:
Fever
Icterus
Anemia
Cyanosis
Convulsions

Ophthalmia neonatorum	Gonococcus (most frequent cause) Streptococcus pneumococcus, colon, diphtheria or influenza bacilli	Acute severe inflammation of eyes or conjunctiva characterized by: Redness or swelling of the lids Purulent discharge becoming profuse Granular appearance of conjunctiva Clouding of the cornea One or both eyes may be affected	*Prophylactic* One drop of 1% AgNO₃ in each eye Penicillin ophthalmic ointment (100,000 U per gram) *or* Aqueous penicillin drops, 5,000 U per ml. Isolation Protection of sound eye if only one eye affected *Symptomatic* Cold compresses may be ordered Irrigation of eyes	Isolation precautions Observation Administration of treatment as ordered	Favorable if treatment instituted early

COMPLICATION	ETIOLOGY	SIGNS AND SYMPTOMS	TREATMENT	NURSING CARE	PROGNOSIS
			with normal saline q. 1 hour or more frequent if necessary Daily smears for diagnosis Antibiotics orally, locally or intramuscularly		
Thrush	A.P. Discomforts of Pregnancy *Monilia albicans* (*Candida albicans*) (*see* vaginal discharge) May be transmitted by nipples, vagina or careless hygiene	White patches over the tongue and buccal surfaces Microscopic exam of smear establishes diagnosis	*Prophylactic* Avoidance of trauma to infant's mouth either in immediate postpartal care or nursery care Stress personal hygiene of mother's hands at nursing Cleanliness of mother's nipples and of bottles and nipples *Symptomatic* Swab the mouth with 25% solution of sodium borate in glycerine Swab or paint the mouth with gentian violet 1% aqueous solution	Daily inspection of infant's mouth Hand, bottle and nipple precautions	Favorable

				Suspension of nystatin, 100,000 u/cc, 10 gtts. 4 × daily after feeding
Icterus neonatorum (physiologic jaundice)	Inadequate liver function and destruction of red blood cells during first week of life	Appearance of jaundice on 3rd-5th day of life	Observation	Favorable (usually lasts only a few days)
Erythema toxicans (newborn rash)	Not known	Blotchy erythematous rash usually appearing on back, shoulders or buttocks	Observation	Favorable (usually disappears in a few days)

THE PARENTS TAKE THE BABY HOME

Anticipatory Guidance

In the early stages of growth and development, satisfactory emotional experiences are of great importance. The infant already knows the frustration of being hungry and the satisfaction of being fed. His first social contact has been with the people who held him for his feedings. The parents will need to know how to satisfy their baby's hunger and how to provide experiences that satisfy a younger baby.

Feeding Technics

All babies swallow air. This can cause colic. The baby should be kept warm and held securely in an upright position to help him get rid of the air. This takes patience and time. This must be done, as often as necessary, before, during and after feeding.

Hunger pains are irregular for about 3 months, so the baby should be fed when he is hungry, every 3 to 5 hours. He soon will settle down to a routine, but it may seem at first that he wants to eat all the time. The parents must be warned to meet their child's needs and not to worry about what the neighbors and relatives think.

Experiences That Satisfy

Things to look at, grasp and reach for.

People who talk, sing and smile at the infant.

An environmental temperature that provides warmth without overheating, 72-80°.

Being held, rocked and comforted.

Being fed by a relaxed person who is gentle and who takes the time to hold the baby.

Section 4

Nursing of Children

GROWTH AND DEVELOPMENT

Growth denotes increase in size by cell multiplication. Development indicates differentiation in structure and function.

First Year

LENGTH

a. Birth length: 19-21 inches
b. Length at 6 months: 25-27 inches (grows 1 inch a month)
c. Length at 1 year: 29-31 inches (grows ⅔ inch a month)

WEIGHT

a. Birth weight: 7½ pounds (average)
b. Six months: doubles birth weight
c. One year: triples birth weight

HEAD CIRCUMFERENCE

a. Birth: approximately 14 inches
b. One year: approximately 18.8 inches

SUTURES

a. Cranial sutures are open at birth, and the spaces between them are called fontanels. This allows for growth of the skull and, although the spaces close as the child gets older, they do not ossify until early adulthood
b. At 3 months, the posterior fontanel is no longer felt
c. At 18 months, the anterior fontanel is no longer felt

(*Continued on p. 468*)

453

GROWTH AND DEVELOPMENT
ONE MONTH TO ONE YEAR

1 TO 3 MONTHS	4 TO 6 MONTHS	7 TO 9 MONTHS	10 TO 12 MONTHS

PHYSICAL
Neurophysical Muscular
  Control

At birth can raise head for a short time when prone but not when supine. Head lag continues through the 2nd month, but the baby is able to hold it somewhat erect when he is pulled to a sitting position.

At 2 months can hold a rattle but does not wave it. Smiles and wiggles when spoken to softly. Uses thumb to squeeze when he grasps.

At 3 months, rolls from side-to-side but not over. Can lift head when supine. Plays with hands. Reaches for object. Pushes with feet against floor when held.

At 4 months the baby has more control of his head and can move it from side to side easily. His interest in his environment is increasing. He holds a toy that is placed in his hands and looks at it attentively, even exploring it with his tongue and his eyes. He can be propped in a sitting position for 10 or 15 minutes at a time.

At five months the baby should not have head lag when pulled to a sitting position. He now incorporates eye control with hand and arm control and will reach out to grasp things that he sees. He is not able to grasp things when lying on his back unless they are approximately 1 inch from his hand.

At 6 months he has less desire to suck and more willingness to try drinking from a cup. He can "transfer" an

At 7 months a baby can lift his head from the bed quite well. This is a big step in attaining independent sitting position. He now looks at small objects and tries to pick them up, but he can only rake them by spreading his fingers over the objects and trying to close them. He usually picks up small objects only if they stick to his fingers. He likes to bang things up and down on a firm surface as he has just added vertical movements to his list of accomplishments. He can sit alone for short periods before falling forward and supporting his trunk with his hands and arms.

At 8 months he can pull himself to a sitting position and sit unsupported. He is still practicing picking up small objects, but his thumb and index finger come to-

Creeps at 10 months but will probably have individual style. Uses his fingers to poke and to push, pokes his own eyes, ears and mouth.

At 11 months he likes to take things out of containers but still has difficulty releasing them. Between 11 and 12 months he has fun practicing releasing and then throws everything on the floor.

At 1 year he can stand alone.

Senses

Vision

At 1 month the baby stares at large bright objects.

Between 1 and 2 months he sees things out of the corner of his eye first and sees things in the room only if they move.

At 2 months he catches sight of objects in the midline and follows them past the mid-line.

Eye muscles are stronger in the 3rd month, although there may still be evidence of squint at times. He spends long periods looking at his hands.

gether in only crude approximation. He is beginning to have better and more co-ordinated movements of his legs at this age.

A 9-month-old can propel himself forward by creeping and hitching. He can pull himself to a standing position with assistance but has difficulty sitting himself down. He uses thumb and index finger to pick up objects and likes to finger-feed himself. Waves "bye-bye," likes to poke finger into holes and to bang objects.

Vision

At 4 months control of eye muscles is achieved as well as central vision. Stares at objects and people even if they do not move. Sees color. Follows objects from side to side in a full 180° arc.

At 5 months he looks when someone enters the room. Spends a great deal of time "looking."

Eye-hand coordination has developed so that a baby can pick up an object on sight if it drops within reach.

object from one hand to the other, and this is one of the most important aspects of behavior to assess his maturity at this age. He can roll completely over and can sit without being propped for 30 minutes or longer.

Vision

Between 7 and 8 months a baby who has had social stimulation and good physical care is interested in his environment and will move toward things that he sees. Likes using his motor ability. By 9 months he sees into the 3rd dimension.

Vision

By 1 year his eyes are co-ordinated, and he shows pleasure or displeasure at what he sees.

GROWTH AND DEVELOPMENT (Continued)
ONE MONTH TO ONE YEAR (Continued)

1 TO 3 MONTHS	4 TO 6 MONTHS	7 TO 9 MONTHS	10 TO 12 MONTHS
Touch The sense of touch is highly developed at birth, but it is thought that the sense of pain is not as well developed. Sensitivity to heat and cold is rapid. **Hearing** The auditory sense is well developed at birth, but the mechanical need for air in the middle ear is necessary before the infant hears. This usually takes 24 hours, after which the infant responds to a whisper. A 2-month baby shows evidence of hearing by changing facial expression. **Smell** The sense of smell seems to be developed to the degree that the infant seeks the mother's nipple. The rooting reflex is used in reference to the action that the infant uses to "root" with his lips and tongue for milk. A slight			

touch on the cheek causes the infant to open his mouth, and a slight touch on the lips causes him to suck.

Taste

The sense of taste is developed to the extent that the infant likes sweet things and gets used to certain formulas.

Sleep

Newborn to 1 month: releases into sleep by sucking. Sleeping is not completely quiet.

At 3 months he stays awake for longer periods.

By 5 months, a baby sleeps through the night without awakening for feeding.

After 6 months, a baby has longer periods of wakefulness.

At 7 months, the baby takes 2 naps a day.

Nap in the morning is shorter. Babies sometimes like to postpone going to bed at this time, as they are preoccupied with their locomotor abilities. They are fearful, too, of being separated from their parents. Babies cannot regulate their own bedtime and need limits set by an understanding mother.

Elimination

The infant's kidneys are nearly twice the size of adults when related to body weight. The body is not as efficient in controlling excretion of water and chemicals until after the 1st year. Baby voids about 18 times a day. Babies fed on cow's milk will have yellow, putty-like stools which do not cling to

Bladder capacity becomes larger as the baby grows.

The character of the bowel movements changes as new foods are added to the list.

GROWTH AND DEVELOPMENT (Continued)
ONE MONTH TO ONE YEAR (Continued)

1 TO 3 MONTHS	4 TO 6 MONTHS	7 TO 9 MONTHS	10 TO 12 MONTHS
the diaper. One to 4 stools are passed a day with an average of 1 or 2. Breast-fed babies have 1 to 8 stools a day (average 2 to 4), and stools are usually pasty, mushy, sour-smelling and light yellow in color.			
LANGUAGE Has differential cry for discomfort, pain and hunger at 1 month. He coos at 8 weeks. He uses syllables and mostly front vowels when crying at 2 months.	The baby laughs out loud and also initiates social contacts for himself by smiling spontaneously at 4 months. By 5 months, he squeals out loud as he produces high pitched sounds, and by 6 months vocalizes several well-defined syllables.	At 7 months he begins to use his lips to form syllables. He combines single syllables at 8 months, but they have no meaning. He recognizes meaning in the speech of others at 9 months and recognizes his own name. He also shows that he knows the meaning of "no."	At 10 months, he means "Ma-Ma," when he says it. He can usually say 3 words. He is associating words with gestures and plays "pat-a-cake" without being shown first.
EMOTIONAL AND PERSONALITY DEVELOPMENT The baby learns to trust people in the infant period. He is completely dependent on adults for survival, and the quality of the satisfying	At 4 months, he laughs spontaneously and initiates social contact. He notices other members of the family beside his mother and doesn't	At 7 months he is fearful of strangers and, because of his increasing motor ability, he can move away when strangers approach.	The baby at 10 months can detect his mother's feeling from the tone of her voice. His interest in standing and walking make it difficult for

experiences that he has helps to strengthen the foundation of his personality structure. He requires feeding and love, likes to be held, and uses crying as a means of communication. Sucking is his best means of self-comfort.

At 1 month, he begins to smile and at 3 months shows interest in the adult's face and responds quickly to social stimulation. (Bowlby's work has shown that it is important from this time on to have a constant mother or mother-substitute to care for the baby.)

NURSING IMPLICATIONS

Hold the baby for feeding and place him on his side p.c. to prevent aspiration.

The baby becomes enraged if restrained suddenly but gains security if wrapped securely. He is upset by sudden loss of support and may react by Moro reflex.

Baby at this age may respond to infection and emotional disturbances by diarrhea and vomiting. Formula should be sterilized, and baby

mind seeing strange people or being left in strange places. Some sources say that a baby recognizes his mother's face at this time.

Most sources agree that by 5 months a baby recognizes the voice and face of the person who cares for him (mother). He shows more interest in other people, especially children. He begins to protest if some pleasure is taken from him and resents being left alone in a room.

He begins to show fear of strangers at 6 months, and his behavior might begin to change at this age as he changes from a passive joyful baby to a more active one.

A baby of this age needs the opportunity to see people. He also enjoys looking at things. Toys strung across the bed provide an opportunity to look at and to grasp objects. If toys are tied to the bed use short string to prevent accidents.

He is physiologically ready for solid food but may resist at first because of the new consistency and taste. There is no one way to offer new

Separation from his mother is a frightening and threatening experience for him.

His increasing activity poses more problems for the mother of an 8-month-old.

One month later he begins to show more signs of memory and may cry, laugh or imitate when appropriate stimuli are used.

(Mother might play a more active role in the care of her hospitalized infant as the baby is more fearful.)

He needs an opportunity to practice new abilities—vocalizing, grasping, watching and locomotion—as well as an opportunity to be near people, to listen to music and to imitate simple games.

He is so interested in his environment that he is easily distracted from doing things

the mother to hold him as she did before.

He continues toward independence and shows this in his attempt to help, when being dressed. He begins to obey simple commands, but, on the other hand, the mother has to impose some limits which he might resist.

This baby needs a safe area in which to play and interesting toys to keep him busy.

He should practice walking on a firm surface, otherwise his feet will tend to turn outward.

In the convalescent period he will welcome a change in environment. Being wheeled in a stroller or sitting in a high chair affords a change in activity.

He needs careful supervi-

GROWTH AND DEVELOPMENT (Continued)
ONE MONTH TO ONE YEAR (Continued)

1 to 3 Months	4 to 6 Months	7 to 9 Months	10 to 12 Months
should be kept away from people with infection.	foods, but they are sometimes accepted more readily if some formula is offered first as he has a limited capacity to wait for satisfaction at this age.	that people want him to do, i.e, eating, unless the environment is quiet. If weaning has been started at home, the baby will probably regress when hospitalized or ill at home. He will probably refuse the cup and need to suck as he did previously. Sucking relieves tension.	sion, and accident prevention is again stressed.
Baby needs approximately 2½ ounces of fluid and 50 calories per pound. Care should be taken that records are accurate as baby does not respond as a more mature organism to changes in blood balance.			The nurse working in all areas should be aware of developmental milestones and should refer patients to proper resources if she suspects the need.
Tension is relieved by sucking on a pacifier, and this offers some measure of contentment if he is on "nothing by mouth," takes his feeding too quickly or is sleepless.	Safety continues to be important, but, as the child's abilities increase, one must be alerted to possible consequences of new behavior.	As the baby learns to pick up small objects, nurses and mothers must take care to remove them as "everything goes into the mouth" at this age.	
His temperature regulating mechanism is immature, and he may react to sudden changes by skin mottling and shivering. He begins to perspire in the 1st month.	Immunizations are usually started in this age group. A baby may have more drooling before the first teeth appear and have a need to bite on something hard to relieve his pain and discomfort.		
His skin is sensitive, and he is prone to rashes and burns. Care should be taken to change wet clothing. Hot water bottles should be avoided as they are potentially dangerous.			

He cries when he is hungry, uncomfortable or wants to be held. Holding the baby at this age does not spoil him.

(It is difficult for a mother to be separated from her baby at this age, and she may be jealous of the nurse who is caring for the baby.)

GROWTH AND DEVELOPMENT (Continued)
TODDLER, PRESCHOOL, SCHOOL AGE

TODDLER (1-2½ YEARS)	PRESCHOOL (2½-5 YEARS)	SCHOOL AGE (6-12 YEARS)
PHYSICAL *Height:* Grows about ½ inch a month between the 1st and the 2nd year, and only 2 inches between the 2nd and the 3rd year. *Weight:* Gains 5 pounds between the 1st and the 2nd year. *Teething:* Has 20 teeth by 2½ years. *Neuromuscular:* Child progresses from an unsteady wide-base gait and protruding abdomen to a more grown-up steady gait. He continues to perfect the skills of walking, running, jumping and climbing. His large muscles are developing rapidly, but he is using his small muscles too—he tries to undo buttons, etc.	*Height:* Grows about 5 inches between 2½ and 5 years. *Weight:* Body is losing baby look and becoming longer and thinner. Child gains 10 pounds between 2½ and 5 years. *Neuromuscular:* Muscular co-ordination is improving as the child develops skill in running, galloping, jumping and skipping.	Individual differences and sex influence the height and weight. Girls begin to have a growth spurt 2 years before the menarche and usually are taller than boys at the same age. Deciduous teeth begin to fall out between 5 and 6, and permanent teeth take their place. By 7 they have more fine motor co-ordination. Eyes are better able to accommodate and children are no longer far-sighted. The 9- and 10-year-old may be beginning prepubescent development and, if so, slow down in activity and become fatigued and appear lazy. If the growth spurt comes later, the child continues to be active. Boys are superior in athletics.
ELIMINATION Toilet training sometimes becomes a power struggle between the toddler and the mother. He is being asked to conform, and he resists in his usual ways; consequently a stressful situation may ensue. Toilet training is usually most effectively begun when a child can walk well and when he realizes the relationship between a puddle and the sensation he	Bed-wetting is usually over at 4 years.	

had prior to the appearance of the puddle. Walking is one indication that myelinization is complete, and sphincters can be controlled. Another clue to readiness is his ability to stay dry for 2 hours.

When toilet training is started, it is wise to apply developmental facts. For example: keeping in mind that his tolerance to frustration is low, he is fearful of new gadgets and his attention span is short. Praise for a job well-done is very worthwhile.

SLEEP

Night-crying is common in the toddler period, and many children may begin to have night-terrors.

Sleep problems are related to ambivalent feelings toward parents, and scolding makes the problem worse. The toddler needs comforting when having sleep problems.

It is important to have a quiet period before bedtime.

Ritualism in sleep is a problem for parents and toddlers because children sometimes keep adding to their rituals, and it becomes necessary to set limits.

It is important to examine the amount of sleep a child gets during the whole day, including naps. The amount of sleep, a child gets cannot be left up to him, and although he may resist going to bed, he needs limits set by parents. He may have fears which keep him

The child still makes small requests at bedtime which may be an indication of basic behavior patterns.

The amount of sleep a preschooler gets ranges from 18 hours a day at 2½ years to about 12 hours a day at 5 years. Naps get shorter as the child gets older, and at 4 years he may just rest or play quietly.

His imagination may be so vivid at this age that he may resist going to sleep. He may have night-terrors.

Ritualism at bedtime is decreasing.

School age children need between 10 and 12 hours of sleep a day, and their needs may vary.

Exciting TV programs disturb sleep, sometimes for days.

If a child has difficulty getting up in the morning, he probably needs to go to bed earlier. Parents must set limits.

GROWTH AND DEVELOPMENT (Continued)
TODDLER, PRESCHOOL, SCHOOL AGE (Continued)

TODDLER (1-2½ YEARS)	PRESCHOOL (2½-5 YEARS)	SCHOOL AGE (6-12 YEARS)
from falling asleep. Example: fear of being left alone, fear of the dark and fear of wetting the bed. He may find comfort in taking some familiar toy to bed.		

EATING

TODDLER (1-2½ YEARS)	PRESCHOOL (2½-5 YEARS)	SCHOOL AGE (6-12 YEARS)
This is a period of slow growth, and the appetite decreases (physiologic loss of appetite). He likes to feed himself and eats a full family diet. He manages a cup fairly well but likes to throw it on the floor when he is finished. He may go on "food jags." This is the time when many feeding problems start because of the toddler's independent spirit and small appetite. He needs a quiet period before mealtime as he is highly excitable and easily distracted. He sometimes is too tired to feed himself, but he doesn't want anyone to feed him either.	He likes plain foods served attractively. He has definite food likes and dislikes and seems to prefer the foods that he knows best. He dislikes gummy foods and likes foods that he can pick up with his fingers. At 4 he can feed himself without spilling, but table manners are still a problem.	School age children may find it difficult to find time to eat—they are so busy doing other things. They also go on "food jags" and consume very little beside peanut butter sandwiches or one of their other favorites. Emotions affect their appetites and food consumption. Disagreeable subjects should not be discussed at mealtime. Overweight and underweight may be problems in this age group.

SPEECH

TODDLER (1-2½ YEARS)	PRESCHOOL (2½-5 YEARS)	SCHOOL AGE (6-12 YEARS)
If speech isn't learned here, a child is apt to become emotionally disturbed because he can't express himself. At first he uses a single word to express a situation and then progresses to simple sentences. He can understand	Vocabulary increases 600 words yearly. His ability to communicate word speech is improving steadily, but he sometimes understands things and can ask about things just enough to misunderstand them.	By 6 years, he has command of practically every sentence structure, and the length of the sentence increases up to the age of 9½ years. His vocabulary is as large as the vocabulary of the adults in his environment.

much better than he can speak, but when he is faced with a stressful situation, he uses gestures and cannot talk. He usually learns to talk after he can walk and needs stimulation from the environment. After he learns to talk, he talks constantly and is almost compulsive about speech.

PLAY

He progresses from solitary play to parallel play, but he cannot play with others or share his toys or anyone else's.

He has a favorite soft toy which he carries about with him and hugs repeatedly.

He likes push-and-pull toys and large boxes that he can crawl in and out of. Water- and sand-play are fun, and he loves to pour things back and forth.

The toddler likes rough play, but he may become overstimulated and need help to calm down.

EMOTIONAL AND PERSONALITY DEVELOPMENT

The young toddler is gradually realizing that he is a separate person from his mother. He has a desire for independence and demonstrates this by being negative and having temper tantrums when he is thwarted. He can't stand too much frustration and sometimes adult demands are more than he can cope with, and, again, he has temper tantrums. He has ambivalent feelings to-

Linked with developmental tasks. It centers around physical activity and progresses from parallel play to group play and games. He is imaginative and likes dramatic play. Girls imitate their mother's household activities; boys imitate their father's. Preschoolers like to paint, build with blocks, read picture books and play in rhythm. They chatter while they play.

The preschooler is full of imagination, energy and a zest to find the "why" of his world. He sets unreachable goals for himself. He is independent and sees himself as a person who wants to be like his parents. His motor abilities improve, and he uses his powers of locomotion to explore. He can use language much better, too, and between language and locomotion his world enlarges.

Stuttering is found in 1 per cent of children of school age, and it is usually caused by emotional tension.

Twice as many boys suffer from speech defects.

Group activities begin to interest the child rather than individual play.

The gang age appears at approximately 8 years. The gangs are composed of members of the same sex. Gangs are formed by the children themselves, as they learn that jealousies, temper tantrums, gloating, etc., will not be tolerated by others. They develop responsibility, helpfulness, good humor and independence.

In the early school years the child cannot lose games gracefully; he may use subtle cheating to win but gradually learns the value of fair play. His social insight increases each year.

The school age child is turning to the outside world for patterns from which to establish a scale of values. For this he turns to his contemporaries and other adults, especially teachers. He continues to try to be independent of his parents and uses outside authority to prove his parents' fallibility.

He continues to develop his conscience and is avid for self-control and self-

GROWTH AND DEVELOPMENT (Continued)
TODDLER, PRESCHOOL, SCHOOL AGE (Continued)

TODDLER (1-2½ YEARS)	PRESCHOOL (2½-5 YEARS)	SCHOOL AGE (6-12 YEARS)
ward his mother, the great need for independence and the great need for her love. Ritualism is important to him for security—the home routines for eating, playing and sleeping should remain undisturbed as much as possible for his peace of mind. He is unable to control his emotions and may need adult guidance to help him control crying or laughing. He is still closest to his mother and fears separation.	He can't help frightening himself with his thoughts, sometimes, because he is so imaginative. His conscience is developing. He is learning to distinguish between right and wrong, but, because he doesn't clearly understand the difference between what is real and what is fantasy, he sometimes misunderstands.	discipline. These traits are sometimes missed by parents and other adults because he seems to want to defy them and also shows disrespect. A school age child is concerned with doing and achieving. He wins recognition by producing things and derives satisfaction by completing tasks. He enjoys doing things with people and needs to have a feeling of his worth and equality for opportunity. At this time, he may begin to be aware of discriminating influences which may thwart his efforts and which may have lasting harm if he feels that he will be judged by the color of his skin, his background and/or social status rather than for his own abilities and eagerness to learn and to produce.

NURSING IMPLICATIONS

Separation from mother is very stressful for a toddler who is hospitalized. He cannot reason or understand that she will come back, and, consequently, rooming-in or long daily visiting hours are important for his well-being. If this cannot be managed, one nurse should be assigned to him for continuity of care. He cannot relate to more than one person at a time, and he easily becomes confused when he is ill and hospitalized. He should have his favorite toy from	The preschooler needs repetitive simple explanations. He doesn't understand sly remarks with double meaning and takes things literally. His questions should be answered simply, and clues to misunderstanding watched for. Limits should be set for discipline so that he has freedom to accomplish his tasks in a socially acceptable way, but he usually needs limits set by the adults in the situation. He should not be frightened into doing things, because he is so	A school age child likes to be given a chance to talk things over. He likes to help in making reasonable decisions for himself. He expects to have explanations made to him. His need to achieve, compete and be with his friends is interfered with when he is sick or hospitalized. He needs sympathetic guidance and understanding at difficult points. He takes cues for his behavior from his peers, and if a group of school agers

home, and something that belongs to his mother for comfort, too.

He cannot understand reasons for things, and long explanations just confuse him. Treatments should be done efficiently with comforting words repeated over and over. Equipment should be kept at a minimum. He needs physical contact with a comforting person when he is under stress and usually seeks it. He regresses in all areas of development but mostly in the one he was perfecting when admitted to the hospital.

He needs close supervision, as he is into everything and doesn't understand danger.

He likes to do things for himself, and a positive approach and distraction are good ways of coping with his independence before he gets negativistic. Don't treat negativism with negativism.

The toddler becomes more anorexic in the hospital, but usually eats more if he can feed himself, although he needs adult supervision and guidance. He may regress to bottle-feeding for a time. Because he refuses to eat when one approach is used, don't give up; use others, but don't use force.

If he has a nickname, use it. Use his name often when speaking to him—he doesn't always respond to "you," etc. Speak in short sentences phrased positively.

Never practice a procedure or appear unsure of a technic when working with a toddler—they are sensitive and need security.

imaginative and his emotions are so intense.

He understands time in relation to his day's activities.

Sibling rivalry is high at this age, and the child needs guidance and love if his mother has a baby when he is a preschooler.

If his body is covered by dressings or casts, he may imagine that part of him has been removed and be very anxious. He usually likes to look when dressings are being changed.

He may be afraid of the dark and need to keep the light on at night.

Although he dislikes being separated from home, this is not as stressful in the preschool period as it was in the toddler period.

are together in a ward, they might have to have their interests channeled. Things that he can construct give him satisfaction. Singing and playing simple musical instruments help relieve pent-up emotions. Card games and other competitive board games hold his interest. He likes to read adventure stories, animal stories and stories about heroes.

Boys and girls are antagonistic toward each other but may tease and try to get each other's attention in later school years.

They are usually very modest and like privacy.

He is interested in his own body. Consequently, it is a good time to teach about health. Prepubertal body changes should be explained.

Dental supervision is important.

Accident prevention should be stressed. Children of this age are apt to take dares.

(*Continued from p. 453*)

DENTITION

Lower central incisors are the first teeth to erupt and usually appear at approximately 6 months

REFLEXES

a. *Moro, tonic neck and grasp reflexes* begin to disappear between 6 and 8 weeks and should be gone by 4 months
b. *The Babinski reflex* is positive but does not become clinically significant until the end of the 2nd year
c. *Retrusion tongue reflex* disappears between the 1st and the 2nd month

PREMATURE CARE

A premature infant should have nursing care arranged to meet his needs as related to his specific immaturity. Weight is only one (although a fairly accurate) criterion for determining the degree of immaturity.

Immediate Nursing Care

Protect the head. When breathing is established, keep the baby horizontal and on his side.

Provide a clean, warm, isolated environment.

High humidity has been thought to be beneficial.

The infant should be baptized, if his parents so desire.

One per cent silver nitrate drops (1) should be instilled into each eye.

Hykinone, 2 mg., should be given.

Maintain adequate respirations. If baby becomes cyanotic, or if respirations are difficult, the baby may need:

Suction. If a machine is available, the pressure should be between 120 and 140 mm. Hg. Some form of suction must be planned.

Oxygen. It should be administered at a flow of not more than 2 L./min. When the baby is in the confined space of an incubator, an oxygen analyzer should be used every 8 hours to be sure that the concentration doesn't go higher than 34 per cent, unless a higher percentage is ordered. Blindness can occur if the baby gets too much oxygen. A small amount of oxygen often is essential to relieve acute respiratory distress, but should be discontinued as soon as the distress is relieved.

Caffeine sodium benzoate 0.03 Gm. (½ gr.)

Artificial respiration. This may be given by a resuscitator, or by a rhythmical see-saw motion. Keep body straight and raise head as you lower feet. NEVER use chest compression or abdominal squeezing.

Give nothing by mouth for at least 24 hours. The first feedings are usually 5 per cent glucose before the formula is given. The formula should be low in fat and suited in amount and calories to ensure a satisfied baby. (Begin formula in very small amounts, increase slowly to approximately 120 cal./Kg. at 1 week.) The baby's ability to suck is indicative of his ability to swallow. If sucking is vigorous, usually he can take bottle feedings; if he is weak and listless, he will need tube feedings.

All prematures should be placed where they will receive the best care. If they are transferred to a hospital away from the mother, the father should be permitted to visit so that he can see the care that his child receives. The nurse should be sure that he obtains adequate knowledge about his baby so that he and his wife can be satisfied that their baby is getting the best care available. All premature infants should be considered on a "danger list" until an appraisal indicates that they are mature enough to live, and they demonstrate ability to gain weight.

Observations should be made in the first 24 hours to detect evidence of serious congenital anomalies, jaundice, edema, hemorrhage, or skin eruptions.

General Nursing Care

Prevent asphyxiation. Adequate respirations must be maintained at all times. It is usual to leave the clothes off, except for a diaper, when the baby is in an incubator, so that the nurse can be constantly on the alert for signs of asphyxiation.

The same emergency treatment discussed under immediate care can be given to a baby.

The baby should be placed on his side after feedings (alternating the side), even though the nurse assumes he is adequately "burped." A premature infant can re-gurgitate at any time, and aspiration is a real danger.

Prevent infection. A separate nursery and individual equipment with personnel free from infection should be provided. All personnel should wash their hands with germicidal soap. Visitors should be prohibited, except for viewing the baby through a protective barrier.

Linen for the premature infant should be autoclaved or brought from the laundry in a closed carrier.

Maintain a stable body temperature. There is no known "normal" body temperature. The level of body temperature of very small premature infants will depend on the temperature of the incubator. In the past, it was necessary to provide a very warm (90° F.) environment. Today, the ideal environmental temperature is uncertain. It is important to provide the warmth necessary to keep the infant's body temperature from fluctuating, whatever this might be. A constant level is the aim. On admission to a nursery, the premature infant usually is placed in an incubator that has been preheated to 85° F. and to which humidity is added. The amount of humidity needed may depend on the immaturity of the infant. How beneficial a high humidity is for the infant whose respirations are adequate depends on what future studies reveal. The bed temperature and the baby's temperature (axillary) should be checked every hour until the temperature remains level. When this is established, the 2 temperature readings are made before each feeding.

Conserve the infant's energy by planning the activities that are essential, leaving time for adequate rest.

Tube or nipple feedings depending on the infant's ability to suck and swallow. If nipple-fed, elevate the baby's head; if tube-fed, have the baby well on his side.

Weigh only twice a week.

Baths. Until the infant is out of the incubator, the skin should be carefully checked at each feeding time, especially the creases, and washed p.r.n. with cotton and warm water. When the infant is out of the incubator, soap-and-water baths are given after the cord has healed. The nurse should observe and record: any discharge from eyes, nose or ears, color of the sclerae, skin color and condition, the cord and condition, type of respirations, color and consistency of stools, urination, and infant's vigor (alert or listless).

FLUID AND ELECTROLYTE BALANCE IN CHILDREN

(The general principles are covered in the
Medical-Surgical Section)

Fluid requirements: Infants require, proportional to a unit of body weight, three times the adult fluid intake.

Normal fluid requirements in ml./Kg. body weight/24 hrs. (+ or − 30 ml.)

Infant—150 ml./Kg.

Toddler—100 ml./Kg.

Older child—50 ml./Kg.

Reasons given for the relatively larger fluid requirements in early childhood:

Cause is not fully understood

The surface area in early childhood is relatively greater in relation to body weight than in adulthood

There is a higher metabolic rate

The kidneys are less able to concentrate urine

The pituitary gland is immature

Relatively common causes of dehydration and of electrolyte imbalance in childhood:

Diarrhea—loss of cations and fluid in the stools leads to dehydration and acidosis

Vomiting—loss of anions and fluid in vomitus may result in dehydration and alkalosis

Diabetes—acidosis and milder dehydration results from the accumulation of ketone bodies in the blood and from polyuria

Aspirin intoxication—respiratory acidosis results (the child breathes rapidly and deeply, blowing off excessive amounts of carbon dioxide)

DIARRHEA

Diarrhea is a common symptom in childhood and, in infancy, can be a particularly serious one. With severe diarrhea, the infant's fluid and electrolyte balance is upset by the loss of water and basic electrolytes in the stools. If the diarrhea does not cease, and if replacement therapy is not instituted, the infant progresses to dehydration, metabolic acidosis, shock and death. Severe episodes of diarrhea are usually thought to be of infectious origin. The common offending organisms are varied: viral, *Escherichia coli*, *Salmonella*, *Shigella*.

Tests done to determine etiology and extent of acid-base imbalance

Stool culture
Blood Na, K, Cl, CO_2 and pH

Medical Management

Discover etiologic factors and eradicate
Rest the gastrointestinal tract
Correct the dehydration and the acidosis
Resume oral feedings, progressing gradually from clear fluid, dilute protein milk or skim milk, regular diet

Nursing Responsibilities During the Acute Phase

Strict isolation technic
Observation, reporting and recording
  Manifestations of Dehydration
    Dry skin, poor tissue turgor
    Depressed fontanels
    Dry mucous membranes
    Facies, sunken eyes, pinched, anxious expression
    Oliguria, concentrated urine
    Loss of weight . . . DAILY WEIGHT SHOULD BE RECORDED
    Ashen pallor
  Manifestations of Acidosis
    Deep, rapid respirations
    Cherry-red lips
    Lethargy, progressing to coma
  Manifestations of Shock
    Ashen or gray color
    Cold, clammy skin

Rapid pulse rate
Vital signs
    Axillary temperature
    Apical pulse
    Respirations
Intake and Output
    Accurate record of intravenous (I.V.) fluids received
    Frequent observation of infant with I.V.
        Rate of flow
        Signs of infiltrations, patency of tubing
        Response of infant
    Urination
        Frequency
        Amount
        Concentration
    Stools
        Frequency
        Size
        Consistency (loose, watery)
        Color (yellow, green)
        Content (mucus, blood)
Mouth Care
    Mucous membranes dry
    Sterile swab and water for mouth
    Cold cream on lips
Buttocks Care
    Corrosive stools irritate the skin
    Wash buttocks after every stool
    Expose to air and light p.r.n.
    Use ointment p.r.n.
Care of the Infant (receiving intravenous and nothing orally)
    Intravenous fluids, given frequently through a scalp vein
    Restraint of upper extremities necessary
    Infant needs opportunity to suck
    Infant needs physical contact, needs to be held, talked to, free of restraint when feasible
    Infant needs change of position

RESPIRATORY CONDITIONS

Otitis Media

Fifty per cent of upper respiratory infections (U.R.I.) are accompanied by otitis media in infants and young children.

Eustachian tube in infants is short and wide so that infection ascends quickly. This changes as child grows older; then otitis media is less frequent.

Any organism may cause difficulty.

SIGNS AND SYMPTOMS

Fever and irritability with U.R.I. are outstanding symptoms in infants
May pull on ear
May be swelling behind ear
Older children have definite earache
Drainage after rupture

TREATMENT

Aspirin, codeine and luminal for pain and restlessness
Antibiotics
Nose drops
Ear drops
After myringotomy—need dry wipes and occasional irrigation

Mastoiditis

At birth there is no pneumatization of temporal bone, only mastoid antrum present. Pneumatization begins during 1st year and is not complete to tip until 5 years. Mastoid antrum infected in all otitis media. When there is inadequate drainage, infection extends further to mastoid.

Organism—anything causing otitis media.

SIGNS AND SYMPTOMS

Postauricular edema
Pain and tenderness over mastoid
Sagging posterior wall of external meatus
Fever, toxicity and leukocytosis
Thick and poor drainage from ear

TREATMENT

Antibiotics. Many will clear up without surgery.
Mastoidectomy—simple or radical.

Cervical Adenitis

Lymph nodes draining nasopharyngeal region become
overwhelmingly infected
More common in early years
Most often due to hemolytic streptococcus

SIGNS AND SYMPTOMS

Usually fever
Swelling of lymph nodes of neck with tenderness.
May have stiff neck
May go on to become hot, red and fluctuant. Has
gone on to abscess formation

TREATMENT

Antibiotics
Wet or hot packs locally
Codeine and luminal
Incision and drainage when fluctuant—unless con-
traindicated

Infections of the Larynx

SPASMODIC CROUP (*Catarrhal Spasm of Larynx*)

U.R.I. irritates laryngeal muscle that responds by
spasm, producing croup.
Signs and symptoms are hoarseness, "barky" cough.
Usually not croupy during day, but at night de-
velops respiratory distress with stridor and re-
tractions.
Usually lasts 2 to 3 days and then recovers. Have
mild fever, depending on severity of U.R.I.
Treatment
All, except very mildest cases, are admitted to
hospital. Prognosis very difficult to predict except
by continued observation.
Steam—can be either hot or cold
Sedation—very important in spasmodic croup
Antibiotics

Close observation for progression of respiratory distress

Emetic such as ipecac may relieve spasm by reflex action

ACUTE LARYNGOTRACHEOBRONCHITIS

Refers to more serious type of "croup." Is severe infection of respiratory tree and usually involves all parts. Here, obstruction in the larynx is not due to spasm, but is actual swelling and congestion in wall of larynx, leading to complete obstruction. Is one of the most terrifying diseases in pediatrics.

May accompany U.R.I. or childhood disease.

Signs and Symptoms

May be fulminating or may gradually get more severe. Children usually very sick; have fever, leukocytosis. Voice hoarse or lost.

Severe respiratory difficulty: increased respirations, retractions, stridor, cyanosis, fast pulse, increasing fatigue.

Treatment

Steam (hot or cold)

Antibiotics

Sedation: may be dangerous to sedate child because it may mask symptoms.

Tracheotomy is indicated. Tracheotomy not desirable if it can be avoided, but, on the other hand, do not wait until the child is exhausted.

Post-tracheotomy essentials

Special nurses "around the clock" for indefinite period

Steam (either with or without Croupette)

Suction

Bronchoscopy

EPIGLOTTITIS DUE TO HEMOPHILUS INFLUENZAE (TYPE B)

Influenzae type B. Always accompanied by septicemia.

Signs and Symptoms

Sudden onset of fever, prostration and rapid development of obstruction. On examination, child has large swollen epiglottis. Child may die of obstruction in 4 hours.

Treatment

Tracheotomy—necessary to save child's life
Antibiotics

Bronchi

ALLERGIC

Asthma (*See* Medical-Surgical Section)

FOREIGN BODY

Worst thing to aspirate is vegetable material (e.g. nuts) because severe inflammatory reaction is set up called "vegetal bronchitis."

Within 12 hours after aspiration of peanuts into lungs there will be fever, cough and signs of consolidation. Will lead to abscess formation.

Very dangerous to give anything containing peanuts to small children.

Treatment

Bronchoscopy, *stat*. Antibiotics.

Nursing Care

Observation: report signs of increasing respiratory obstruction or fatigue, tachycardia, fever, increasing cyanosis, increasing retraction and restlessness.

Support and reassurance for child and parents. Child will be very frightened and anxious and should have someone with him to offer support. Allow him to assume most comfortable position. Do not restrain or disturb unnecessarily. Try to help him to conserve strength.

Hydration. Try to maintain good oral intake unless degree of respiratory distress makes this unwise. Supplementary fluids may have to be given.

Post-tracheostomy care—(*See* Technics).

BLOOD DISEASES IN CHILDREN

Child differs from adult in:

Polycythemia at birth—gradually falling to normal.

Relative anemia at 6 to 10 weeks; therefore, 12 grams of hemoglobin at birth is anemia; at 2 months it is normal.

Peripheral blood more apt to contain immature forms.

Relative lymphocytosis until about 3 years of age.

All elements are affected in disease process. When need for blood is great, spleen and liver enlarge and serve as centers of extramedullary hematopoiesis.

Anemia—3 Classifications

BLOOD LOSS FROM ANY SOURCE

Acute hemorrhage

Chronic hemorrhage

Chronic blood loss results in *iron-deficiency anemia* and will respond to treatment with iron.

DECREASED PRODUCTION

Iron-deficiency anemia

Premature and twins

Children born of anemic mothers

Nutritional anemia

Pernicious anemia

Rare in children

Toxins

Endogenous; e.g., nephritis

Exogenous; e.g., poisons, sulfonamides, Dilantin, Chloromycetin

Infections

Common cause of anemia

Aplastic anemia

Production of cells stops. May have definite cause or may be idiopathic.

Myelophthisic anemia

Marrow crowded out by other pathologic process: e.g., leukemia, malignancies, "marble bones."

INCREASED DESTRUCTION

In all hemolytic anemias, the increased destruction is manifested by appearance of breakdown products of hemoglobin, evidence of hyperactive regeneration.

Congenital Hemolytic Anemias

FAMILIAL HEMOLYTIC ICTERUS (OR ANEMIA)

Heredity plays role

Abnormal-shaped cells—spherocytes; increased fragility; spleen destroys them.

Some members have spherocytosis and increased fragility without disease.

Bilirubin gallstones

Have hemolytic crises which consist of anemia, jaundice, enlarged spleen, fever and chills, abdominal pain, joint pain

Treatment

Splenectomy effective. Cells still fragile, but destruction does not take place.

Cause

Not known

Prognosis

Good, after splenectomy

SICKLE CELL ANEMIA

Abnormal cell type—shape of sickle

Negroes: white cases extremely rare

Sickle cells present in 5 to 7 per cent of Negroes, only 1 in 40 have disease of anemia; active and latent sickling can be differentiated

Onset in childhood—much more serious than other anemias.

Crises: jaundice, fever, pain anywhere, heart enlarged with murmurs, spleen enlarged, convulsions and coma, anemia, apt to get infections.

Bone marrow hyperplastic to keep up with above; changes are noted on x-ray examination.

Treatment: symptomatic. Transfusion at time of crises.

COOLEY'S ANEMIA (Mediterranean Anemia)

Occurs mainly in Mediterranean ethnic groups —Italians, Greeks.

Erythroblastic overproduction in bones—young cells—more fragile. Young cells not filled with hemoglobin.

Usually 1st year of life; pale, slightly icteric, enlarged spleen and liver; enlarged heart with murmur; characteristic bone changes.

Treatment: TRANSFUSION. Keep these children living on borrowed blood. Spleen may be so large that it has to be removed because of its weight and to partially decrease erythrocyte destruction.

Other Blood Diseases

HEMOPHILIA—(*See* Medical-Surgical Section)

PURPURA—(*See* Medical-Surgical Section)

LEUKEMIA

Incidence

Relatively common. May occur at any age, may be congenital. Race and sex are not factors.

Pathology

Bone marrow replaced by leukemic cells.

Signs and Symptoms

In children, usually is acute form with rapid onset.

Pallor and anemia

Enlargement of spleen, liver and lymph nodes

Fever

Pain in bones

Bleeding tendency

Susceptibility to infections

Laboratory

Bone marrow diagnostic. White blood cell count (wbc.) may be very high or very low.

Treatment

6-Mercaptopurine	may produce remis-
Aminopteron and	sions lasting as long
Amethopterin	as 18 to 24 months
Cortisone and ACTH	

HYPOPLASTIC-APLASTIC GROUP

Aregenerative anemia

Involves only RBC. May be familial.

Failure of red cell production in bone marrow.

Must transfuse every 1 to 2 months for years.

Occasionally may recover. Hg. and RBC. remain at fair level and need no further transfusion.

Symptoms are those due to anemia only.

Nursing Care

Nursing care in blood diseases is directed toward support for the child and for the family throughout the short or long period that the condition persists. Because of repeated episodes of some type of crisis, usually bleeding, which occur periodically, the child has numerous hospitalizations, and, as he grows older, he realizes that he has a chronic condition for which there apparently is no cure. Over the years, these children have become well acquainted with each other as they meet frequently in the hematology clinics or on admissions to the hospital. The sudden disappearance of one child can mean only one thing to the others, although they seldom ask any questions or seem in any doubt as to the explanation. For both the child and the family in these difficult circumstances, the presence of friendly, understanding nurses and doctors in familiar surroundings is a source of comfort and help. In the acute or terminal stage, constant nursing is necessary. Many of the patients have profuse and persistent bleeding in a number of areas. Mouth care is often indicated; sponges gently administered to lower fever, careful positioning to prevent skin breakdown and the maintenance of a good fluid intake are important. The most effective measure of relief to the child is the administration of sedatives in whatever doses the doctor prescribes. Throughout this ordeal, the presence of a sympathetic nurse near the child and his parents is a great help to them when the end comes.

DISEASES OF THE NERVOUS SYSTEM

Peculiarities in Early Life

Development of central nervous system (C.N.S.) is not complete at birth. Higher centers not in use.

Child with complete absence of cerebral hemispheres may react in normal way at birth and exhibit normal reflexes.

Mental deficiency usually not detected until later.

Same is true of spastic paralyses that are not diagnosed until later.

Lesions of C.N.S. in neonatal or intra-uterine period will lead to much more widespread damage than the same injury at a later date. This is because development is not complete.

Infant's C.N.S. is more sensitive to stimulation; e.g., children may have a convulsion with febrile episode, etc.

Any injury is repaired with scar tissue only. No regeneration of nerve tissue.

Congenital Abnormalities of the C.N.S.

HYDROCEPHALUS

Anatomy

Cerebrospinal fluid is produced by the choroid plexus in the ventricles. It flows from the lateral ventricles, the 3rd and the 4th ventricle into the subarachnoid space of the brain and the spinal cord. It is absorbed into the venous sinuses.

Definition

Hydrocephalus is an abnormal accumulation of cerebrospinal fluid, under pressure, within the ventricular system. The condition may be apparent at birth, become apparent in the first few months of life, or be associated with certain disease conditions early in childhood.

Etiology

An obstruction to the normal circulation of cerebrospinal fluid anywhere along its course caused by

Congenital atresias or stenosis in ventricular system

Infection

Hemorrhage

Neoplasms

Overproduction of fluid?

Underabsorption of fluid?

Diagnosis

Clinical picture

Periodic measurement of head circumference

Abnormally large proportionately

Growing at abnormally fast rate

X-ray

Sutures wide

Fontanel wide

Injection of dye into ventricular system to determine the presence of block.

Summary of Infant's Responses to Chronic Increased Intracranial Pressure.

Head circumference disproportionately large and increasing at abnormally fast rate

Bulging and enlarged anterior fontanel

Widened sutures

Venous dilatation

"Sunset" eyes

Irritability

Vomiting

Retarded development in all areas

Treatment and Prognosis

Of the children with hydrocephalus, 40 to 50 per cent have the potential for spontaneous arrest. If the process is not arrested, the child eventually succumbs from intercurrent infection, malnutrition or collapse of vital brain centers. Treatment is based on the possibility of spontaneous arrest and is aimed at tiding the child over until that time. Cerebro-spinal fluid is shunted via a catheter from a ventricle to one of the numerous areas in the body such as pleural cavity, peritoneal cavity, ureter, etc., where it may be absorbed. The hope is that by relieving intracranial pressure and thereby allowing for the rapid brain growth that occurs in the first few years of life, when the hydrocephalic process arrests, the child will be mentally intact. Shunting procedures to date have had only fair success.

The Nursing Care of an Infant with a Ventriculo-Pleural Shunt

FACTORS TO CONSIDER

Common complications following this procedure:
Accumulation of nonabsorbed cerebrospinal fluid in pleural cavity
Obstruction of lumen in shunting catheter
Meningitis
Hydrocephalic infants have a continuous need for good skin care and frequent change of position to prevent pressure sores on scalp.

POSITION AND FEEDING

Semi-Fowlers to facilitate drainage
Hold for feeding
Feed slowly; bubble well
Record intake
Record behavior

OBSERVE AND REPORT IMMEDIATELY

Increased respiratory rate and/or dyspnea
Uneven expansion of chest wall
Vomiting, tense fontanel, poor suck
Increased irritability or sudden decrease in responsiveness
Fever

PLAY STIMULUS APPROPRIATE TO DEVELOPMENTAL LEVEL

SPINAL CORD ABNORMALITIES (neural tube closes over and fuses in mid-line to form adult structure)

Spina Bifida Occulta

Incomplete fusion of vertebral lamina

Very common anomaly and usually causes no symptoms

Meningocele

Spina bifida with protrusion of meninges through it

Occurs most commonly in lumbosacral or cervical areas; protruding tumor covered by skin.

No spinal cord involvement, so there are no neurologic manifestations

May rupture and develop meningitis

Early operation advisable.

Myelomeningocele

Usually in lumbosacral area

Consists of spinal cord elements in meningocele

Usually have neurologic involvement

Paralysis of lower extremities

Incontinence of urine and feces

Loss of sensation

Nursing Care

Measures to prevent infection from feces, urine or other contamination

Protection from any trauma to the area

Frequent turning of the child from side-to-side and positioning

Bradford frame may be used in conjunction with adequate restraint and support

Holding for feeding whenever possible with plenty of time allowed for affectionate handling

Mongolism

A congenital condition of mental deficiency with certain pathognomonic clinical features that make recognition possible at birth. This category constitutes 7 to 10 per cent of the institutionalized mental defectives.

ETIOLOGY

Obscure, although it has been recently demonstrated

that mongols have 47 rather than the normal 46 chromosomes

INCIDENCE

Estimated at 2 to 3 per 1,000 births (Benda)

DIAGNOSIS

Appearance

HEAD

Skull—small, flattened anteriorly and posteriorly

Eyes—osseous orbits small
Lateral upward slope
Epicanthal fold of inner angle (disappears by 10 years)
Brushfield spots—white spots on irides present in infancy

Nose—short with flat bridge

Mouth—oral cavity small
Tongue usually protruding
Tongue fissured and furrowed by 6 months
Teeth—small, late erupting, malaligned

NECK

Short, broad
Laxity of muscles on lateral aspects

HANDS

Short, square
Short, incurved 5th finger
Simian line (single transverse palmar crease)

FEET

Wide-spaced 1st and 2nd toes

MUSCULAR HYPOTONIA

Hyperextensible joints
Protruding abdomen

X-RAY

2nd phalanx of 5th finger rudimentary in 40 per cent of mongoloid children
Characteristic alteration in bony pelvis

DEFECTIVE DEVELOPMENT

Facts Relevant to Prognosis
Few reach a mental age of 6 years
Average I.Q. = 35 to 50
Susceptible to infections, particularly in infancy
High incidence of associated cardiac anomalies
Majority have cataracts by 17 years of age

Microcephaly

Newborn infant has an abnormally small skull, and the brain has failed to develop
Condition results in severe mental retardation

Premature Synostoses of the Skull

Deformity of the head caused by premature closure of the sutures
Damage to brain and eyes is frequent

Treatment

Surgery to enlarge intracranial space

Meningitis

An inflammation of the meninges. The child responds with fever, signs of meningeal and encephalitic irritation, signs of increased intracranial pressure and possible shock.

COMMON CAUSATIVE ORGANISMS

Pneumococcus, staphylococcus, streptococcus, meningococcus, *Hemophilus influenzae,* tubercle bacillus, *Escherichia coli,* virus, e.g., Coxsackie, ECHO

DIAGNOSIS

Contributory findings
Clinical picture
Altered cell, protein and sugar content in the cerebrospinal fluid
Positive nasopharyngeal and blood cultures
Diagnostic findings
Culture of organism from cerebrospinal fluid

NURSING OF CHILDREN

MEDICAL MANAGEMENT

Identify organism by smear and culture

Prompt intensive therapy to eradicate the organism

Medication

Antibiotics appropriate for organism

Isoniazid, para-aminosalicylic acid and streptomycin for tubercular infection

Route

Intravenous

Intrathecal (occasionally)

Orally, after acute phase

Strict isolation until therapy renders patient's condition noninfectious.

PROGNOSIS

Dependent on organism

Dependent on promptness of therapy

Common forms of residual damage: deafness, blindness, mental retardation, hydrocephalus

SUMMARY OF CHILD'S PHYSICAL RESPONSES

Fever

Meningeal signs

Nuchal rigidity

Kernig's sign (the leg cannot be passively extended at the knee when the thigh is flexed to a right angle at the hip)

Brudzinski's sign (an involuntary flexion of the thigh when the neck is flexed)

Increased intracranial pressure

Infant

Irritability

Poor suck and cry

Tense fontanel

Vomiting

Child

Headache

Vomiting

Papilledema

Blurred vision, diplopia, nystagmus

Encephalitic irritation
  Changes in sensorium
  Seizures

Coma

Shock
  Waterhouse-Friderichsen syndrome, associated
    with meningococcal septicemia, is characterized
    by shock, generalized purpura and hemorrhages.

ADMISSION

The infant may present with fever, irritability and
  tense fontanel.
The older child will usually present with the classic
  meningeal signs. Physicians view this admission
  as a medical emergency and know that the
  promptness with which they start therapy will, to
  a large extent, influence the child's prognosis. The
  nurse should consider the following factors:
The following will be needed immediately:
  An isolation unit
  Equipment for lumbar puncture, nose and throat
    culture, blood culture
  Equipment for I.V. fluids and medication
  Restraints
The parents will be anxious.
If conscious, the child will be confused and fright-
  ened.

NURSING RESPONSIBILITIES DURING THE ACUTE PHASE

Age of child
  See Growth and Development Section for impli-
    cations for nursing care for specific age groups

Vital signs
  Prompt reporting of any change

Fever
  Fluids as tolerated P.O.
  Sponging (*See* Technics)
  Antipyretics, as ordered
  Mouth care (*See* Technics)

Intravenous medications and fluids
    Careful regulation of I.V. to:
        Maintain constant blood level of antibiotics
        Maintain hydration
        Prevent overloading of circulatory system
    Restraints to ensure noninterference with I.V. therapy
Respirations
    Maintain airway
        Suction and oxygen available
        Position on side, tongue forward
        Have tongue blade available
    Prevent aspiration
        Position on side
        N.P.O. with vomiting, dysphagia or coma
        Suction p.r.n.
    Report any change in rate or in depth immediately
Seizures: see section on Seizures for description and responsibilities
Coma
    Positioning and turning
    Skin care
    Prevention of aspiration
    Relief of urinary and fecal retention p.r.n.
    Prevention of any deformities: range of motion, support to parts
Nursing observation, recording and reporting
    GENERAL APPEARANCE
        Posture, color, respirations, fontanel, skin turgor, petechiae
    CHILD'S EXPRESSIONS OF
        Fears
        Perceptual impairments
        Pain
    LEVEL OF CONSCIOUSNESS
        Oriented, excited, somnolent, stuporous, comatose
    MOTOR BEHAVIOR
        General
            Posture; muscle tone; movement—rate, amount, organization, strength limitations, seizures

Eyes
Focus; pupil dilation—degree and equality; co-ordination and range of movement
Ability to swallow
Bowel and bladder
Continence or retention
Responsiveness to the parents' and the child's need for emotional support

SEIZURES

Types

GRAND MAL

There is sudden loss of consciousness and postural tone that may be preceded by an aura. The total body musculature stiffens (tonic phase) before going into the clonic phase of patterned, rhythmical jerking. The spasms also involve the facial muscles and the muscles of respirations so that the child may have an accumulation of oral secretions, cyanosis from respiratory inadequacy and a weak irregular pulse. In the postictal phase the child may have a headache, muscular aches, confusion and a strong desire to sleep.

PETIT MAL

The child experiences a brief loss of awareness without any motor component. The child may appear to be having a brief staring spell.

PSYCHOMOTOR

These seizures are episodes of bizarre, automatic, purposeless behavior that appear strikingly out of context. The episode may be preceded by an aura. There is clouding of consciousness during the episode. After the seizure there may be no memory of the bizarre behavior and there may be confusion and drowsiness.

FOCAL

Reflect dysfunction of a local area of the brain, sensory or motor. Consciousness and postural tone may be retained while involuntary convulsive movements pro-

491

gress from the distal to the proximal part of an extremity or while the patient has a bizarre sensory experience. Focal seizures may progress to a generalized convulsion, grand mal seizure.

FEBRILE

These are grand mal seizures that occur in 6 to 8 per cent of children under 3 years of age in response to the rising temperature associated with an infection. These children are otherwise seizure free. At the time of the febrile seizure, effort is directed at preventing an episode of status epilepticus. The subsequent management of the child includes using antipyretic measures when the child shows evidence of fever and may include prophylactic anticonvulsant therapy until the child is 3 years old.

STATUS EPILEPTICUS

A series of grand mal convulsions in which the patient does not recover from one convulsion before the onset of another. The convulsion must be stopped. Paraldehyde, rapid-acting barbiturates intramuscularly (I.M.) or I.V. and general anesthesia may be used in an effort to terminate the convulsions. There is danger that while in status epilepticus the patient may suffer cerebral hypoxia and brain-cell damage.

Overview: *see* chart, p. 494

Nursing Care

READINESS

Placement of child for easy observability
Suction and oxygen available
Tongue blade at bedside
Padded crib rails
Helmet on older child p.r.n.

DURING SEIZURE

Tongue blade inserted prior to tonic phase or during a moment when jaws are relaxed
Do not attempt to move or to hold patient
Remove dangerous objects from environment

Suction and oxygen p.r.n.
Provision for quiet and rest postictally

OBSERVATION AND RECORDING OF TOTAL BEHAVIOR PRIOR TO, DURING AND AFTER THE SEIZURE. SPECIAL ATTENTION TO:

Nature of aura if present
Movements
　Type
　Extent of body involved
　Onset—focal elements or generalized
　Termination—generalized relaxation of total body musculature or relaxation beginning in one part and spreading
　Sequence in both instances
Duration of
　Aura
　Tonic phase
　Total seizure
　Postictal state
Respiration, pulse rate and color
Eyes
　Pupil dilatation
　Position
Incontinence and time of occurrence
Memory, consciousness, co-ordination and disposition postictally

FACTORS TO CONSIDER IN PLANNING TOTAL NURSING CARE

Medication
　Of all children with recurrent seizures, 80 per cent can be controlled by anticonvulsant drugs.
　Medications must be taken regularly.
Community resources available.
The meaning of the illness to the child and the parent.
Continuity of care: school nurse and teacher.
Community attitude
　Awareness of above as reflected in camp, educational and employment restrictions placed on the child or adult with this diagnosis.
　Nurse's role as an educator.

	PETIT MAL	GRAND MAL	PSYCHOMOTOR	FOCAL
AGE OF ONSET	Always in childhood	At any age	At any age	At any age
FREQUENCY	4 + 20 to 100/day	1 + Sporadic	1 to 2 + Sporadic	2 +
DURATION	Less than 30 seconds	Greater than 60 seconds	Greater than 60 seconds	Greater than 60 seconds
AURA	None	+ or −	+ or −	+ or −
MOTOR ELEMENTS	None	+	Purposeless	+ or −
POSTICTAL	None	+	Usually	+ or −
ELECTROENCEPHALOGRAM (EEG)	+	+ or −	+ or −	+ or −
TREATMENT	Tridione (trimethadione)	Phenobarbital Dilantin (diphenylhydantoin) Mysoline (primidone)	Dilantin Mysoline	Dilantin

CEREBRAL PALSY

This is a group of diseases that affect control of voluntary motor system and have their origin in various parts of the brain.

Clinical Manifestations

Spasticity
    Hemiplegia
    Diplegia
    Quadriplegia
Athetosis
Tremor and rigidity
Ataxia or flaccidity

Types and Their Supposed Lesions

MOTOR CORTEX

Spasticity: muscles of lower extremities contract under tension; i.e., when you try to extend the triceps, the spastic biceps interferes and you can't extend the arm.

Hemiplegia: most common both arm and leg
Monoplegia: single extremity
Spastic quadriplegia: all extremities involved
Spastic diplegia: legs (scissors gait)
Spastic paraplegia: must differentiate from spinal cord lesions

Flaccidity: always associated with some spasticity
Mental retardation associated

BASAL GANGLIA

Rigidity: differentiate from spasticity by absence of stretch reflex and presence of resistance of both flexor and extensor muscles.

Athetosis: may involve any or all of the extremities. Marked by bizarre nonrepetitive movements (involuntary). Tension may result from attempts to control motion. May be interference with eye motion and hearing. May mask normal intelligence.

CEREBELLUM

> *Ataxia:* marked by disturbances in balance, co-ordination and control of voluntary movement.
> *Mixed lesions:* frequently encountered.

Etiology: Brain Damage

PRENATAL

Result of viral or noxious agents during time of organogenesis in fetal life
Maternal rubella
Toxoplasmosis
Syphilis
May be genetically determined

AT TIME OF BIRTH

Hemorrhage or anoxia
Premature infant's skull is particularly liable to trauma
Skull fracture, tentorial tears, intracranial and subdural bleeding
Traumatic delivery
Anoxia may be cause, but congenital defect may have been responsible for the anoxia
Severity of injury does not correlate with degree of future involvement

POSTNATAL

Kernicterus
Intracranial infections. Now, with antibiotics, children survive infections which were formerly fatal, only to have this residuum.
Pertussis, measles, meningitis
Encephalitis
Brain abscess, tumors, subdural hematoma
Injury, anesthesia, poisons (lead and CO.)

Treatment

The earlier the better because of the emotional and mental needs of the family and the child.

RE-EDUCATION

Physical therapy: passive movement of spastic muscles

Occupational therapy

Speech training

Teaching relaxation

Teaching balance

OPERATIVE PROCEDURES (mostly for spastics)

Tendon lengthening

Tenotomy

Neurectomy

Arthrodesis

Tendon transplantation

There is no cure for cerebral palsy. Teaching of the parents is essential in order that they, in turn, will teach the patient. There is an unwarranted sense of shame still attached to this disease. Re-education of the parents and the members of the community is necessary to remove this stigma.

It is difficult to determine the I.Q. of these children because no tests have been devised which consider the speech and the motor-skill difficulties present due to the cerebral damage.

NEPHROSIS IN CHILDHOOD

Nephrosis in childhood is characterized by intermittent gross edema (anasarca) associated with proteinuria, hypoproteinemia (gamma globulin and albumin) and an elevated serum cholesterol. The child may have hematuria, hypertension and an elevated nonprotein nitrogen (NPN), but not necessarily.

The condition usually starts in the toddler period but may occur at any age (very rare in infancy). The incidence and the etiology of the disease are unknown, but there are several theories, among them being: antigen-antibody reactions, psychological factors and hereditary factors.

Presenting symptoms usually are: insidious onset of edema, generally beginning with hands, ankles and eyes and progressing to anasarca. Sometimes there is a history of an upper respiratory infection. As weight increases, child may have hydrothorax, ascites and, as a result of one or both, shortness of breath. Diarrhea and vomiting may occur with abdominal pain giving evidence of peritonitis. These children are prone to infections, especially pneumonia, peritonitis and cellulitis.

Untreated cases have spontaneous remissions and exacerbations of the illness. The treatment at present is steroid therapy. Steroids are given in divided doses daily until diuresis occurs (usually the 10th to 14th day) and then intermittent steroid therapy is continued until patient has recovered. Potassium in some form is given with steroids. Prophylactic chemotherapeutic agents sometimes are given intermittently. In the future chlorothiazide may be used more extensively as a diuretic.

Laboratory Findings

URINE

Albumin 3 to 4 +. This decreases as general condition improves.

Microscopic examination reveals casts, occasional RBC.

BLOOD

Complete blood count (c.b.c.) shows anemia and, usually, an elevated w.b.c.

Erythrocyte sedimentation rate is elevated.

Nonprotein nitrogen is normal or slightly elevated.

Cholesterol level is grossly elevated.

Protein electrophoretic pattern (PEP) shows low serum albumin.

If nose and throat culture is positive, blood culture is then indicated.

Before starting steroid therapy, Mantoux test is done.

Treatment

GENERAL MEASURES

Rest, as tolerated

Unrestricted diet without added salt. Children usually are anorexic and become more so with a more more restricted diet. However, diet changes depend on the doctor's orders.

Intake and output

Weight—daily record

Treatment of any infections

Blood pressure—daily record. In acute stage, may be recorded more frequently.

Nursing Care

Consider growth and development of child and the nursing implications.

Parent education. Answer questions as helpfully as possible so that they understand how to care for the child at home.

PHYSICAL CARE

Edema. Turn frequently to change position. Pressure areas develop quickly because of poor circulation. Head should be elevated to facilitate breathing and to lessen edema of the eyelids. Scrotum may have to be supported by pillows or a "Bellevue Bridge" support.

Skin. Cleanse and dry well, especially between folds. Cotton, if changed often, may be used in the groin area to prevent cellulitis which might result from skin surfaces rubbing together. Do not use adhesive tape unless absolutely necessary.

Intake and Output. Measure and save urine (if ordered). Chart the type of fluid the child is drinking.

Elimination. Observe and chart the amount and the type of stools

Diarrhea ⎤
Vomiting ⎟ Should be reported—may be sign of a
Pain   ⎟   complication
U.R.I.   ⎦

Irritability. Usually observed

Anorexia. Food should be as appetizing as possible —see implications for nursing care.

Observation. In addition to the above:

Take blood pressure as ordered
Progress of edema—weigh daily
Signs of complications

CELIAC DISEASE

Clinical picture shows inability to digest fat and starch, poor motility of gut, enlarged abdomen, atrophied muscles and episodes of diarrhea and of dehydration.

Etiology
Unknown.

Clinical Findings
Usually starts during 2nd year of life. Children often have increased or frequent stools before this.
They become listless and fail to gain on a normal diet.
May have episodes of diarrhea.
Often are very irritable.
After a variable period, they have full-blown picture in which there is extreme emaciation—especially of trunk, buttocks and extremities; large distended abdomen; skin hangs in folds; marked irritability.
May have what is known as celiac crisis. This is most apt to occur with upper respiratory infections; patients develop severe diarrhea and become rapidly dehydrated. May die if not treated promptly.

Laboratory Examination
The finding of fat and starch in the stool is diagnostic.

Treatment
CRISIS: parenteral fluids and treatment of infection.
DIET: aqueous multivitamin preparations and vitamin B complex are given; iron and vitamin K may be ordered by the physician; high protein and the use of simple carbohydrates and starches is determined by the age and the condition of the patient depending on the phase of the disease.

Prognosis
May continue over long period of time, but most of these children do well.

CYSTIC FIBROSIS OF THE PANCREAS

Cystic fibrosis of the pancreas is a relatively common hereditary disease. A decade or so ago many children died in infancy of pneumonia and malnutrition while the diagnosis of cystic fibrosis was unsuspected. It is a disease of the exocrine glands in which the mucous-secreting glands of the bronchi and the nasal passages, the sweat glands and the digestive glands are affected in somewhat different ways.

DIGESTIVE GLANDS

The pancreas and the intestinal tract produce a very thick secretion, blocking the ducts which drain the secretions into the intestines. The name cystic fibrosis of the pancreas describes the condition, as the ducts are dilated and surrounded by scar tissue. Digestion is impaired and the child loses about 50 per cent of the fat and protein and 15 per cent of the carbohydrate ingested. Fat-soluble vitamins are lost, resulting in a deficiency in vitamins A, D, E and K. Slow growth, a large appetite and bulky stools are characteristic of pancreatic malfunction.

Ten per cent of all infants with the disease are born with meconium ileus, and a large number of these succumb at birth.

MUCOUS GLANDS

The mucus is abnormally thick and children have difficulty clearing their bronchi, resulting in emphysema, bronchiectasis and chronic bronchopneumonia. They are more susceptible to respiratory infections, especially bronchitis, and each new infection increases respiratory changes.

SWEAT GLANDS

The sweat glands are affected and produce sweat that contains excessive amounts of salt. This can be dangerous during hot weather as children lose large amounts of salt and develop heat prostration.

Diagnosis

Stool examination—large amounts of fat.
Sweat test—excessive amount of salt.

(*Continued on p. 505*)

CYSTIC FIBROSIS OF THE PANCREAS

EARLY PHASE	CHRONIC PHASE	TERMINAL PHASE
SYMPTOMS		
Acute respiratory infections	All symptoms of acute phase plus:	Severe respiratory distress
Coughing	Cyanosis	Anorexia
Large frothy stools	Barrel chest	
Rectal prolapse	Clubbing of the fingers	
Vomiting with coughing	Pallor	
Malnutrition	May develop:	
Retarded growth	Cardiac decompensation	
Good appetite	Spontaneous pneumothorax	
Abnormal salt loss	Atelectasis	
	Diabetes mellitus (rare)	
	Duodenal ulcer	
	Portal hypertension	
	Cirrhosis of the liver	
MEDICAL INTERVENTION	Continue treatment as in the acute phase and add treatment of complications.	Symptomatic and palliative
Medications		
Antibiotics		
Pancreatin		
Aerosol		
Vitamins		
Oxygen		
May have intermittent positive pressure re-breathing mask (IPPB) for short periods with aerosol.		
Diet		
High protein, high caloric, low fat, moderate starch. Supplementary salt		
Postural drainage		
Breathing exercises		
Tapping or clapping posterior and lateral chest while patient is in postural drainage position to help loosen secretions		

NURSING CARE
Nursing care geared to the age of the child

Giving Medications
  Antibiotics
    Knowledge of drugs needed, many research drugs are being used.
    Usually better when given between meals as child coughs and vomits when excited.
  Pancreatin
    Give at mealtimes. Mix with palatable substance and administer immediately.
  Cotazyme
    Digests more fat than pancreatin, but is more expensive
  Aerosol
    Be confident and know how to administer before approaching child. Children are sensitive to nurses' insecurity.

Diet
  Encourage between meal feeding for high caloric content. Fluid intake should increase during summer along with salt. Tolerance for fat may increase with age, and diet will be adjusted accordingly.

Aerosol
  Postural drainage will probably precede aerosol.
  The head of the bed is raised and the child is placed in Trendelenburg position on the inclined bed. Chest tapping may be ordered for a specific period of time before aerosol while the child is in postural drainage position.
  Watch for increased dyspnea and fatigue during the procedure and notify the doctor of undue reaction.

Nursing care continues as in the beginning phase, but new antibiotics and treatments may be added.

Nursing care continues to be the same, but the child is more lethargic and dyspneic.

Usually refuses food and fluid and needs intravenous feeding.

CYSTIC FIBROSIS OF THE PANCREAS (Continued)

EARLY PHASE	CHRONIC PHASE	TERMINAL PHASE
Support Go to the child when he coughs. Support his chest when he coughs as you would a post-operative chest surgery patient.		*Support* Child tends to stay in orthopneic position and even leans forward supporting himself on his arms for long periods. May want to lean on a tray rack or shelf to rest and may even sleep leaning on a padded tray rack.
Prevent Infection Gamma globulin is given if the child is exposed to measles to prevent severe complications.		
Exercise Normal activity as tolerated. Deep breathing is encouraged.		
Education of parents should include: Most of the above plus: Physical care of their child Financing the cost of medications and hospitalization Questions about the hereditary nature of the disease The amount of exercise and normal activity the child may be allowed Prevention of infection Stress that these children live to adulthood	Those of the early phase plus: Problems of vocation for the child Additional stress of emerging complications Depression of the older school-age child or of the adolescent	

Duodenal drainage: if under 100 units of trypsin
per ml. = positive for cystic fibrosis
higher viscosity in cystic fibrosis
10 to 15 per cent have normal trypsin.

Vitamin A and carotene—decreased

Chest x-ray—emphysema and microcardia

Head x-ray—show pansinusitis

Dietary Management

High protein, low fat, low starch

Diets with added vitamin supplements

Vitamins A, D, C in water-soluble form

Vitamin B complex

Vitamin E

Pancreatin given with each meal

Extra salt is added; amount varies with season and
environment

SURGICAL CONDITIONS

Thyroglossal Cyst

Embryology of thyroid formation: progression from
back of tongue to permanent position during fetal
life.

May leave cyst or fistulous tract in mid-line of arch.

Symptoms:

Recurrent abscess at mid-line of neck

Bad taste on back of tongue

Treatment—excision of cyst or fistulous tract. Often
difficult neck dissection.

Branchiogenic Cyst

Embryology: remnants of "gill slits" or branchiogenic
clefts.

May be cysts or fistulous tracts anywhere along
lateral aspect of neck.

Often bilateral.

Symptoms: usually repeated abscesses in same place
or a mass.

Treatment: surgical excision.

Tracheo-esophageal Fistula

Anatomic anomaly
> Atresia of esophagus
> Fistula from lower segment of esophagus to trachea
> usual type

Signs

> *Nurse is usually the first one to notice.*
> Immediate vomiting of all food given by mouth. Regurgitation through nose and mouth, often with cyanosis and choking.
> Intermittent cyanosis and dyspnea. Whenever mucus accumulates in the proximal pouch, it runs over into the trachea and the lung.
> Frothy mucus at mouth often needing frequent suction. (*Nurse should recognize these symptoms and report immediately.*)
> Prognosis
> Unless there is prompt surgical intervention, all will die of bronchopneumonia. These infants should not be fed and should not have barium. It all goes right into the lungs and produces aspiration pneumonia.
> Diagnosis is made by passing a catheter under fluoroscope and instilling 1 ml. of Hypaque.
> Surgery is done as direct anatomic repair. Gastrostomy usually is done 2 days later so that feedings may be given by that method while allowing the esophagus to heal.

Nursing Care

> Preoperative
>> Do not feed baby. Keep flat or in position ordered by doctor. Usually, the baby is in an Isolette because many are under 2,500 grams.
>> Should be suctioned frequently—at least every 15 minutes—to prevent aspiration and puddling of secretions.
> Postoperative
>> Position carefully. Do not disturb chest tube in situ. Change position every 2 hours.

Suction every 15 minutes. Use catheter which has been marked to show how far the anastomosis is from the mouth or the nose.

Watch for signs of respiratory distress: retractions, gasping, nasal flaring. Suction; then give oxygen.

Patient will have N.P.O. for several days. Intravenous therapy for this time.

Gastrostomy usually is done on the 2nd or 3rd day after the anastomosis, and gastrostomy feedings are started shortly thereafter. If no gastrostomy is done, the child will start on P.O. feedings by dropper on about the 5th postoperative day.

Great skill is necessary in giving the gastrostomy feeding.

They usually are given through a Murphy drip setup so as not to have distention and a possible strain on the anastomosis.

The stomach is aspirated before the feeding. The amount is measured and, if it is over 5 ml. subtracted from the feeding and then reefed so as not to lose the gastric juices.

The gastrostomy tube is usually left open attached to an Asepto syringe to prevent any distention or possible vomiting.

Pacifiers should not be given unless ordered. It is thought that the sucking and the swallowing puts a strain on the anastomosis.

The feedings are increased very gradually until the child is taking all feedings by mouth. It is necessary to note any signs of respiratory distress or abdominal distention during the entire postoperative period.

Pyloric Stenosis

(Congenital idiopathic hypertrophic pyloric stenosis)
Most common of congenital anomalies

Hypertrophy of circular muscle at pylorus diminishes size of lumen. Forms complete obstruction due to swelling mucous membrane. May be slight at first and gradually get worse until no food gets through.

Etiology unknown.

Symptoms (Same as those of high obstruction of gastrointestinal tract)

Vomiting usually starts at about 2 weeks of age, rarely earlier.

Typical vomiting is projectile and contains no bile. Child hungry after vomiting.

Small and infrequent stools

Dehydration and loss of weight

Alkalosis

Physical findings

Usually male—80 per cent.

Dehydrated. Often alkalotic.

Tumor in right upper quadrant of abdomen (R.U.Q.)

Peristaltic waves from left to right.

Treatment: Usually surgery. Results are *very good.*

Medical therapy has higher mortality. This consists of thickened feedings and the use of antispasmodics, atropine or scopolamine derivatives

Preoperative: Hydration

Surgery: Fredet-Ramstedt operation (longitudinal section of circular muscle allowing enlargement of lumen)

Postoperative: Fluids and gradual increase in feedings.

Mortality: Practically nil in good surgical hands. No recurrence.

NURSING CARE

Preoperative

Usually N.P.O. for several hours before operation. May require I.V. fluids or hypodermoclysis.

Chart vomiting carefully. Note type, amount, color, time.

Postoperative

Child is picked up for all feedings. Turn on alternate sides after feeding. Support in proper position with rolled pad.

Keep patient's bed flat at all times after reaction from anesthesia.

Feedings and fluids:

Feedings are given very slowly starting with 5 per cent glucose water solution—30 ml. 3 hours after feedings q3h for 2 feedings.

Dilute formula is then started at 30 ml. and gradually increased until on the 7th day the baby is getting 120 ml. of standard formula every 4 hours.

Multi-vitamins 0.6 ml. O.D. are started on the 5th postoperative day.

Malrotation of Gut and Volvulus

In fetal life the gut rotates until the cecum is in the R.L.Q. and is fixed to the posterior abdominal wall.

In malrotation, the cecum does not complete this prenatal journey and may remain in the R.U.Q. This may cause incomplete obstruction of the duodenum due to pressure. The pressure, in turn, causes the mesentery to be pulled from its position. Because the mesentery is not fixed to the posterior wall of the abdomen, volvulus (twisting of the intestines) may occur. Volvulus leads to obstruction of the lumen of the gut, obstruction of the blood vessels, strangulation and resultant gangrene of the intestinal wall.

SYMPTOMS:

Incomplete duodenal obstruction: vomiting bile, failure to gain weight, etc.

Volvulus: sudden complete obstruction with vomiting, dehydration, shock, etc.

TREATMENT:

Surgical release of volvulus immediately. Give proper preoperative care from both the medical and the nursing viewpoints.

There is not very much that can be done about a mobile cecum or gut, but it does not usually recur after surgery.

Atresia of Bile Ducts

SIGNS AND SYMPTOMS:

Jaundice from birth or early in the infant's life. Clay-colored stools. Bleeding due to vitamin K deficiency. Poor absorption of fat-soluble vitamins. These babies will die of cirrhosis in 1 to 2 years unless the condition is corrected surgically. Unfortunately, in most cases it is impossible to do anything surgically.

DIFFERENTIAL DIAGNOSIS (*jaundice in newborn*):

Syphilis, erythroblastosis fetalis, icterus neonatorum, sepsis, toxoplasmosis, hepatitis.

Imperforate Anus

This occurs in 1 in every 5,000 births and often is accompanied by other congenital anomalies. In the development of the urogenital sinus in the embryo, the proctodeum breaks through in the 8th week. If there is an imperfect development at this time, an imperforate anus may result. There are 4 types: low obstruction of the gastrointestinal tract, and rectal, vaginal or urethral fistulae, the fistulae comprising 55 per cent of these cases.

TREATMENT:

If of a very simple type, it may be treated by dilatation of the anus. At times, a temporary colostomy is done until other procedures can be attempted.

Usual operation is an abdominal perineal "pull-through." This is very difficult surgery and should never be undertaken except by well-trained surgeons.

Omphalocele

Contents of abdominal cavity protrude into the root of the umbilical cord or through a defect in the skin of the anterior abdominal wall. Mass may contain much of the intestines and liver and is covered with delicate membrane.

Treatment:

Surgical repair before sac ruptures and infection sets in.

Prognosis:

Guarded: often associated with other congenital anomalies.

510

Acute Appendicitis

INCIDENCE

Most common lesion requiring abdominal surgery in childhood.

The older the child the more common is appendicitis, although it may occur in babies. (Rare in first year, uncommon in second year, but after that progresses to adult incidence.)

PATHOLOGY

Same as adult—inflammation of mucosa, vascular engorgement, edema, hemorrhage, ulceration, purulent exudate in lumen, involvement of deeper layers, thrombosis, gangrene and rupture.

Peritoneal reaction with fluid develops and then becomes infected after (or before) rupture.

Checking of inflammation depends on walling off
Adults—omentum is used
Children—omentum, short and thin. Cannot cover inflamed appendix so they develop peritonitis more easily.

Cathartics dangerous—increase peristalsis and intraluminal pressure, result in perforation.

ETIOLOGY—unknown

U.R.I. often precedes or accompanies—⅕ cases.
Obstruction plays role.

SYMPTOMS

Diagnosis is difficult unless one knows how to examine children who are harder to evaluate than adults and cannot give an adequate description; the child can't tell you. Most common in R.L.Q.; malrotation causes pain in R.U.Q.; generalized in peritonitis.

Vomiting—rarely absent. May be only once or may be frequent.

Fever—usually 100° to 101°. May be higher, especially if peritoneum is involved. May be normal.

Usually constipated but may be normal or may have diarrhea.

511

SIGNS

Tenderness—appendix longer, may be anywhere, severe with rebound in peritonitis

Muscle spasm—marked in rupture

LABORATORY

Leukocytosis—12,000 to 20,000. Polys: 85 to 95 per cent, higher if peritonitis is present

Urinalysis to rule out pyelitis

TREATMENT

Surgery

A gentle enema is not dangerous in differential diagnosis

Stomach should be empty ⌐

Preoperative medication

Rupture with peritonitis

Operation if early

Appendectomy

Drainage

Localized abscess

Operation—appendectomy with drainage

Antibiotics and chemotherapy

POSTOPERATIVE CARE

Simple Appendicitis

Children do very well

Clear fluids after first day, gradually giving (in days following) full fluids and soft diet

Sutures out on 5th day

Discharged on 7th day

Ruptured Appendix

Child is hard to care for, usually delirious and thrashing around

Surgery and appendectomy

Continuous drainage, M-A type—nothing by mouth

Fowler position—prevents subdiaphragmatic abscess

Sedation—morphine for rest, quiet and pain

Drains—loosened on 5th day, completely removed
after 7th or 8th day

Chemotherapy—antibiotics, penicillin and streptomycin.

Intussusception

DEFINITION—telescoping of one segment of bowel into
more distal segment.

One of most important surgical emergencies in infancy and childhood, fairly common.

Death rate high if not diagnosed early.

Results in both obstruction and strangulation of gut.

ETIOLOGY

In adults usually caused by mechanical factors—
polyp, cancer, etc.

In childhood, only 5 per cent have mechanical
cause; others are idiopathic.

Usual at time solids are started. Cause may be
related to increased intestinal peristalsis.

INCIDENCE

Three to 11 months of age—75 per cent of cases

62 per cent males and 38 per cent females

Usually fat, healthy males.

SYMPTOMS

Colicky abdominal pain which disappears and then
recurs

Vomiting

Later in course, symptoms of shock, pallor, sweating, collapse and dehydration

Bloody stools in majority of cases

May not occur in first 12 to 14 hours

Typical bloody mucoid material ("currant jelly")

SIGNS

Depend on duration of symptoms—normal or shock
or dehydration

Abdominal mass (sausage-shaped) in majority. Not
tender; may be anywhere in abdomen.

Rectal—blood on finger, mass in rectum.

TREATMENT

In early cases, reduction by barium enema (guided by fluoroscopy) is often successful.

If late, or if nonsurgical treatment is unsuccessful, operation is required.

Intussusception is reduced simply by gentle pressure.

If reduction is impossible, resection is necessary.

PROGNOSIS

Good if treated early—within 24 hours
Increasingly poor as time goes on
STAT EMERGENCY.

Preoperative

Fluids
Empty stomach

Postoperative

May develop fever, diarrhea, occasionally peritonitis
Once reduced, very seldom recurs

Hernias

INGUINAL HERNIA—all of congenital origin, not acquired as seen in adults.

Always indirect type, and represents fetal outpocketing of peritoneum through inguinal canal.

Right testis descends at later date than left so processus closes off later. Therefore, right inguinal hernias are more common than left.

Symptoms

May be seen at birth or soon after; most are discovered at 2 to 3 months when child begins to cry more vigorously and pushes intestine out into sac. May be small at internal ring or may be large, filling entire scrotum. Usually contains only small intestine but may contain bladder.

Incarceration

Very frequent—especially in first 6 months of life.
Painful swelling. Reflex vomiting.

Treatment: sedation, positioning, pressure, operation.

Prognosis

May close up in first few months of life, *but this is rare.*

Best to keep it collapsed and hope for spontaneous closure; very rare.

Treatment

Avoid constipation, crying and coughing.

Yarn truss. No other truss is safe.

Operation—only treatment if it doesn't close spontaneously. Is tolerated very well.

HYDROCELE (very similar to congenital inguinal hernia)

If processus vaginalis closes off at neck, fluid accumulates and produces hydrocele.

If inferior portion only is open, hydrocele of tunica results.

If higher up—hydrocele of cord.

Frequently seen in infants and children.

Symptoms

Local soft swelling in scrotum and a round spermatic cord.

Transilluminates light.

Usually no discomfort even though it may become very large.

Treatment

Small ones usually disappear during first year of life.

Natural process continues.

Those that persist or appear after 1 year usually require surgery because they do not heal spontaneously after this time.

Surgery easy. Only rarely recur.

UMBILICAL HERNIA

Common in young children; usually in Negroes. Results from muscular and fascial defects of abdominal wall where blood vessels of umbilical cord went through.

Usually just skin and peritoneum. May be more than umbilical hernia, i.e., diastasis recti.

Twice as common in girls.

Usually small in infants; may become larger. Rarely contains anything except intestine or omentum. Rarely incarcerated.

Symptoms: Swelling or "bulge" that attracts immediate attention.

Treatment

Remember, most will disappear with normal growth, and most need no strapping.

If large, strap with adhesive and pull tight. Coins and trusses do no good. No value to strapping after 1 year.

If it persists, surgical repair is the only treatment, but only after 2 years of age.

CONGENITAL HERNIA OF DIAPHRAGM

Child born with opening in diaphragm between abdominal cavity and pleural cavity. Entire abdominal contents may be in chest.

Newborn child shows cyanosis, dyspnea and vomiting.

Treatment: surgical repair—*urgent.*

Cryptorchidism *(Undescended Testicles)*

Part of same process discussed above.

Develops high in posterior abdomen and then descends. May stop anywhere along the way. Always associated with inguinal hernia.

COMPLICATIONS

Cosmetic deformity

Diminished spermatogenic activity if kept under high temperatures (out of the scrotum).

May have malignant changes.

TREATMENT

In most cases descent will continue during childhood.

Hormone therapy—gonadotropic hormone given.
Expensive, painful and bothersome.
Results inconclusive.

Operation—best therapy
Best between 4 and 7 years of age.
Always do herniorraphy also.

Congenital Megacolon (Hirschsprung's Disease)

Due to aganglionic segment of gut, usually low, large bowel. As a result peristalsis is absent, feces cannot pass, and the proximal gut dilates and hypertrophies tremendously trying to force feces through. Thus the dilated gut is really the normal part, and the narrow gut is abnormal.

SYMPTOMS

Abdominal enlargement
Constipation—may go weeks without a stool (paradoxical diarrhea)
Later may have severe abdominal distention, anorexia, malaise, etc.

SIGNS

Tremendous enlargement of abdomen
Enlarged colon usually can be felt

TREATMENT

Try medical control: diet, enemata, etc.
Best treatment is surgery in all but mildest cases.
Abdominoperineal "pull-through" operation is done to remove in toto the aganglionic segment. Without complete removal, operation is unsuccessful.

Osteomyelitis (Acute Hematogenous)

DEFINITION. An infection in bone

ETIOLOGY. Blood-borne organisms. Most are caused by *Staphylococcus aureus*. In younger infancy may be caused by streptococcus, *Hemophilus influenza, type B,* pneumococcus, *Escherichia coli,* etc.

Contributing Factors. Trauma plays a definite role by causing disruption of fine bony trabeculae with resulting hemorrhage; blood-borne organisms may lodge in these areas. Common sites—upper end of tibia, lower end of femur, upper end of humerus, etc. Multiple foci may develop. The disease is more common in boys than in girls, and most cases occur in the 2 to 15 year age group.

Many people may have transient bacteremias, especially if carbuncles, boils or other infections are present. These organisms enter the nutrient artery of the bone and then pass to the ends of the arteries, usually forming infected thromboses which shut off the blood supply to the bone. This is the focus of the septicemia.

Osteomyelitis (Septicemia)

SYMPTOMS

> *Severe.* May be fulminant septicemia with high fever, chills, prostration and positive cultures (usually with *Staphylococcus aureus*). May be no signs of local lesions until later when pain and tenderness develop.
>
> *Mild.* May or may not have positive blood culture. Fever, localized pain and tenderness and limitation of motion.

DIAGNOSIS

> History and physical examination
> Blood culture
> X-rays—usually do not show anything for 8 to 10 days

TREATMENT

> Penicillin and other chemotherapy
> Traction and immobilization
> Surgery necessary in some cases—less frequent since advent of penicillin

THE GENITOURINARY TRACT

Exstrophy of the Bladder

The posterior and the lateral surfaces of the bladder

are exposed, and the urethral outlets are visible. There is continual dripping of urine, and the exposed mucous membrane is very sensitive and easily irritated by clothing or dressings. The condition is accompanied by wide separation of the pubic bones and results from the failure of union between the two sides of the lower abdomen producing a fissure in the mid-line from the umbilicus to the genitalia.

Treatment: surgery aimed at providing satisfactory means of receiving and discharging urine, relieving discomfort caused by the exposed mucous membranes, remedying the appearance and the structure of the genitalia, and, in the male, constructing a urethral tube to permit reproductive activity.

Hypospadias

A congenital anomaly in which the urethra does not extend the entire length of the penis and opens on its lower surface.

Treatment: surgery.

Epispadias

A rare congenital anomaly in which the opening of the urethra is on the dorsal surface of the penis.

Treatment: surgery.

Phimosis

A narrowing of the preputial opening so that retraction of the foreskin cannot take place.

Treatment: circumcision—the surgical removal of that part of the foreskin that covers the glans.

Hydronephrosis

This is a dilatation of the kidney pelvis and calyces, caused by obstruction.

Symptoms: interference with the flow of urine, infection and renal insufficiency.

Treatment: medical management of the renal insufficiency and infection when present, and relief of the obstruction by surgery.

Wilms's Tumor

Highly malignant tumor of kidney seen in early life.

It usually produces no symptoms; the abdominal mass is often so big that the parents see it and seek advice. Once discovered, it should not be palpated and should be removed as soon as possible (danger of spread). Post-operatively, the child should be given radiation therapy. The prognosis is guarded.

CONGENITAL MALFORMATIONS OF THE HEART

Among the many and varied types of congenital heart lesions, the following are most commonly seen.

Patent Ductus Arteriosus

Failure of the duct, present in the fetus between the pulmonary artery and the aorta, to close at birth or by the age of 3 months.

SIGNS AND SYMPTOMS

Retarded growth and development
Frequent upper respiratory infections
Presence of typical machinery-like murmur over pulmonary artery
Cardiac output increased and subsequent enlargement of the left side of the heart.

SURGICAL TREATMENT

Ligation and division of the ductus, usually performed after 2 to 3 years of age; may be done at *any* time.

Tetralogy of Fallot

Most common variety of cyanotic heart disease which can be treated by surgery.

ANATOMY

Stenosis of the pulmonary artery or valve
Overriding of aorta at its origin in the heart
Ventricular septal defect
Hypertrophy of the right ventricle

SIGNS AND SYMPTOMS

Cyanosis
Polycythemia
Heart murmur
Easy fatigability
Squatting
Clubbing of the fingers and toes
Enlarged heart on x-ray

TREATMENT

Surgery: establish a patent ductus to "detour" blood
into the lungs for oxygenation.
Blalock-Taussig operation: anastomosis of subclavian artery to the pulmonary artery.
Potts procedure: side-to-side anastomosis between
aorta and pulmonary artery.
Open-heart surgery to repair defects directly.

Pulmonic Stenosis

Valvular stenosis with fusion of cusps—they do not
open properly and it is difficult for the heart to eject
blood into the pulmonary artery.

TREATMENT

Closed Brock valvulotomy for infants
Open-heart procedure for older children

Coarctation of the Aorta

A narrowing of the aorta in a short segment just
distal to the point of emergence of the left subclavian
artery.

SIGNS AND SYMPTOMS

Hypertension in arms
Low blood pressure in legs

DIAGNOSIS: confirmed by aortogram

TREATMENT: surgical excision of the constricted segment and anastomosis of the free ends. Operation
should be done between 8 and 15 years of age.

NURSING OF CHILDREN

Nursing Care

Important aspects of postoperative nursing care are:
Temperature control.

Check pulse and respirations. If respirations are labored or child is retracting, suction; change position.

Watch color: report any change. Child is usually in oxygen with high humidity.

Careful checking of intravenous fluids: strict control of amount given.

Watch dressing for any drainage.

Chest tubes will be in place. Watch for any fluctuation.

(*See* Care of Patient with Cardiac Surgery in Medical Surgical Section.)

CLEFT LIP AND PALATE

Cleft lip and palate are fairly common congenital anomalies resulting from a failure of the lip and/or palate to fuse in embryonic life. The exact cause is unknown. They occur in 1 in 750 to 1,000 births.

Cleft lips range from a slight notch in the vermilion of the lip to a cleft which extends through the lip to the nostril. They may be unilateral or bilateral. If unilateral, they occur most frequently on the left side.

Cleft palate may range from a simple bifid uvula to a completely cleft palate extending from the uvula forward through the tooth ridge anteriorly.

A child can have a cleft lip or a cleft palate or both.

Cleft lips are usually repaired during the 2nd or 3rd months of life or when the baby weighs approximately 10 pounds.

Cleft palates are repaired somewhat later, depending upon the policy of the individual surgeon.

Management of All Cases

EARLY

Full explanation to parents of what the anomaly is and what their role will be in protecting the child from colds and other infections to which these children are prone.

Cautioning parents not to overprotect their child.

Complete explanation of the future for their child.

Long-term condition

Surgical repair

Speech therapy

Orthodontic therapy

Agencies from which they may receive financial help

PREOPERATIVELY

CBC and urinalysis

Blood typing done since surgery is in a vascular area and hemorrhage may occur.

Preoperative photograph for comparison studies after surgery. Remember to get written permission from child's guardian.

Check for signs of respiratory or ear infections which are very common in these children.

Make sure child is adequately nourished and in good fluid and electrolyte balance.

Accustom child to postoperative routine.

Elbow cuffs worn to prevent child from getting hands near face and mouth.

For repair of cleft lip—feed baby high calorie, high protein, full fluid diet by Asepto syringe with rubber tip.

For repair of cleft palate—feed child high calorie, high protein, full fluid diet by cup.

POSTOPERATIVELY

Make sure adequate drainage is insured.

If suctioning is necessary, suction only through nose. DO NOT SUCTION AGAINST SUTURE LINE.

If endotracheal anesthesia is used during operation, a Croupette may be used for a few hours postoperatively.

Sedation may be necessary for 48 hours postoperatively.

Elbow restraints applied immediately postoperatively.

NURSING OF CHILDREN

Points of Emphasis

NUTRITION

Cleft lip—feed by Asepto syringe with rubber tubing for infant and young child. For older child, one may use a straw. DO NOT USE CUP as this would cause fluid to flow over suture line.

Cleft palate—feed by cup only to prevent anything from coming into contact with the suture line.

CLEANLINESS

Do not touch suture line unless so ordered by doctor.

If doctor orders lip suture line to be cleansed, hydrogen peroxide mixed with equal amount of sterile water may be used. This may be applied to the suture line gently with a sterile swab. Try not to let excess fluid flow over lip sutures.

Always follow cup feedings with a drink of water to help cleanse palatine suture line.

PREVENT UNHAPPINESS AND CRYING

Must prevent crying to prevent tension on suture lines.

Give extra tender loving care.

Remove restraints (ONE AT A TIME) to enable child to exercise and to develop his muscles. Stay with him and play with him.

RESTRAINTS

Elbow restraints to be kept on continuously, even during sleep.

If removed, stay with child—remove only one at a time.

Prevent child from getting hands or food or playthings to mouth.

Watch child carefully so that he will not chew paint from crib rails or playpen rails. The paint may cut into the suture line.

Never brush child's teeth while he is still in the hospital.

Give the child NO LOLLIPOPS AT ANY TIME. Before discharge, instruct parents in care of child with restraints and give guidance as to adequate diet.

TONSILLECTOMY AND ADENOIDECTOMY

Tonsillectomy in children is usually an elective procedure as treatment for some of the following conditions.

Frequent tonsillitis or pharyngitis (frequent seat of acute and chronic infectious processes)

Recurrent or persistent cervical adenopathy

Pathologic tonsils

Mechanical obstruction due to hypertrophy

Recurrent otitis media

Some Contraindications for Surgery

Acute upper respiratory infections

Acute local infectious process

Hemophilia and other blood dyscrasias

Pulmonic diseases or vascular anomalies in tonsillar region

During time of epidemics

Preoperative Preparation

CBC and urinalysis

Bleeding and clotting time

Check to make sure child is afebrile and free from infection

State of good hydration

Check history for any allergies to medications

Check history for any bleeding tendencies

Postoperative Care

KEEP AIRWAY CLEAN AND CLEAR

Remove thick sanguinous drainage with tissue. Suction if necessary

Positioning. Allow child to assume natural position with head turned to side.

NURSING OF CHILDREN

OBSERVATIONS

Bleeding is chief complication. May be gradual or dramatic.

Signs of bleeding are:

Spitting bright red blood

Frequent swallowing

Vomiting *large* amounts of dark blood

Change in pulse—increased rate, threadiness, irregularity

Embarrassed respirations. May be due to edema of the uvula and may require tracheostomy for relief.

Infection—manifested by elevated temperature.

MAINTENANCE OF HYDRATION

Cracked ice and water as soon as nausea subsides.

Progress to *bland* fluids.

Child may refuse fluids to postpone swallowing. This must be encouraged in order to keep throat limber. Sucking on a lollipop may encourage swallowing.

NEED FOR REST

Prevent excessive activity—bed rest with bathroom privileges

Prevent excitement

May require sedation for restlessness

NEED FOR DISTRACTION

Pain and sore throat may cause child to cry, thus increasing danger of hemorrhage

Allow quiet activity in bed—games and reading

Special Emphasis

DO NOT SUCTION ROUTINELY. Maintain airway and adequate drainage by positioning. If suction is necessary (i.e., if patient is gurgling from secretion), turn head to side and place suction catheter between cheek and molars. Keep suction pressure 120-140 mm. Hg when catheter is pinched shut.

Keep tonsil hemorrhage tray with tonsil fossa plugs and tracheostomy set near at hand for emergency use.

Have adequate light available; either strong lamp, electric headlight or good flashlight.

CONGENITAL DISLOCATION OF HIP

Clinical Manifestations

When unilateral, congenital dislocation of the hip can be recognized by the classic signs: Asymmetry of skin folds, shortening of the limb, limited abduction of the affected hip, push-pull instability and palpable displacement of the femoral head from its normal position in the groin deep to the femoral pulse. Diagnosis is confirmed by roentgenograms. If the dislocation is bilateral, the only clinical signs are: broadening of the perineum, instability and palpable distortion of anatomy on both sides.

Treatment

The treatment may be nonsurgical or surgical. In either procedure, the child is placed in a hip spica cast. Not only should the nurse be concerned with the comfort and the well-being of the patient, but she must also give constant care to the cast if it is to maintain its primary function of hip immobilization.

After application of the plaster, it should be supported with pillows or sand bags to prevent breaking if stress is noted. Keep it exposed to the air to accelerate drying. Some doctors recommend the use of a heat lamp for drying. However, before using one, consult the doctor in charge; he may have definite ideas to the contrary.

Nursing Care

DAILY CARE

Bathing with close observation under cast edges for blemishes or skin irritations. Gauze moistened with 70 per cent alcohol cleanses accessible skin under the cast. After the skin is thoroughly dry, a good baby talcum, used sparingly, helps to relieve irritation.

Care of the toes can be accomplished with applicators moistened in 70 per cent alcohol.

Observation of circulation, color, function and sensation of toes. Reporting any abnormality to the doctor.

Checking for proper maintenance of position and pressure from cast.

Checking for unusual odors. Daily sniffing with nose down to the cast helps detect unwanted odors. Remember that the child cannot tell you; you must feel and sense all your patient's discomfort for him. Never be surprised if a crayon or a small toy is found lodged in some obscure spot under the cast. Skin irritation, to the point of sloughing, can be caused by such foreign bodies, if they are not found in time.

TOILET CARE OF THE CHILD

For the child who is not toilet trained, thorough skin care after voiding and defecating is essential. Because urine and excreta often get up under the cast, it is necessary to reach far up underneath with gauze and alcohol.

Protection is facilitated by two folded diapers tucked under the edges of the cast, anteriorly and posteriorly; then, a piece of plastic sheeting slightly larger, placed over and under in the same manner.

If the inner lining of the cast becomes quite wet, diapers or soft towels may be used to slip up under the cast anteriorly and posteriorly. These can be removed when all is dry; on the other hand, if changed when necessary, there is no objection to maintaining them for skin and cast protection.

The toilet-trained child can be placed on the bedpan just as the adult is. Care should be taken to turn the patient on the unaffected side, the bedpan placed so the buttocks rests on the posterior portion of the pan, then turned to a supine position with head, back and encased leg supported with pillows.

Turning and Positioning Patient

A small child can be picked up and placed from supine to prone position. A larger child should be gently pulled, on the affected side, to the edge of the bed. The nurse then places one arm under the shoulders, supporting the head with her arm. With the other arm under the buttocks, she grasps the cast on the opposite side and lifts and rolls the patient to the desired position. When the child is supine, a small pillow can be placed under the head. Whether supine or prone, the toes need protection from pressure.

The patient can be in the playpen for variation or in a large baby carriage for going outdoors.

Care of the Cast

Before the cast is applied, stockinette, according to size and height of child is prepared to resemble a sleeveless sweater. It is slipped over patient's head with arms in place, stockinette brought down over full extent of torso to the point where anterior and posterior portions of stockinette can be held together with safety pin, thus, covering and protecting the entire perineal area. Proper size stockinette is then put on each leg according to the area encased in plaster.

After the cast is applied, most doctors will check with nurse to determine the proper cutting of cast anteriorly and posteriorly to facilitate toilet care. All rough and sharp edges can be removed by beveling with a sharp plaster knife. The stockinette can then be smoothly anchored over the raw edges of plaster with 3 thicknesses of 3 inch plaster bandage.

Stains can be removed by scrubbing with Bon Ami followed by a coating of talcum powder to whiten. Odors from excreta can be removed by scrubbing with hydrogen peroxide, then powder. It may be necessary to reinforce the plaster occasionally with one or two rolls of plaster, particularly if scrubbings have been frequent. Any indication of a break in the cast over the affected hip is serious; it must be re-enforced by the doctor as soon as detected.

RECOMMENDED IMMUNIZATION PROGRAM

AGE	
2 months	Diphtheria, pertussus, tetanus #1; Poliomyelitis #1
3 months	Diphtheria, pertussus, tetanus #2; Polio #2
4 months	Diphtheria, pertussus, tetanus #3
5 months	Smallpox vaccination
10 to 12 months	Polio #3
18 months	Diphtheria, pertussus, tetanus booster
22 to 24 months	Polio #4
5 to 6 years	Diphtheria=tetanus toxoid booster Smallpox vaccination
9 to 10 years	Diphtheria=tetanus toxoid booster Tetanus booster every 3 years thereafter, or as a booster with injury Diphtheria booster every 3 years thereafter, if Schick test is positive.

Section 5

Normal and Therapeutic Diets

Adapted From the Diet Manual of
The Presbyterian Hospital
in the City of New York

NORMAL REGULAR DIET

Purpose

To provide the essentials for good nutrition. This diet provides approximately 70 Gm. of protein and 2,000 calories. Minerals and vitamins meet the standards for adults in the Recommended Dietary Allowances of the Food and Nutrition Board of the National Research Council.

General Rules

Include the following foods daily
  Whole milk—1 pint
  Eggs—1
  Meat, fish or fowl (3 oz.)
  Cheese, meat, fish or fowl—1 oz.—or 1 egg
    (Dried peas, beans or peanut butter can be used
    occasionally)
  Potato, rice, noodles, macaroni or spaghetti—1 serv-
    ing
  Vegetables—3 servings, 1 green or yellow
  Fruit—2 servings, 1 orange or grapefruit
  Butter or fortified margarine—3 servings, 1 tbsp.
  Bread or cereal, whole-grain or enriched
  Other foods to provide adequate calories.

Suggested meal plans in this section are for the hospitalized patient. Any meal plan for an individual not in the hospital should be adapted to his food habits, his

NUTRITIONAL REQUIREMENTS

Food and Nutrition Board, National Academy of Sciences-National Research Council
Recommended Daily Dietary Allowances,* Revised 1963
Designed for the Maintenance of Good Nutrition of Practically All Healthy Persons in the U.S.A.
(Allowances are intended for persons normally active in a temperate climate)

	Age† (Yrs.)	Weight Kg.	(Lbs.)	Height Cm.	(In.)	Calories‡	Prot. (Gm.)	Calc. (Gm.)	Iron (Mg.)	Vit. A (I.U.)	Thiam. (Mg.)	Ribo. (Mg.)	Niacin (Mg. Equiv.§)	Asc. Acid (Mg.)	Vit. D (I.U.)
Men............	18–35	70	(154)	175	(69)	2,900	70	0.8	10	5,000	1.2	1.7	19	70	...
	35–55	70	(154)	175	(69)	2,600	70	0.8	10	5,000	1.0	1.6	17	70	...
	55–75	70	(154)	175	(69)	2,200	70	0.8	10	5,000	0.9	1.3	15	70	...
Women.........	18–35	58	(128)	163	(64)	2,100	58	0.8	15	5,000	0.8	1.3	14	70	...
	35–55	58	(128)	163	(64)	1,900	58	0.8	15	5,000	0.8	1.2	13	70	...
	55–75	58	(128)	163	(64)	1,600	58	0.8	10	5,000	0.8	1.2	13	70	...
	Pregnant (2nd and 3rd trimester)					+ 200	+20	+0.5	+ 5	+1,000	+0.2	+0.3	+ 3	+30	400
	Lactating					+1,000	+40	+0.5	+ 5	+3,000	+0.4	+0.6	+ 7	+30	400
Infants‖......	0–1	8	(18)			Kg. × 115 ±15	Kg. × 2.5 ±0.5	0.7	Kg. × 1.0	1,500	0.4	0.6	6	30	400
Children.....	1–3	13	(29)	87	(34)	1,300	32	0.8	8	2,000	0.5	0.8	9	40	400
	3–6	18	(40)	107	(42)	1,600	40	0.8	10	2,500	0.6	1.0	11	50	400
	6–9	24	(53)	124	(49)	2,100	52	0.8	12	3,500	0.8	1.3	14	60	400
Boys.........	9–12	33	(72)	140	(55)	2,400	60	1.1	15	4,500	1.0	1.4	16	70	400
	12–15	45	(98)	156	(61)	3,000	75	1.4	15	5,000	1.2	1.8	20	80	400
	15–18	61	(134)	172	(68)	3,400	85	1.4	15	5,000	1.4	2.0	22	80	400
Girls........	9–12	33	(72)	140	(55)	2,200	55	1.1	15	4,500	0.9	1.3	15	80	400
	12–15	47	(103)	158	(62)	2,500	62	1.3	15	5,000	1.0	1.5	17	80	400
	15–18	53	(117)	163	(64)	2,300	58	1.3	15	5,000	0.9	1.3	15	70	400

* The allowance levels are intended to cover individual variations among most normal persons as they live in the United States under usual environmental stresses. The recommended allowances can be attained with a variety of common foods, providing other nutrients for which human requirements have been less well defined. See text for more detailed discussion of allowances and of nutrients not tabulated.

† Entries on lines for age range 18–35 years represent the 25-year age. All other entries represent allowances for the midpoint of the specified age periods, i.e., line for children 1–3 is for age 2 years (24 months); 3–6 is for age 4½ years (54 months), etc.

‡ The table on the reverse side of this sheet shows the calorie adjustment to be made for weight and age of men and women.

§ Niacin equivalents include dietary sources of the preformed vitamin and the precursor, tryptophan; 60 mg. of tryptophan represents 1 mg. of niacin.

‖ The calorie and protein allowances per Kg. for infants are considered to decrease progressively from birth. Allowances for calcium, thiamine, riboflavin and niacin increase proportionately with calories to the maximum values shown.

Adjustment of Calorie Allowances for Adult Individuals of Various Body Weights and Ages*
(At mean environmental temperature of 20 C. (68 F.) assuming average physical activity)

Men					Women				
Desirable Weight		Calorie Allowances†			Desirable Weight		Calorie Allowances†		
Kg.	Lbs.	25 Yrs.(1)	45 Yrs.(2)	65 Yrs.(3)	Kg.	Lbs.	25 Yrs.(4)	45 Yrs.(5)	65 Yrs.(6)
50	110	2,300	2,050	1,750	40	88	1,600	1,450	1,200
55	121	2,450	2,200	1,850	45	99	1,750	1,600	1,300
60	132	2,600	2,350	1,950	50	110	1,900	1,700	1,450
65	143	2,750	2,500	2,100	55	121	2,000	1,800	1,550
70	154	2,900	2,600	2,200	58	128	2,100	1,900	1,600
75	165	3,050	2,750	2,300	60	132	2,150	1,950	1,650
80	176	3,200	2,900	2,450	65	143	2,300	2,050	1,750
85	187	3,350	3,050	2,550	70	154	2,400	2,200	1,850

* This table and the Recommended Dietary Allowances are reprinted from the 6th Revised Edition, Report of The Food and Nutrition Board, National Academy of Science, National Research Council Pub. No. 1146, Washington, D.C., 1964.
† Adjustment of calorie allowances for individuals of different weights and ages have been calculated from simplified formulas for the age-range periods as follows: (1) $727 + 31W$; (2) $650 + 28W$; (3) $550 + 23.5W$; (4) $525 + 27W$; (5) $474 + 24.5W$; (6) $400 + 20.5W$.
Values have been rounded to the nearest 50 calories. To convert formulas for weight in pounds, divide factor by 2.2.
These formulas were developed on the premise that 25 per cent of the energy expenditure is independent of weight and 75 per cent is directly proportional to body weight. The factors are derived by dividing 75 per cent of the calorie allowance by the reference weight for each group.

working hours, his economic status and other factors that may affect his selection of food or his meal hours.

An example of this may be: the man who carries a lunch might have a sandwich, fruit, cake and milk (thermos) instead of the standard luncheon in the text.

SUGGESTED MEAL PLAN

Breakfast

    Fruit
    Cereal (whole-grain or enriched) with milk and sugar
    Egg
    Whole-wheat or enriched roll or toast
    Butter or fortified margarine
    Hot beverage with cream and sugar

Luncheon or Supper

    Cheese, meat, fish or eggs
    Potato or substitute
    Vegetable
    Salad with dressing
    Whole-wheat or enriched bread
    Butter or fortified margarine
    Fruit
    Milk

Dinner

    Meat, fish or fowl
    Potato or substitute
    Vegetable
    Whole-wheat or enriched bread
    Butter or fortified margarine
    Dessert
    Milk

Between meal nourishments should not be necessary. If the patient is hungry a bedtime feeding of milk, cocoa or fruit juice may be given.

HIGH CALORIC DIET

Purpose

To provide an adequate diet higher in calories than the normal requirement.

General Rules

Some patients may take 3 large meals, others may take more food if given 3 average meals and 2 or 3 nourishments.

Nourishments should be given at such times that they do not interfere with the appetite for the next meal.

The following additions to the regular diet will provide approximately 24 Gm. of protein and 1,000 calories:

Breakfast

1 slice bread, 1 teaspoon butter
1 tablespoon marmalade

Luncheon

1 slice bread, 1 teaspoon butter
1 tablespoon marmalade

Dinner

1 slice bread, 1 teaspoon butter

Between-Meal Nourishment

Afternoon—chocolate milk, crackers
Evening—1 glass milk, frosted cake

For the patient who finds it difficult to take the regular diet plus the additional foods, it may be necessary to plan meals smaller in volume and more concentrated in food value.

LOW CALORIC DIET

Purpose

To provide a low caloric diet that contains the essentials for good nutrition.

General Rules

Include the following daily:
Milk—1 pint
Meat, fish, fowl or cheese—5 oz.
Egg—1
Butter or fortified margarine—3 tsp.
Whole-grain or enriched cereal or bread—1 serving

535

Vegetables*—3 to 4 servings, 1 dark green or yellow
Fruit*—3 servings, unsweetened, 1 citrus

Other foods to provide the calories desired, preferably bulky ones to satisfy appetite.

AVOID the following foods or use in limited amounts, as the caloric allowance permits:

Beverages and soups made with cream, butter, whole milk, cereal or sugar

Cereals, including bread, rolls, crackers, noodles, rice, spaghetti, macaroni, waffles and pancakes

Rich or sweet desserts, such as cake, cookies, pudding, pastry and ice cream

Sweetened, canned or stewed fruit

Vegetables high in carbohydrate such as sweet potato, corn, dried peas, lima or kidney beans, parsnips (may be used as a substitute for potato or bread)

Fat meat and fish, such as fresh pork, ham, bacon, sausage, sardines or other fish canned in oil

Cream—sweet and sour

Chocolate (cocoa may be used sparingly)

Sauces and gravies

Fried food, including potato chips and doughnuts

Oil and salad dressings, including mineral oil

Sweets, such as sugar, candy, jelly, jam, marmalade, syrup, honey and molasses

Nuts

Bottled beverages, such as ginger ale, pop, cola beverages, beer, wine and other alcoholic beverages

ALLOW as desired: clear broth, lemon juice, bouillon, vinegar, raw celery, carrots, lettuce, radishes, noncaloric carbonated beverages, tea, coffee, lemonade (no sugar), saccharine or other noncaloric sweeteners.

* *See* lists, pp. 548-549.

SUGGESTED MEAL PLAN

FOR 1,200 CALORIES

Breakfast

Fruit—fresh or unsweetened—1 serving
Egg—1
Whole-wheat or enriched roll or toast—1 slice

Butter or fortified margarine—1 tsp.
Coffee or tea with milk and artificial sweetener

Luncheon or Supper

Lean meat, fish or cheese—2 oz. (or 2 eggs)
Vegetable—1 serving
Salad with lemon or vinegar
Butter or fortified margarine—1 teaspoon
Fruit (unsweetened)—1 serving
Milk—1 glass

Dinner

Lean meat, fish or fowl—3 oz.
Vegetable—2 servings
Butter or fortified margarine—1 teaspoon
Fruit (unsweetened)—1 serving
Milk—1 glass

Between-Meal Nourishment

None is given unless the patient complains of hunger; then lemonade without sugar, tea with lemon, or bouillon is allowed. Milk may be omitted from the meals and used for between-meal nourishment.

FOR 1,000 CALORIES

Use the 1,200-calorie diet as a basis. Substitute skim milk for whole milk.

FOR 1,500 CALORIES

Use the 1,200-calorie diet as a basis. Add
  Potato—1 medium
  Butter or fortified margarine—2 tsp.
  Bread—2 slices
NOTE: It is suggested that vitamin supplements would be desirable for the 1,000-calorie diet.

HIGH PROTEIN DIET

(APPROXIMATELY 100 GM. OF PROTEIN)

Purpose

To provide the essentials for good nutrition and to increase the protein to at least 100 Gm.

537

DIET

General Rules

Supplement the regular diet with extra complete protein foods as meat, fish, fowl, cheese, milk and eggs.

SUGGESTED MEAL PLAN

Breakfast
Fruit
Cereal with milk and sugar
Eggs—2
Whole-grain or enriched toast
Butter or fortified margarine
Hot beverage with cream and sugar

10 A.M.
Milk

Luncheon or Supper
Cream Soup
Meat, fish or cheese—large serving (3 oz.)
Potato, rice, noodles, spaghetti or macaroni
Salad
Whole-grain or enriched bread
Butter or fortified margarine
Fruit
Milk

Dinner
Meat, fish or fowl—large serving (3 oz.)
Potato
Vegetable
Whole-grain or enriched bread
Butter or fortified margarine
Dessert
Milk or cocoa

8 P.M.
Eggnog

HIGH CELLULOSE DIET

Purpose

To encourage regular elimination by stimulating muscle tone.

General Rules

Provide a diet higher in vitamins, carbohydrate and residue than the normal standard.

Supplement the normal diet with:

2 servings fruit

2 servings vegetable (use 2 raw daily)

2 servings whole-wheat bread

Jelly, jam, marmalade, sugar or hard candy at each meal.

Force fluids unless otherwise ordered.

Buttermilk may be substituted for whole milk.

Emphasize good health habits.

Regular hours for meals

Sufficient sleep

Regular time to visit toilet

MODERATELY LOW FAT DIET

(APPROXIMATELY 65 GM. FAT)

Purpose

To provide the essentials for good nutrition using easily digested foods that are low in fat and seasonings.

General Rules

Include the following daily, limiting the amounts whenever indicated:

Whole milk—1 pt. (no more)

Lean meat, fish or fowl, or pot cheese—2 servings (5 oz.) (no more)

Egg—1 (no more)

Butter or fortified margarine—3 tsp.

Whole-grain or enriched cereal or bread—2 servings

Fruit—2 servings, 1 to be orange or grapefruit

Potato—1 or 2 servings

Vegetables—2 to 3 servings, one dark green or yellow

Other carbohydrate foods to provide adequate calories.

Note: Additional skim milk may be used as desired.

Avoid

Beverages and soups made with cream, butter or whole milk (except that allowed on diet)

Rich desserts, such as pastry, puddings, cakes (except angel food), ice cream (except sherbet and ice)

Fat meat and fish such as pork, sausage, sardines or any fish canned in oil

Cream—sweet and sour

Cheese—except pot or uncreamed cottage

Chocolate (cocoa may be used)

Fried food

Sauces and gravies

Salad dressings, including mineral oil dressing

Nuts

Excess spices or condiments

Unless tolerated by the patient:

    Melons and raw apples

    Strongly flavored vegetables, such as cabbage, broccoli, cauliflower, Brussels sprouts, onions, turnips, radishes, cucumbers, green peppers, dried peas and beans

SUGGESTED MEAL PLAN

Breakfast

Fruit

Whole-grain or enriched cereal with milk (½ cup) and sugar

Egg—1

Whole-wheat or enriched roll or toast

Butter or fortified margarine—1 tsp.

Coffee or tea with milk and sugar

Luncheon or Supper

Uncreamed cottage cheese, lean meat or fish—2 oz.

Potato, rice, noodles, spaghetti or macaroni—without fat

Vegetable—without fat

Salad with vinegar or lemon

Whole-wheat or enriched bread

Butter or fortified margarine—1 tsp.

Fruit

Milk—1 glass

Dinner

Lean meat, fish or fowl—3 oz.
Potato—without fat
Vegetable—without fat
Whole-wheat or enriched bread
Butter or fortified margarine—1 tsp.
Fruit, gelatin, ices or angel food cake
Milk—½ glass

Between-Meal Nourishment

None is given routinely: If desired, fruit juice, tomato juice or tea with lemon may be given.

STRICT
(NOT MORE THAN 25 GM. FAT)

If not more than 25 Gm. fat is desired, substitute skim milk for whole milk and omit the butter. Jelly may be used on bread in place of butter. This diet may be low in Vitamin A. When it is continued for longer than 2 weeks, a concentrate should be prescribed.

MODERATELY LOW FAT, HIGH CARBOHYDRATE, HIGH PROTEIN DIET

(60 GM. FAT, 350 GM. CARBOHYDRATE, 125 GM. PROTEIN)

Purpose

To provide a diet with decreased fat and increased carbohydrate and protein.

General Rules

Include the following foods daily:
Milk—skim—5 cups
Lean meat, fish, fowl or uncreamed cottage cheese—
2 large servings, 4 oz. each
Egg—1
Potato—2 or more servings
Vegetables—2 to 3 servings, 1 dark green or yellow
Whole-grain or enriched bread or cereal—7 servings
Butter or fortified margarine—3 tsp.

Fruits—3 or more servings, 1 citrus

Sugar—3 tbsp. or more

Jelly, honey or marmalade—3 tbsp. or more

Desserts as water ices, plain gelatin desserts, puddings made with skim milk and angel cake may be used.

For a higher protein diet, dry skim milk solids, egg white or gelatin may be added to allowed foods. Protein hydrolysates may be given if ordered by the physician.

If additional carbohydrate is desired, crackers or bread, jelly and hard candy may be given between meals.

AVOID the same foods listed for the Low Fat Diet.

SUGGESTED MEAL PLAN

Breakfast

Fruit

Whole-grain or enriched cereal with sugar

Egg—1

Whole-wheat or enriched bread—2 slices

Butter or fortified margarine—1 tsp.

Jelly—1 tbsp.

Milk, skim—1 cup

Sugar—4 tsp.

Coffee

Luncheon or Supper

Uncreamed cottage cheese, meat or fish—4 oz.

Potato, rice, noodles or macaroni—no fat

Vegetable—no fat

Salad with vinegar or lemon

Whole-wheat or enriched bread—2 slices

Butter or fortified margarine—1 tsp.

Jelly—1 tbsp.

Fruit

Milk, skim—1 cup

Midafternoon

Milk, skim—1 cup

Dinner

Lean meat, fish or fowl—4 oz.

Potato—no fat

Vegetable—no fat
Whole-wheat or enriched bread—2 slices
Butter or fortified margarine—1 tsp.
Jelly—1 tbsp.
Fruit, gelatin, water ices or angel food cake
Milk, skim—1 cup

Evening

Milk, skim—1 cup

LOW SODIUM DIET

STRICT LOW SODIUM DIET
(APPROXIMATELY 250 MG. SODIUM)

Purpose

To provide a diet containing approximately 250 mg. of sodium or 11 milliequivalents of sodium.

General Rules

Prepare all the food without salt and soda, and do not allow a salt shaker on the tray.

Include the following daily only in the amounts allowed (see lists of foods allowed):

Low-sodium milk—1 pt.
Meat, fish or fowl—2 servings (5 oz.)
(2 oz. unsalted pot cheese may be used instead of 2 oz. meat.)
Egg—1
Sweet butter—1 tbsp. or more
Cereal (see list)—1 serving
Unsalted bread or matzoth—3 slices
Fruit—3 servings or more
Vegetables—3 servings (see list to avoid)
Potatoes, or substitute—1 to 2 servings
White sugar—1 tbsp. or more
Jelly—3 tbsp. or more

Allow the Following

CEREALS

Ralston
Wheatena

Cornmeal
Pettijohn's
Farina (unenriched)
Oatmeal
Rice
Puffed wheat and rice
Shredded wheat
Macaroni and spaghetti

FISH

Fresh cod
Fresh halibut
Oysters
Fresh salmon
Bluefish
Catfish
Trout

Use as Desired

Tea, coffee, sugar, jelly, jam, marmalade, honey, oil, unsalted cooking fats, unsweetened chocolate, cornstarch, flour, plain gelatin, tapioca granules, plain matzoth, unsalted nuts, fruit juice, coca-cola.

Do not use salt in cooking or on food afterwards.

Avoid the Following

Canned, salted or smoked meat as ham, bacon, sausage, corned beef, liverwurst, chipped beef, frankfurters or fish, as herring, salmon, tuna fish, sardines, lox

Frozen fish fillets

Powdered eggs

Any cakes, muffins, cookies, pastry, crackers, pretzels, biscuits or hot breads made with baking powder, soda (baking) or salt

Ice cream

Puddings or other desserts made with milk and eggs

Commercial ready-made mixes as rolls, gingerbread, cake, pie crust

All prepared cereals except shredded wheat, puffed rice and puffed wheat

Beets, beet greens, kale, spinach, celery, sauerkraut. and frozen peas, lima beans, succotash, mixed vegetables and mixed peas and carrots

All canned vegetables except those canned without salt

Canned soup or bouillon cubes

Cheese, except low-sodium cheese

Salted butter or margarine

Cantaloupe

Kidney

Commercial salad dressing

Baking soda in any form

Salted nuts or peanut butter

Candy and candy bars

Relishes, olives, pickles, catsup, chili sauce

Tomato paste, commercial tomato sauce or any other commercial meat sauces

If desired, the following may be used for seasoning:

Pepper	Ginger	Onion juice
Paprika	Nutmeg	Bay leaves
Lemon	Dry mustard	Poultry seasoning
Vanilla	powder	Green pepper
Allspice	Curry powder	Vinegar
Cinnamon	Sweet butter	Cream—2 tbsp.
	Garlic	only

Use no prepared seasoning salts, such as onion, garlic or celery salt.

NOTE: This diet contains approximately 70 Gm. of protein. If higher protein is desired, the sodium will be increased. If the low-sodium milk is omitted, the protein is decreased 15 Gm., and the diet is inadequate in calcium and riboflavin.

Supplements may be indicated when the diet is followed for a period of time.

Salt substitutes may be used only if ordered by the physician. Some "salt substitutes" contain sodium and cannot be used (e.g., sodium formate and sodium malate).

DIET

Medications containing sodium should not be used.

When this diet is used for congestive heart failure, the following vegetables, which cause distention for some people, should be omitted:

Lima beans	Cauliflower
Broccoli	Cucumber
Brussels sprouts	Onions
Cabbage	Rutabagas

Suggested Meal Plan

All food is prepared without salt or soda, and salt is not served on the tray.

Breakfast
Fruit
Cereal
Egg—1
Unsalted bread or toast with sweet butter and jelly
Low-sodium milk
Hot beverage with sugar

Luncheon or Supper
Cheese—unsalted, meat, fish or fowl (2 oz.) or 2 eggs
Potato, rice, spaghetti or macaroni
Vegetable or salad with unsalted French dressing or mayonnaise
Unsalted bread with sweet butter and jelly
Fruit
Low-sodium milk

Dinner
Meat, fish or fowl—3 oz.
Potato
Vegetable
Unsalted bread with sweet butter and jelly
Fruit
Hot beverage with sugar

Between-Meal Nourishment

None is given routinely. Fruit juices may be used if desired.

MODERATE LOW SODIUM DIET
(APPROXIMATELY 500 MG. OR 22 MILLIEQUIVALENTS SODIUM)

For a moderate low sodium diet, use the same general rules as for the strict low sodium diet, but substitute 1 pint regular milk for the low sodium milk.

DIABETIC DIETS

Diabetic patients differ greatly in their dietary needs; therefore, no recommended diets are given. The physician will prescribe the relative amounts of protein, fat and carbohydrate; he will designate also the desired distribution of the carbohydrate in the 3 meals and other feedings, if any.

For those who are calculating such prescribed diets, simplified Exchange Lists prepared by the American Diabetic Association and the American Dietetic Association in co-operation with the Diabetes Branch of the Public Health Service are given.

LIST 1. MILK EXCHANGES

CARB.—12 GM., PROTEIN—8 GM., FAT—10 GM.,
CALORIES 170

	MEASURES	GM.
Milk, whole*	1 cup	240
Milk, evaporated	½ cup	120
Milk, powdered*	¼ cup	35
Buttermilk*	1 cup	240

* Add 2 fat exchanges if these are fat free.

LIST 2. VEGETABLE EXCHANGES

These vegetables may be used as desired in ordinary amounts. Carbohydrates and Calories negligible.

Asparagus	Lettuce	"Greens"
Broccoli	Mushrooms	Beet
Brussels Sprouts	Okra	Chard
Cabbage	Pepper	Collard
Cauliflower	Radishes	Dandelion
Celery	Rhubarb	Kale
Chicory	Sauerkraut	Mustard
Cucumbers	String Beans,	Spinach
Escarole	young	Turnip
Eggplant	Summer Squash	
	Tomatoes	

With these vegetables, 1 serving equals ½ cup equals 100 Gm.

Carb.—7 Gm., Protein—2 Gm., Calories—36

Beets	Peas, green	Squash, winter
Carrots	Pumpkin	Turnip
Onions	Rutabaga	

LIST 3. FRUIT EXCHANGES
CARBOHYDRATE—10 GM., CALORIES—40

	MEASURE	GM.
Apple	1 sm. (2″ diam.)	80
Applesauce	½ cup	100
Apricots, fresh	2 medium	100
Apricots, dried	4 halves	20
Banana	½ small	50
Berries:		
Straw., Rasp., Black.	1 cup	150
Blueberries	⅔ cup	100
Cantaloupe	¼ (6″ diam.)	200
Cherries	10 large	75
Dates	2	15
Figs, fresh	2 large	50
Figs, dried	1 small	15
Grapefruit	½ small	125

	MEASURE	GM.
Grapefruit juice	½ cup	100
Grapes	12	75
Grape juice	¼ cup	60
Honeydew melon	⅛ (7″ diam.)	150
Mango	½ small	70
Orange	1 small	100
Orange juice	½ cup	100
Papaya	⅓ medium	100
Peach	1 medium	100
Pear	1 small	100
Pineapple	½ cup	80
Pineapple juice	⅓ cup	80
Plums	2 medium	100
Prunes, dried	2 medium	25
Raisins	2 tbsp.	15
Tangerine	1 large	100
Watermelon	1 cup	175

LIST 4. BREAD EXCHANGES

CARBOHYDRATE—15 GM., PROTEIN—2 GM.,
CALORIES—68

	MEASURE	GM.
Bread	1 slice	25
Biscuit, Roll	1 (2″ diam.)	35
Muffin	1 (2″ diam.)	35
Cornbread	1 (1½″ cube)	35
Flour	2½ tbsp.	20
Cereal, cooked	½ cup	100
Cereal, dry (flake and puffed)	¾ cup	20
Rice, grits, cooked	½ cup	100
Spaghetti, noodles, etc., cooked	½ cup	100
Crackers, Graham (2½″ sq.)	2	20
Oyster	20 (½ cup)	20
Saltines (2″ sq.)	5	20
Soda (2½″ sq.)	3	20
Round, thin (1½″ diam.)	6-8	20

LIST 4. BREAD EXCHANGES—(*Continued*)

	MEASURE	GM.
Vegetables		
Beans and Peas, dried, cooked	½ cup	90
(lima, navy, split pea, cowpeas, etc.)		
Baked beans, no pork	¼ cup	50
Corn	⅓ cup	80
Parsnips	⅔ cup	125
Potatoes, white, baked, boiled	1 (2″ diam.)	100
Potatoes, white, mashed	½ cup	100
Potatoes, sweet, or yams	¼ cup	50
Sponge cake, plain	1 (1½″ cube)	25
Ice cream (omit 2 fat exchanges)	½ cup	70

LIST 5. MEAT EXCHANGES

PROTEIN—7 GM., FAT—5 GM., CALORIES—73

	MEASURE	GM.
Meat and poultry (medium fat)	1 oz.	30
(beef, lamb, pork, liver, chicken, etc.)		
Cold cuts (4½″ sq., ⅛″ thick)	1 slice	45
Frankfurter	1 (8-9/lb.)	50
Fish: cod, mackerel, etc.	1 oz.	30
Salmon, tuna, crab	¼ cup	30
Oysters, shrimp, clams	5 small	45
Sardines	3 medium	30
Cheese, cheddar, American,	1 oz.	30
Cottage	¼ cup	45
Egg	1	50
Peanut butter*	2 tbsp.	30

* Limit use or adjust carbohydrate.

LIST 6. FAT EXCHANGES

FAT—5 GM., CALORIES—45

	MEASURE	GM.
Butter or margarine	1 tsp.	5
Bacon, crisp	1 slice	10
Cream, light, 20%	2 tbsp.	30
Cream, heavy, 40%	1 tbsp.	15
Cream cheese	1 tbsp.	15
French dressing	1 tbsp.	15
Mayonnaise	1 tsp.	5
Oil or cooking fat	1 tsp.	5
Nuts	6 small	10
Olives	5 small	50
Avocado	⅛ (4″ diam.)	25

FOODS ALLOWED AS DESIRED

(NEGLIGIBLE CARBOHYDRATE, PROTEIN AND FAT)

Coffee	Rhubarb
Tea	Mustard
Clear broth	Pickle, sour
Bouillon	Pickle, dill—unsweetened
Gelatin, unsweetened	Saccharine
Rennet tablets	Pepper
Cranberries	Spices
Lemon	Vinegar

SAMPLE DIABETIC DIET CALCULATION

Calculation of a prescribed diabetic diet and the sample meal pattern for that diet is given, showing the use of the lists presented above.

Diet Order: Protein—80 Gm., Fat—80 Gm., Carbohydrate—170 Gm.

Carbohydrate divided:

Breakfast 40; Lunch 50; Dinner 70; Bedtime 10

DIET

Foods	Amount	Protein	Fat	Carbo-hydrate
BREAKFAST				
Fruit	2 portions	..	..	20
Egg	1	7	5	..
Carbohydrate exchange	1	2	..	15
Fat exchange	1	..	5	..
Milk	½ cup	4	5	6
	Total	13	15	41
LUNCHEON				
Protein exchange	2	14	10	..
Vegetable:				
As desired Group A	..	..	..	..
Carbohydrate Exchange	2	4	..	30
Fat exchange	1	..	5	..
Fruit	1	..	..	10
Milk	1 cup	8	10	12
	Total	26	25	52
DINNER				
Protein exchange	3	21	15	..
Vegetable:				
As desired Group A				
Group B	1 portion	2	..	7
Carbohydrate exchange	3	6	..	45
Fat exchange	2	..	10	..
Fruit	1 portion	..	..	10
Milk	½ cup	4	5	6
	Total	33	30	68
EVENING				
Milk	1 cup	8	10	12
	Complete Total	80	80	173
	Calories—1732			

Sample Meal Plan for Calculated Diet Given

BREAKFAST
Fruit	2 (see list)
Egg	1
Bread or toast	1 slice
Butter or margarine	1 tsp.
Milk	½ cup
Coffee	

LUNCHEON
Sandwich:	
bread	2 slices
butter or mayonnaise	1 tsp.
cheese	2 oz.
Tomato—sliced	1
Milk	1 cup
Fruit	1 (see list)
Tea or coffee	

DINNER
Meat, fish or fowl	3 oz.
Potato, mashed	½ cup
Vegetables	
Group A	as desired
Group B	½ cup
Butter or margarine	2 tsp.
Bread	2 slices
Milk	½ cup
Fruit	1 (see list)

EVENING
Milk	1 cup

552

PREGNANCY AND LACTATION

NORMAL DIET

Purpose

To provide the essentials of good nutrition for mother and infant during the prenatal and the postnatal, lactating period.

General Rules

Include the following daily:

Milk—1 qt. (1½ qt. for lactation)

Egg—1 or 2

Meat, fish, fowl—1 large serving (3 to 4 oz.)
Use liver once or twice a week.

Cheese, meat, fish or fowl, 2 oz., or 2 eggs

Vegetables—2 or more servings; 1 serving should be green or yellow; 1 serving should be raw

Fruit—2 or more servings; 1 should be large serving of orange, grapefruit or tomato (extra large during lactation)

Whole-grain or enriched white bread or cereal—4 servings

Potato—1 serving

Butter or fortified margarine—6 tsp.

Vitamin D—400 units from reinforced milk or vitamin supplement

Water—6 to 8 glasses

SUGGESTED MEAL PLAN

Breakfast

Orange or grapefruit

Egg—1

Whole-grain or enriched toast, or roll

Butter or fortified margarine

Tea, coffee, milk or cocoa

Luncheon or Supper

Choice of cheese, dried peas, beans, peanut butter, fish or meat—2 oz. or 2 eggs

Whole-grain or enriched bread

Butter or fortified margarine

DIET

Vegetable or salad or both
Fruit or dessert
Milk
Tea or coffee, if desired

Dinner

Meat, fish, fowl or liver—3 to 4 oz.
Potato or, occasionally, rice, noodles or macaroni
Vegetables
Salad
Whole-grain or enriched bread
Butter or fortified margarine
Dessert or fruit
Milk
Tea or coffee, if desired

Midafternoon and Evening

Milk
NOTE: Milk may be flavored with chocolate, coffee or vanilla

1,800-CALORIE, RESTRICTED SALT DIET

Purpose

To provide the essentials for normal nutrition during pregnancy with a diet that is restricted in calories and limited in sodium content to 1 to 1.5 Gm.

General Rules

Do not use salt in food preparation.
Do not add salt afterwards.

INCLUDE THESE FOODS DAILY:

Milk—1 qt.
Egg—1
Lean meat, fish, fowl or liver—3 to 4 oz.
Unsalted cottage cheese, fish or meat—2 oz. (or 2 eggs)
Vegetables—2 large servings or 4 small servings (1 should be green or yellow; 1 should be raw)
Unsweetened fruit—3 servings (1 to be a large serving of orange or grapefruit)

Sweet butter—3 tsp.

Potato—1 small

Whole-grain or enriched bread or cereal—3 servings

Vitamin D—400 units from reinforced milk or vitamin supplement

Avoid

Foods high in sodium. (*See* list under Low Sodium Diet.) Pregnancy restricted salt diet may use regular bread.

High-caloric foods. (*See* list under Low Calorie Diet.)

SUGGESTED MEAL PLAN

Breakfast

Unsweetened orange or grapefruit—1 serving

Egg—1

Whole-wheat or enriched bread or cereal—1 serving

Sweet butter—1 tsp.

Tea or coffee —without sugar

Luncheon or Supper

Meat, fish, unsalted cottage cheese—2 oz., or 2 eggs

Vegetables—1 or 2 servings

Whole-grain or enriched bread—2 slices

Sweet butter—1 tsp.

Unsweetened fruit—1 serving

Milk—1 glass

Dinner

Lean meat, fish, fowl or liver—3 to 4 oz. (not fried, no gravy, no sauces)

Potato—1 small

Vegetables—1 or 2 servings (1 to be a salad, omit oil)

Sweet butter—1 tsp.

Unsweetened fruit—1 serving

Milk—1 glass

Midafternoon and Evening

Milk—1 glass

DIET

HIGH CARBOHYDRATE DIET—FREQUENT SMALL FEEDINGS

(FREQUENTLY USED FOR HYPEREMESIS GRAVIDARUM)

Purpose

To provide a diet high in carbohydrate and low in fat that will be digested and assimilated easily.

General Rules

FIRST TO THIRD DAY

6:00 A.M. or on Awakening
  Saltines—2, with 1 or 2 tsp. jelly
  Hard candy or loaf sugar if desired

Breakfast
  Cereal—½ cup, with sugar
  Milk for cereal if desired, *or*
  Dry toast and jelly

Midmorning
  Crackers—2, with 1 or 2 tsp. jelly
  Hard candy or loaf sugar, if desired

Luncheon or Supper
  Salty broth—½ cup, or tomato juice
  Toast—1 slice, *or* 2 crackers
  Gelatin dessert or fruit

Midafternoon
  Crackers—2, and 2 tsp. jelly
  Gelatin dessert or fruit

Dinner
  Salty broth
  Plain potato
  Canned fruit or gelatin

8:00 P.M. and 10:00 P.M.
  As at midmorning or midafternoon

During the Night
  If the patient is awake, give nourishments as at midmorning or midafternoon.

SOFT DIET

Purpose

To provide the essentials for good nutrition using foods that are soft in consistency and omitting rich and strongly flavored foods that may cause distress.

General Rules*

Include the following foods daily:

Milk—1 pint

Egg—1

Tender meat, fish or fowl—3 oz.

Soft cheese, tender meat, fish or fowl—2 oz. or 2 eggs

Potato or substitute—1 serving

Butter or fortified margarine—3 tsp.

Strained whole-grain cereals or enriched bread—3 servings

Soft fruit—2 servings

Orange or grapefruit juice—1 serving

Cooked vegetable—2 servings (see list)

Other foods as allowed to provide adequate calories

Typical Foods Allowed

All beverages and strained soups

Bread, crackers and cereal

White, fine whole-wheat and rye bread without seeds

White crackers

Dry cereals, such as cornflakes, Rice Krispies, puffed rice and Pablum

Fine white cereals, such as farina, Cream of Wheat, cornmeal, hominy grits, rice, noodles, spaghetti and macaroni

Strained coarse cereals, such as oatmeal

Desserts

Custard, blanc mange, tapioca, rice and bread pudding; cake, cookies, frozen and gelatin desserts all without nuts, cocoanut or fruits not on *avoid* list.

Fruit

* If greater restrictions are required, serve ground meat and strained vegetables.

Cooked and canned soft fruit, without seeds and skin such as apricots, applesauce, peaches, pears, plums; fruit juices, ripe banana and orange and grapefruit sections without membrane

Vegetables

Cooked vegetable such as asparagus, beets, carrots, peas, spinach, string beans, squash without seeds

Mashed sweet potato

White potato without skin, any way except fried

Meat

Tender meat, poultry, fish and shellfish

Milk and eggs

Cheese

Mild, soft cheese, such as cream, cottage and grated American cheese in sauce

Avoid

Coarse dark bread; whole-grain crackers; coarse dark cereals unless strained

Rich pastries and any dessert containing nuts, cocoanut or fruits not on *allowed* list

Raw fruit except juice, ripe banana, orange and grapefruit sections

Tough meat with gristle and bone and fat pork. Salted and smoked meat and fish

Excessive seasoning

Raw, coarse and strong-flavored vegetables

SUGGESTED MEAL PLAN

Breakfast

Soft fruit or fruit juice
Cereal
Egg
Butter or fortified margarine
Toast
Beverage

Luncheon or Supper

Egg, mild soft cheese, tender meat or fish
Potato or substitute
Cooked vegetable (see list)

Bread
Butter or fortified margarine
Soft fruit
Milk

Dinner

Tomato, orange or grapefruit juice
Tender meat, fish or fowl
Potato (without skin)
Cooked vegetable (see list)
Bread
Butter or fortified margarine
Dessert
Milk

Between-Meal Nourishments

None given except upon request. If desired, milk, cocoa or fruit juice may be given.

BLAND DIET REGIMEN

The regimen consists of four stages. Progression from one stage to the next is made only upon order of the physician.

Purpose

To give frequent small feedings of foods that will avoid irritation of the gastrointestinal tract and will provide frequent dilution and neutralization of gastric secretion.

BLAND DIET 1

Ninety ml. (⅓ cup), half milk and half light cream given every hour from 6 or 7 A.M. to 9 or 10 P.M. Continue through the night if necessary.

BLAND DIET 2

1. Give 180 ml. (¾ cup), half milk and half light cream at 6 A.M., between meals, at 8 P.M., and every 4 hours during the night if necessary.

2. Three small meals, not to exceed 6 oz. (¾ cup) are selected from the following list of foods:

soft-cooked eggs
baked or soft custard
eggnog
junket
plain gelatin dessert
plain cornstarch puddings
butter or fortified margarine
sugar in small amounts
refined or strained cereals
strained cream soup
rice
white potato—no skin
white bread, toasted
saltines and soda crackers
milk toast
salt to make food palatable

SUGGESTED SCHEDULES

	BLAND 2	BLAND 3
6 A.M.	Milk and cream*—6 oz.	
Breakfast	Strained oatmeal—½ cup Sugar—1 tsp. Milk—½ cup	Strained oatmeal—½ cup Sugar—1 tsp. Milk—½ cup Soft cooked egg Toast—1 slice Butter—1 tsp.
Midmorning	Milk and cream—6 oz.	Milk—1 glass Saltines—2
Lunch or Supper	Cream soup—½ cup Saltines—2 Gelatin dessert—¼ cup	Cream soup—⅔ cup Cottage cheese—2 or 3 oz. Strained fruit—⅓ cup
Midafternoon	Milk and cream—6 oz.	Milk—½ glass Saltines—2 Dessert
Dinner	Soft-cooked egg White toast—1 slice Butter—1 tsp. Dessert—½ cup	Soft cooked egg White potato, no skin— 1 small Orange juice—⅓ cup Dessert (not fruit)—½ cup
8 P.M.	Milk and cream—6 oz.	Milk—1 glass Saltines—2

* This mixture is half milk and half light cream (commercial "Half and Half" may be used).

BLAND DIET 3

Substitute whole milk for the half-milk half-cream, and increase the amount of each feeding from 6 oz. to 10 to 12 oz. In addition allow the following foods not included on Bland Diet 2:

cottage, cream and pot cheese
macaroni, noodles or spaghetti with butter
grapefruit, orange or tomato juice—1 serving
cooked strained applesauce, apricots, peaches, pears, plums, prunes—1 serving

AVOID ALL OTHER FOODS including tea, coffee, coffee substitutes, carbonated beverages, meat broths, spices, *condiments*.

BLAND DIET WITH 6 FEEDINGS

General Rules

Include the following daily:

Milk—4 to 6 glasses
Meat, fish or fowl (ground unless tender)—1 serving (3 oz.)
Eggs—2, or 1 egg and another serving of meat, fish or soft cheese
Butter or fortified margarine—3 servings (½ oz.)
Strained whole-grain cereal or enriched white bread —2 servings
Strained fruit—1 serving
Orange or grapefruit juice—1 glass
Strained vegetable—1 serving, in addition to 1 serving or more of potato

Other foods as allowed to provide adequate calories.
Include between-meal nourishments consisting of white crackers with butter or fortified margarine and 1 glass of milk.
NOTE: Whole fruit and whole vegetables are given only on the order of a physician.

TYPICAL FOODS ALLOWED

Coffee or tea—½ cup with ½ cup hot milk—not in excess of once a day

DIET

Cream soups—made without stock
Breads, crackers and cereals
  Enriched white
  White crackers
  Dry cereals, such as corn flakes, Rice Krispies and
    puffed rice
  Fine cooked cereals, such as enriched farina, Cream
    of Wheat, cornmeal, hominy grits, rice, noodles,
    spaghetti and macaroni, infant cereals
  Strained coarse cereals, such as oatmeal and petti-
    johns
Desserts—Custards, cornstarch, tapioca, rice or bread
puddings, plain cake, cookies, frozen and gelatin des-
serts—all without nuts and whole fruit
Fruit
  Strained cooked apples, pears, peaches, prunes,
    plums, apricots
  Banana
  Strained orange, grapefruit, pineapple, apple, prune
    or tomato juice
Vegetables—strained cooked

Beets	Sweet Potato	Squash
Carrots	Corn	Spinach
Lima Beans	Asparagus	Tomato
Peas	String Beans	Celery

White potato (serve without skin)—any way except
fried
Meat—Beef, veal, lamb, liver, fowl, fish, oysters,
canned salmon and tuna (without bones, gristle and
excessive fat)—ground unless tender
Milk
Eggs—any way except fried
Cheese—mild soft cheese such as cream, cottage and
grated American cheese in sauce
Miscellaneous (in moderate amount if well tolerated)

Jelly	Honey	Molasses
Syrup	Plain Candy	Sugar

Enough salt to make food palatable.

Avoid

Beverages

Coffee or tea (except in amounts allowed), carbonated drinks, cereal beverages, cola drinks.

Breads, crackers and cereals

Coarse dark cereal

Whole-grain crackers

Coarse dark bread

Fresh or hot breads

Desserts

Rich pastries and any dessert containing nuts or whole fruit

Fruits

Raw fruit except juice and banana

Any not listed

Vegetables

Raw and coarse

Strongly flavored such as cabbage, cauliflower, broccoli, onions, turnips, Brussels sprouts, green peppers

Meat

Gristle, bone and fat

Salted and smoked meat and fish

Pork

Soups—prepared with meat stock

Cheese—strongly flavored

Miscellaneous

Seasonings, spices, condiments, such as mustard, catsup, chili sauce, horseradish, Worcestershire sauce, vinegar, olives, pickles, pepper, garlic

Rich gravies and sauces

Nuts, popcorn, raisins

SUGGESTED MEAL PLAN
BLAND IN 6 FEEDINGS

Breakfast

Fruit juice, strained fruit or ripe banana

Strained whole-grain cereal or enriched white cereal
    with milk and sugar

Egg

DIET

Enriched white toast
Butter or fortified margarine
Bland coffee, cocoa, tea or milk

Midmorning

Milk—1 glass
Saltines—2
Butter or fortified margarine

Luncheon or Supper

Strained cream soup—no stock
Egg, or mild soft cheese, or meat
White potato (no skin), rice, noodles or macaroni
Enriched white bread
Butter or fortified margarine
Strained fruit
Milk

Midafternoon

Same as midmorning

Dinner

Orange, grapefruit or tomato juice
Meat, fish or fowl, ground unless tender
White potato—no skin
Strained vegetable
Enriched bread
Butter or fortified margarine
Dessert (not fruit)
Milk

Night

Same as midmorning

No other nourishments are given routinely. Milk may
be given at any time as requested by the patient.

LOW RESIDUE DIETS

(STRICT)
(APPROXIMATELY CELLULOSE FREE)

Purpose

To restrict the cellulose to a minimum, to prevent
stimulation of peristalsis and to avoid distention.

General Rules

This diet is inadequate in minerals and vitamins and should not be continued for more than 2 weeks.

Typical Foods Allowed

Beverages—milk, cocoa, tea, coffee

Cereals—fine white cereal, including rice, noodles, macaroni and spaghetti; enriched white bread and plain white crackers

Desserts—plain custard, cornstarch, tapioca and rice puddings, plain ice cream, cookies and cake—all without fruit or nuts

White potato—without skin

Very tender ground meat, fish or fowl (serve without grinding if tolerated)

Broth or strained soup

Eggs and mild cheese

Butter or fortified margarine—allow only 1 tsp. per meal

Avoid

Whole-grain cereals and whole-grain bread

Fruits and fruit juices

Vegetables (except potato)

Tough meats

Spices, condiments and highly seasoned food

Fried foods

Excessive amounts of fat and sugar

Nuts

The milk may be boiled to produce a more tender curd. In a patient with a hypersensitive colon this may be indicated.

SUGGESTED MEAL PLAN

Breakfast

Fine enriched white cereal with milk and 1 tsp. sugar

Egg

Enriched white toast

Butter or fortified margarine—1 tsp.

Coffee with milk and 1 tsp. sugar

DIET

Luncheon or Supper

Mild cheese or a substitute of egg, ground tender meat, or fish

White potato (without skin), rice, noodles, spaghetti or macaroni

Enriched white bread

Butter or fortified margarine—1 tsp.

Custard or plain pudding

Milk

Dinner

Ground tender meat, fish or fowl (may be served without grinding if tolerated)

White potato without skin

Enriched white bread

Butter or fortified margarine—1 tsp.

Custard or plain pudding

Weak tea with milk and 1 tsp. sugar

Between-Meal Nourishment

None given except upon request or if it seems advisable to increase the caloric intake. In either case broth, milk, cocoa or tea may be given. One teaspoonful of sugar and 1 or 2 tablespoonfuls of cream may be added to the cocoa or tea.

MODERATE LOW RESIDUE DIET

To the strict low residue diet add:

Citrus juice—1 serving

Vegetable, strained, cooked—1 serving

carrots	string beans
beets	peas
lima beans	squash
spinach	asparagus

Fruit, strained, cooked or canned—1 serving

apricots	pears
apples	plums
peaches	prunes

Or ripe banana

FLUID DIETS

CLEAR

Purpose

To supply fluids, sodium chloride and a small amount of carbohydrate.

Foods Allowed

Broth or bouillon
Tea with lemon and sugar
Ginger ale

Some patients can tolerate these fluids when they cannot take fruit juices. If fruit juices are to be included the physician should order "Clear fluids with fruit juices."

Since this diet does not provide adequate nourishment, it should be changed to a Full Fluid Diet as soon as the patient can tolerate a more liberal diet.

FULL

Purpose

To provide nourishment in fluid form.

General Rules

Give at least 6 feedings daily.

Allow any food in liquid form and in addition: custard, plain cornstarch pudding, junket, gelatin, plain ice cream, fruit ice or sherbet, and soft-cooked eggs.

SUGGESTED MEAL PLAN

Breakfast

Strained orange or grapefruit juice
Strained cereal with hot milk and sugar (if desired)
Soft-cooked egg
Hot beverage with cream and sugar

10 A.M.

Milk, chocolate or malted milk, eggnog or strained fruit juice

DIET

Luncheon or Supper
   Strained soup
   Milk
   Custard, junket, gelatin or ice cream
   Strained fruit juice

2 P.M.
   As at 10 A.M.

Dinner
   Tomato juice or strained fruit juice
   Strained cream soup or broth
   Milk, eggnog or malted milk
   Dessert as at noon
   Hot beverage with cream and sugar

8 P.M.
   As at 10 A.M.

POSTOPERATIVE GASTRIC REGIMEN

Purpose

To test the ability of the stomach to empty and to prevent a feeling of fulness or discomfort by pressure of a full stomach on the wound.

General Rules

Begin with small amounts that are increased as tolerated. All amounts and increases are ordered by the physician.

FIRST DAY

On the first day, give 60 to 100 ml. water every hour, if tolerated.

SECOND DAY

Clear Fluids

Give 30 to 100 ml. (maximum if tolerated) every hour. Fluids that may be given are:
   Broth

Tea with lemon juice and sugar
Lemonade
Ginger ale, if tolerated

THIRD AND FOURTH DAYS

Full Fluid Diet

Give 100 ml. (maximum if tolerated) every hour. Any foods on Full Fluid Diet may be given.

FOURTH OR FIFTH DAYS

Follow the Bland Diet in Six Equal Feedings.
In about 2 weeks, the patient will be able to tolerate the Normal (Regular) Diet.

BLAND IN 6 EQUAL FEEDINGS

This diet contains approximately 12 oz. per feeding. For details *see* Bland Diet.

Breakfast
Strained cereal—⅓ cup
Egg
White toast—1 slice
Butter or fortified margarine—1 tsp.
Milk—⅔ cup
Coffee—½ cup
Sugar—2 tsp.

Midmorning
Fruit juice—⅔ glass
Crackers—4
Butter or fortified margarine—2 tsp.
Milk—1 glass

Lunch
Cream soup—⅔ cup
Ground meat—small serving
Potato, without skin—small
Butter or fortified margarine—1 tsp.
Citrus juice—⅔ glass

DIET

Midafternoon

Plain dessert (no fruit)—½ cup
Plain cookies, small—4
Milk—1 glass
Crackers—4
Butter or fortified margarine—2 tsp.

Dinner

Ground meat—small serving
Potato—small
Strained vegetable—¼ cup
Tomato juice—½ cup
Milk—1 glass
Butter or fortified margarine—1 tsp.

Bedtime

Strained fruit—½ cup
Plain cookies—4
Milk—1 glass
Crackers—4
Butter or fortified margarine—2 tsp.

It must be realized that these are approximate amounts. The amounts must be small and divided throughout the day as equally as possible. Substitutions such as white bread (or toast) may be used instead of crackers for variety. Other than the juices allowed, the diet must not contain more than 1 strained fruit and 1 strained vegetable per day.

TUBE FEEDINGS

Purpose

To provide adequate amounts of nutrients for persons unable to take food by mouth.

There is at least 1 mixture* that, when mixed with

---

* Pareira, M. D., Conrad, E. J., Hicks, W., and Elman, R.: Therapeutic nutrition with tube feeding, J.A.M.A. *156*:810, 1954.

water, supplies nutrients in amounts recommended by the Food and Nutrition Board of the National Research Council. This can be used as a tube feeding or as an oral supplement.

Milk is the basis for most tube feedings with additional carbohydrate foods, protein foods and water-soluble multi-vitamin preparations. Protein hydrolysates sometimes are added to the gastrostomy feeding.

GASTROSTOMY TUBE FEEDING

PROTEIN—74 GM., FAT—77 GM.,
CARBOHYDRATE—195 GM.
APPROXIMATELY 1 CALORIE PER ML.

	MEASURE	GM.
Milk	1½ qt.	1,500
Glucose or sugar	½ cup	120
Eggs	3	150
Sodium chloride	½ teaspoon	2

Water soluble multi-vitamin preparation (as ordered by physician)

DIRECTIONS: Beat the eggs slightly. Add all other ingredients. Strain through fine sieve, pour in bottles, cover, label and place in refrigerator. Tube feeding should be warmed in a double boiler to body temperature before giving.

JEJUNOSTOMY FEEDING

Homogenized milk usually is the basis for this feeding. Hydrolysates of protein and of starch are often used. Details of this feeding are given in the literature.*

* Case, C. T., Zollinger, R. M., McMullen, C. H., and Brown, J. B.: Observations in jejunal alimentation, Surgery *26*:364.

SUMMARY OF VITAMINS

	A	D	E	K	C
Chemical name	(Provitamin) Carotene	Calciferol	Tocopherol	Menadione	Ascorbic Acid
Important food sources	Liver Egg yolk Butter, cream Green and yellow vegetables Fish-liver oil Fortified margarine	Fish-liver oil Irradiated foods Viosterol Butter Egg yolk Liver	Wheat germ Leafy vegetables Vegetable oils Egg yolk Legumes Nuts	Leafy vegetables Pork-liver fat Soybean oil and other vegetable oils	Citrus fruits Strawberries Cantaloupe Tomatoes Sweet peppers Cabbage Potatoes
Stability to cooking, drying, light, etc.	Gradual destruction by exposure to air, heat and drying; more rapid at high temperatures	Stable to heating, aging and storage Destroyed by excess ultraviolet irradiation	Stable to all methods of food processing Destroyed by rancidity and ultraviolet irradiation	Stable to heat and exposure to air Destroyed by strong acids, alkalis and light, oxidizing agents	Unstable to heat and oxidation, except in acids Destroyed by drying and aging
Function: Essential in	Maintaining function of epithelial cells, skin and mucous membranes	Calcium and phosphorus absorption and metabolism	Maintaining function of reproductive and muscular tissues	Clotting of blood necessary in formation of prothrombin	Formation of intercellular substance, cellular oxidation and reduction
Deficiency manifest as	Night blindness Glare blindness Rough, dry skin Dry mucous membranes	Rickets Soft bones Bowed legs Poor teeth Skeletal deformities	Sterility in males (rats) Resorption of fetus (females) Muscular dystrophy in rats and rabbits	Slow clotting time of blood Hemorrhagic disease of newborn Lack of prothrombin	Scurvy Sore mouth Stiff joints Sore and bleeding gums Weak-walled capillaries
Human requirement	*See Recommended Daily Dietary Allowances under Nutritional Requirements*				

Fractions of the Vitamin B Complex

Chemical name	Thiamine (B_1)*	Riboflavin (B_2)*	Niacin and Niacinamide*	Pantothenic Acid	Vitamin B_6 (Pyridoxine)
Important food sources	Pork Liver, meats of organs Whole grains Enriched products Nuts, legumes Potatoes in skin Yeast, wheat germ	Liver, milk Meats, eggs Enriched bread Green, leafy vegetables Yeast	Liver, poultry Meat, fish Whole grains Enriched products Legumes Mushrooms Yeast	Liver Meats of organs Eggs, peanuts Legumes Mushrooms Salmon, whole grains Yeast, wheat germ	Pork Meats of organs Legumes, seeds Grains Potatoes Bananas, wheat germ Yeast
Stability to cooking, drying, light, etc.	Unstable to heat and oxidation	Stable to heat in cooking, to acids and oxidation Unstable to light	Stable to heat, oxidation, acid and alkali	Unstable to acid, alkali, heat and certain salts	Stable to heat, light and oxidation
Function: Essential in	Carbohydrate metabolism, component of tissue enzyme-cocarboxylase	Carbohydrate and amino acid metabolism, component of enzyme system	Carbohydrate and amino acid metabolism, component of enzyme system	Growth and health of all animals Function unknown	Metabolism of **fats** and amino acids
Deficiency manifest as	Beriberi (man) Polyneuritis (animals) Poor appetite Fatigue Constipation	Eye sensitivity Cataract Cheilosis (man) Alopecia (rats)	Pellagra (man) Blacktongue (dogs)	Dermatitis (chicks) Graying of hair (rats)	Acrodynia (rats) Microcytic anemia (dogs) Dermatitis (man) Convulsions (infant)
Human requirement					

*See Recommended Daily Dietary Allowances *under* Nutritional Requirements.

[573]

SUMMARY OF VITAMINS (Continued)

FRACTIONS OF THE VITAMIN B COMPLEX (Continued)

Chemical name	Biotin	Folic Acid	B_{12}	Inositol	Choline
Important food sources	Liver Meats of organs Peanuts, eggs Milk Mushrooms Yeast	Liver Kidney Yeast Salmon, beef Wheat	Liver Kidney Eggs Meat Milk	Liver Brain Muscle meat	Meat Eggs Milk Cereals
Stability to cooking, drying, light, etc.	Very stable to heat, light, acid and mild alkali Unstable to oxidation	Slightly water-soluble Destroyed by light, oxidation, acids, heat and alkali		Stable in acid and alkaline solutions	Water-soluble Destroyed by alkali
Function: Essential in	Growth and respiration of cells	Formation of red blood cells	"Extrinsic" factor in blood regeneration	Enhances lipotropic action of choline	Production of phospholipids and formation of methionine Utilization of fatty acids
Deficiency manifest as	Dermatitis in all animal species	Macrocytic anemia	Pernicious anemia	Lack of growth (rats) Spectacled eyes Poor lactation	Fatty liver Perosis (chick)

APPROXIMATE CALORIC VALUES OF A FEW COMMON FOODS

		Protein	Calories
BREAD			
Bread	1 slice	2 Gm.	65
Muffin	1	4 Gm.	135
Roll	1	3 Gm.	120
Saltines	2	1 Gm.	35
Graham crackers	2 medium	1 Gm.	55
CEREALS			
Cooked, including rice, spaghetti, noodles, macaroni	½ cup	2 Gm.	70
Dry, flaked and puffed	¾ cup	2 Gm.	70
DAIRY PRODUCTS			
Butter	1 tbsp.	..	100
Cheese	1 oz.	..	105
American		7 Gm.	...
Cream		3 Gm.	...
Swiss		8 Gm.	...
Cheese—Cottage	4 tbsp.	10 Gm.	50
Cream—light	2 tbsp.	..	30
Milk	1 cup (8 oz.)	8 Gm.	170
Milk, skimmed	1 cup	8 Gm.	85
Buttermilk	1 cup	8 Gm.	85
Chocolate milk (cocoa) (all milk)	1 cup	10 Gm.	240
Chocolate-flavored milk	1 cup	8 Gm.	185
Egg	1	6 Gm.	75
Eggnog	1 cup	13 Gm.	220
DESSERTS			
Pie, apple	⅑ of 9" pie	2 Gm.	250
Layer cake, icing	3 oz.	5 Gm.	300
Cookie	3" in diam.	2 Gm.	100
Doughnut	1, cake type	2 Gm.	135
Gelatin dessert	½ cup	2 Gm.	80
Ice cream	½ cup	3 Gm.	150-200
Pudding, made with milk	½ cup	4 Gm.	140
Sherbet	½ cup	1 Gm.	120
Custard	½ cup	7 Gm.	145
FRUIT			
Stewed dried (no added sugar)	½ cup	2 Gm.	160
Canned, sweetened	½ cup	..	90
Fresh or unsweetened	See List 3, p. 548		
MEAT, FISH OR POULTRY			
Lean	3 oz.	21 Gm.	220
Medium fat	3 oz.	21 Gm.	285
Bacon	2 slices	4 Gm.	95
VEGETABLES: See List 2, p. 548			
MISCELLANEOUS			
Chocolate syrup	1 tbsp.	..	40
Marmalade, jam, jelly	1 tbsp.	..	55
Mayonnaise	1 tbsp.	..	90
French Dressing	1 tbsp.	..	60
Margarine	1 tbsp.	..	100
Oil—salad or cooking	1 tbsp.	..	125
Sugar	1 tbsp.	..	60
Nuts	2 tbsp. (1 oz.)	2 Gm.	180
Peanut butter	2 tbsp.	8 Gm.	180
Beans, navy, etc. (with pork and sauce)	1 cup	15 Gm.	300

DESIRABLE WEIGHTS FOR ADULTS

Desirable Weights For Women
Ages 25 and Over*

HEIGHT (WITH SHOES) 2-INCH HEELS		WEIGHT IN POUNDS (AS ORDINARILY DRESSED)		
		SMALL FRAME	MEDIUM FRAME	LARGE FRAME
FEET	INCHES			
4	10	92- 98	96-107	104-119
4	11	94-101	98-110	106-122
5	0	96-104	101-113	109-125
5	1	99-107	104-116	112-128
5	2	102-110	107-119	115-131
5	3	105-113	110-122	118-134
5	4	108-116	113-126	121-138
5	5	111-119	116-130	125-142
5	6	114-123	120-135	129-146
5	7	118-127	124-139	133-150
5	8	122-131	128-143	137-154
5	9	126-135	132-147	141-158
5	10	130-140	136-151	145-163
5	11	134-144	140-155	149-168
6	0	138-148	144-159	153-173

* For girls between 18 and 25, subtract 1 pound for each year under 25.

Desirable Weights For Men
Ages 25 and Over*

HEIGHT (WITH SHOES)		WEIGHT IN POUNDS (AS ORDINARILY DRESSED)		
		SMALL FRAME	MEDIUM FRAME	LARGE FRAME
FEET	INCHES			
5	2	112-120	118-129	126-141
5	3	115-123	121-133	129-144
5	4	118-126	124-136	132-148
5	5	121-129	127-139	135-152
5	6	124-133	130-143	138-156
5	7	128-137	134-147	142-161
5	8	132-141	138-152	147-166
5	9	136-145	142-156	151-170
5	10	140-150	146-160	155-174
5	11	144-154	150-165	159-179
6	0	148-158	154-170	164-184
6	1	152-162	158-175	168-189
6	2	156-167	162-180	173-194
6	3	160-171	167-185	178-199
6	4	164-175	172-190	182-204

* Figures from Metropolitan Life Insurance Company, 1960.

INFANT FORMULA

The doctor may prescribe a formula for the infant. He will write specific instructions for the type of formula that is best suited to the nutritional needs of the infant. The following general instructions are given for artificial feeding.

Preparation of Formula

EQUIPMENT

> 8-ounce feeding bottles—sufficient number for the 24-hour period
>
> Nipples—one for each bottle
>
> Nipple caps—one for each bottle
>
> 32-ounce (quart) glass measuring cup or a pitcher (quart size) and an 8-ounce glass measuring cup
>
> Measuring spoon
>
> Tablespoon (for blending ingredients)
>
> Knife
>
> Container of sugar, labeled and used only for formula
>
> Funnel (optional)
>
> 1 bottle brush with tufted head
>
> Rack for holding bottles
>
> Sterilizer—any pot, with a cover, deep enough to hold the rack of capped bottles. (Inverted kitchen bowl or saucepan may be used for the cover.)
>
> Jar with perforated screw cap for nipples used in giving water.

DIRECTIONS FOR TERMINAL STERILIZATION. The formula should be measured and mixed in clean, unboiled equipment. After it has been poured into the feeding bottles, nippled and capped, it is ready to be sterilized.

Never make more than a 24-hour supply of formula at one time.

1. Wash hands.

2. Wash rinsed bottles and caps with a detergent or soap solution, using a brush. *Rinse well,* using lukewarm water. Wash nipples inside and out with a detergent or soap solution by squeezing solution through the holes. A

small brush may be used, if desired. (Force the brush down to the end of the nipple so that all milk is removed.) Rinse in lukewarm running water; squeeze the water through the holes.

3. Place the bottles right side up in the rack.

4. Place the nipples for the water in the jar with the perforated top. Cover the nipples with water and cover with the perforated top. Put the jar in the rack.

5. Cover work surface with a clean towel. Measure the required amount of sugar into the measuring cup or pitcher and add water to the required amount. Stir.

6. Wash the top of an unopened can of evaporated milk. Use a fresh can every day. Add the required amount of milk to the measuring pitcher. Stir.

7. Pour formula into the bottles, measuring the amount by the graduation marks on the bottles.

8. Put the nipples on the bottles, then cover the nipples with the caps. Place the caps on loosely. If using a screw-on cap, screw the cap only half way to allow the steam to escape.

9. Put sufficient *cool water* in the sterilizer to form steam and allow for evaporation. If the cover fits tightly, 1 to 2 in. of water is sufficient. Put the rack and bottles into the sterilizer and cover.

10. Place the sterilizer on the stove and bring to a boil. Allow to boil so that the steam comes out actively for 15 minutes.

11. Cool rapidly by adding warm and then cool water slowly to the sterilizer, being careful not to let the water splash on the bottles. Let the water come to the 6-oz. mark on the bottle. Pyrex bottles may be placed in cool water. When cool, remove the rack from the sterilizer. Gently shake bottles to mix. Push the caps down so that they cover the nipples securely, or screw caps tight.

12. Put all bottles in the refrigerator no later than ½ hour after sterilization.

13. Drain the water from the jar containing the nipples for the water and set the jar aside. Cover perforated cap with wax paper.

THE NORMAL DIETS FOR INFANTS AND CHILDREN

The following diets are adapted from the Diet Manual of The Babies Hospital in the City of New York.

FOR THE INFANT

General Rules

It is important to accustom the infant to the consistency and flavors of solid foods early; then when foods other than milk are essential for adequate nutrition, he will take them willingly.

Start all new foods in small amounts.

Introduce one new food at a time.

Increase quantities according to the appetite of the individual infant.

If an infant does not accept a food, stop giving it for a few days or even weeks and then reintroduce it.

Foods other than formula are often introduced at earlier ages than outlined below, but caution should be exercised in inflicting adult attitudes of intake before foods are essential for nutritional or educational value.

Water and orange juice may be offered by spoon and cup when being introduced. However, milk may not be offered by cup until near the end of the first year. This is a slow, gradual process and should not be forced. It may take several months to accomplish.

For the infant under 5 months, feed at approximately 4-hour intervals, using any convenient schedule.

Suggested Feeding Schedule for the Infant

NOTE: The times listed below are to be used as a guide. Because of individual variations, rigid schedules are not desirable.

6 A.M. Breast feeding, formula or milk
8 A.M. Orange juice (strained) or ascorbic acid
10 A.M. Cereal
Fruit or ripe banana
Breast feeding, formula or milk
A and D concentrate or cod liver oil

2 P.M. Vegetable

Egg yolk, increasing to whole egg (shift to another meal when meat is added), or meat

Potato

Fruit or dessert

Breast feeding, formula or milk

6 P.M. Cereal

Vegetable, if indicated by appetite

Fruit

Breast feeding, formula or milk

10 P.M. Breast feeding, formula or milk

As soon as feasible: Use 4 feedings (approximately 4 to 5 months of age). Offer infant 3-meal schedule for solid supplements. By the 9th or 10th month a larger supper, using an additional serving of protein, may be given.

NORMAL DIET FOR THE INFANT

The foods that the infant needs during his first year, in addition to breast milk, formula or whole cow's milk, are listed below:

SUGGESTED AGES FOR INTRODUCTION	NUTRIENT	DISCUSSION
End of the 1st week	Vitamins A and D	Either 0.3 to 0.6 ml. of a reliable vitamin A and D concentrate *or* 1 to 2 tsp. of cod liver oil. Start with a small amount and increase gradually to normal dosage.
Within the 2nd week	Vitamin C	Begin with 1 tsp. of strained orange juice and 1 tsp. of water. Increase by teaspoonfuls daily until 1 oz. of each is given, then gradually decrease water until 2 oz. of pure orange juice is being given. By 6 months, 3 oz. may be given. *Or*, 25 mg. of ascorbic acid daily, increasing to 50 mg. daily by 6 months.
2 to 3 months	Cereals	Any strained or fine grained enriched cooked or prepared infant cereal may be used. Mix with water or formula. The consistency should be thin initially. Start with 1 to 2 tsp. and increase according to the appetite of the infant.

NORMAL DIET FOR THE INFANT (Continued)

Suggested Ages For Introduction	Nutrient	Discussion
2 to 4 months	Vegetables	Any cooked and strained vegetables, except strongly flavored ones (as cabbage, onions, turnips), or corn and lima beans may be given. Carrots, squash or string beans may be selected to introduce vegetables and usually are taken well.
3½ to 4 months	Egg yolk	Cook egg slowly for 20 minutes. Begin with about ¼ tsp. yolk, increasing gradually to the whole yolk. For ease in eating, moisten with formula or blend with cereal, fruit or vegetable.
6 to 10 months	Whole egg	Soft cooked whole egg may be taken.
6 months	Potato	May be served boiled, baked or mashed.
	Desserts	Soft puddings, gelatin, custard or rennet. May be started earlier if taken well.
	Hard infant biscuits, Zwieback, graham crackers, crisp toast	Offer when the infant is able to hold in his hand or when he begins to cut teeth. Crisp toast may not be taken well until near the end of the 1st year.
9 to 10 months	Cottage cheese, milk toast	May be used at the supper meal, if desired.

FOR THE CHILD OLDER THAN 1 YEAR

General Rules

Vitamin A and D supplement to be used.

Fruit juice, water or milk may be offered between meals. Avoid foods that may interfere with the appetite at mealtime.

Milk intake is variable and may not be more than 1 pint daily during the period of less rapid growth.

Do not keep the child on strained foods too long. When the change to solid food is made, this practice may lead to such feeding difficulties as gagging, vomiting and blowing of food.

When a new food is offered, it should be given in a

small amount and, if possible, in combination with some food which is familiar and acceptable to the child. If the new food is not accepted immediately, do not use force. It is advisable to wait a few days and try again. A child's acceptance of food is variable from time to time and from year to year. There need be no undue concern about food jags, as they soon work themselves out naturally.

The food for the young child should be presented in a form that is easy to manage independently. For example, meat cut into small cubes, fish without bones, potatoes without skins, eggs removed from shells, cherries, prunes or plums without stones, chopped vegetables and fruits, buttered bread, sandwiches in small quarters or strips; milk in light-weight nonbreakable cups (made with a handle large enough for the child to grasp with ease).

Do not attempt to inflict adult standards of table manners when a child is learning to feed himself. It tends only to discourage him. A child should be permitted to feed himself with assistance as soon as he shows an interest in it. This should be encouraged for physical and emotional development.

A child should not be forced or coaxed to eat.

To prevent feeding problems, avoid inflicting adult attitudes about the amount of food to be taken. Also, do not have the child eat given amounts of food either for rewards or to gain parental love.

Remove all toys, games and other distracting objects as a means of increasing the intake of food.

The size of portions is to be determined by the age and appetite of the individual. Small servings should be offered, second portions being available. If no emotional problems are present, a child usually will eat as much as he needs for proper growth and nutrition.

To avoid the chance of aspiration, whole hard peas, kernels of corn, nuts (unless finely ground) or similar foods should not be given to the young child.

Do not offer food when the child is tired or emotionally upset. A short rest before and after meals is helpful.

The child should be seated comfortably and have utensils suitable for his size and stage of development.

Keep mealtime a happy time. Avoid arguments.

DIET

SUGGESTED MEAL PLAN FOR THE CHILD OLDER THAN ONE YEAR

Breakfast

Fruit or fruit juice*
Cereal with milk and sugar
Egg (3 to 7 a week; 1 daily preferred)
Toast or infant biscuit. Bread or roll with butter or margarine when feasible
Milk
Bacon is allowed

Dinner

Ground or finely cut meat, poultry or boneless fish
Potato or substitute
Chopped cooked vegetable
Salad, as carrot or celery sticks, shredded cabbage or greens or diced tomato, when feasible
Bread with butter or margarine when feasible and if appetite is good
Chopped fruit or dessert (pudding, gelatin, rennet, custard, cake, cookies or ice cream)†
Milk

Supper

Ground or finely cut meat, poultry or boneless fish, egg or cheese. May be served in combination with potato or substitute
Chopped cooked vegetable
Dessert or chopped fruit†
Toast or infant biscuit. Bread with butter or margarine when feasible
Milk

* Orange or grapefruit every day in some form.
† Fruit is to be served daily.

BODY MEASUREMENTS FOR GIRLS*

Age	Weight KG. M.	S.D.	Height CM. M.	S.D.	Head Circumference CM. M.	S.D.
Birth	3.2	0.5	49.7	1.9	34.7	1.0
3 mos.	5.9	0.7	59.2	2.1	40.0	1.2
6	7.7	0.8	65.5	2.3	42.9	1.2
9	8.9	1.0	70.2	2.5	44.7	1.2
12	9.9	1.1	74.2	2.7	45.9	1.3
18	11.3	1.4	81.1	3.3	47.4	1.2
			Standing			
2 yrs.	12.5	1.4	86.1	3.2	48.2	1.4
2½	13.6	1.6	91.1	3.4	49.0	1.4
3	14.7	1.8	95.4	3.6	49.3	1.3
3½	15.9	1.9	99.5	3.7		
4	16.9	2.1	103.3	3.9	49.9	1.3
4½	18.1	2.4	107.2	4.2		
5	19.2	2.6	110.6	4.4	50.3	1.3
6	21.9	3.4	117.6	4.7	50.8	1.4
7	24.7	4.0	123.8	5.0		
8	28.1	4.8	129.8	5.3	51.8	1.4
9	31.6	5.8	135.3	5.6		
10	35.4	6.7	141.0	5.9	53.0	1.4
11	40.1	7.7	147.7	6.5		
12	45.5	8.5	154.2	6.8		
13	50.1	8.5	159.5	6.3		
14	54.5	8.4	162.9	5.8		
15	57.4	8.3	164.8	5.5		
16	59.2	8.2	165.5	5.2		
17	60.5	8.2	165.5	5.1		

Age	Weight Pounds M.	S.D.	Height Inches M.	S.D.	Head Circumference Inches M.	S.D.
Birth	7.1	1.1	19.8	0.8	13.7	0.4
3 mos.	13.0	1.5	23.3	0.8	15.7	0.5
6	17.0	1.8	25.8	0.9	16.9	0.5
9	19.7	2.1	27.6	1.0	17.6	0.5
12	21.9	2.5	29.2	1.1	18.1	0.5
18	25.0	3.0	31.9	1.3	18.7	0.5
			Standing			
2 yrs.	27.6	3.0	33.9	1.3	19.0	0.6
2½	30.1	3.6	35.9	1.3	19.3	0.6
3	32.5	3.9	37.6	1.4	19.4	0.5
3½	35.0	4.2	39.2	1.5		
4	37.2	4.6	40.7	1.5	19.6	0.5
4½	40.0	5.2	42.2	1.7		
5	42.3	5.8	43.5	1.7	19.8	0.5
6	48.3	7.6	46.3	1.9	20.0	0.6
7	54.5	8.9	48.7	2.0		
8	61.9	10.5	51.1	2.1	20.4	0.6
9	69.6	12.9	53.3	2.2		
10	78.1	14.7	55.5	2.3	20.9	0.6
11	88.4	17.0	58.1	2.6		
12	100.4	18.8	60.7	2.7		
13	110.5	18.7	62.8	2.5		
14	120.1	18.6	64.1	2.3		
15	126.6	18.4	64.9	2.2		
16	130.5	18.2	65.2	2.0		
17	133.5	18.1	65.2	2.0		

BODY MEASUREMENTS FOR BOYS*

Age	Weight KG. M.	S.D.	Height CM. M.	S.D.	Head Circumference CM. M.	S.D.
Birth	3.4	0.4	50.4	2.0	35.3	1.2
3 mos.	6.5	0.7	61.1	2.3	40.8	1.2
6	8.5	0.8	57.3	2.4	44.0	1.0
9	9.8	1.0	72.0	2.4	45.8	1.0
12	10.8	1.1	76.1	2.5	47.1	1.1
18	12.2	1.2	82.6	2.6	48.8	1.1
			Standing			
2 yrs.	13.2	1.4	87.4	2.9	49.6	1.2
2½	14.3	1.5	92.2	3.2	50.1	1.2
3	15.2	1.6	96.4	3.4	50.4	1.2
3½	16.3	1.8	100.2	3.6		
4	17.3	2.0	104.0	3.8	51.0	1.2
4½	18.4	2.1	107.6	3.9		
5	19.4	2.3	110.7	4.1	51.3	1.2
6	21.9	2.6	117.7	4.4	51.9	1.2
7	24.6	3.2	123.8	4.6		
8	27.7	4.0	129.9	4.9	52.7	1.3
9	31.0	4.9	135.4	5.1		
10	34.8	5.9	141.0	5.5	53.1	1.1
11	38.8	7.3	145.9	6.1		
12	43.2	8.6	151.4	6.8		
13	47.9	9.5	157.5	7.8		
14	54.0	10.1	164.8	8.3		
15	60.0	9.7	171.1	7.3		
16	64.4	9.2	175.2	6.3		
17	66.9	8.9	176.6	5.8		

Age	Weight Pounds M.	S.D.	Height Inches M.	S.D.	Head Circumference Inches M.	S.D.
Birth	7.4	1.0	19.8	0.8	13.9	0.5
3 mos.	14.3	1.5	24.1	0.9	16.1	0.5
6	18.7	1.8	26.5	0.9	17.3	0.4
9	21.7	2.2	28.3	0.9	18.0	0.4
12	23.8	2.5	30.0	1.0	18.5	0.4
18	26.9	2.7	32.5	1.0	19.2	0.4
			Standing			
2 yrs.	29.2	3.0	34.4	1.1	19.5	0.5
2½	31.5	3.3	36.3	1.3	19.7	0.5
3	33.5	3.6	38.0	1.3	19.8	0.5
3½	35.9	4.0	39.4	1.4		
4	38.1	4.3	40.9	1.5	20.1	0.5
4½	40.5	4.6	42.4	1.5		
5	42.8	5.0	43.6	1.6	20.2	0.5
6	48.2	5.8	46.3	1.7	20.4	0.5
7	54.2	7.0	48.7	1.8		
8	61.0	8.8	51.1	1.9	20.7	0.5
9	68.4	10.8	53.3	2.0		
10	76.8	12.9	55.5	2.2	20.9	0.4
11	85.6	16.2	57.4	2.4		
12	95.2	19.0	59.6	2.7		
13	105.7	21.0	62.0	3.1		
14	119.1	22.2	64.9	3.3		
15	132.3	21.4	67.4	2.9		
16	141.9	20.3	69.0	2.5		
17	147.6	19.6	69.5	2.3		

* Holt and McIntosh: Holt's Pediatrics, ed. 12, pp. 1434-1435, New York, Appleton, 1953.

Section 6
Pharmacology

Part I. General Information

DOSAGE

NOTE: All dosages are given in the metric system. For apothecaries' equivalents refer to the table of Approximate Equivalents, pp. 767, 768.

CALCULATION OF DOSES FROM TABLETS

Problem

To give a fractional dose from a tablet of a definite strength.

Rule

Divide the required dose by the strength of the stock tablet. This gives the fraction of the tablet to be given.

Technic

Dissolve the stock tablet in a quantity of water which can be divided evenly by the denominator of this fraction. Give the patient this fraction of the quantity of water in which the tablet has been dissolved.

Example 1

A. How would you prepare strychnine sulfate 1 mg. from a tablet of 2 mg.?

1 mg. divided by 2 mg. equals $\frac{1}{2}$

$\therefore$ Give $\frac{1}{2}$ of the 2 mg. tablet.

PHARMACOLOGY

Dissolve the tablet of strychnine 2 mg. in 2 ml. of water. Give the patient ½ of that or 1 ml.

Example 2

A. How would you give 5 mg. of atropine sulfate from tablets of 6 mg.?

5 mg. divided by 6 mg. equals $\dfrac{5}{6}$

∴ Give 5/6 of the 6 mg.

Since 6 can be divided evenly into 1.2 ml. of solution we dissolve the 6 mg. tablet in 1.2 ml. of sterile water and give the patient 5/6 of it or 1 ml.

Example 3

A. How would you give 2 mg. of strychnine sulfate from tablets of 3 mg.?

2 mg. divided by 3 mg. equals ⅔ tablets

Dissolve 1 tablet 3 mg. in 3 ml. of sterile water and take ⅔ of that or 2 ml.

CALCULATION OF DOSES BY THE FRACTIONAL METHOD

The fractional method of solving any problem in drugs is the following formula:

$$\frac{\text{What You Desire}}{\text{What You Have}} \times \text{Amount of Solution} = \text{Answer}$$

Problem

How many tablets of bichloride of mercury 0.5 Gm. will be required to make 2 L. of a 1:4,000 solution?

$$\frac{\dfrac{1}{4,000}}{0.5} \times 2,000$$

$$\frac{1}{4,\cancel{000}}_{2} \times \frac{1}{0.5} \times \cancel{2,000}^{1} = \frac{1}{1.0} = 1 \text{ tablet}$$

PHARMACOLOGY

SOLUTIONS

In making solutions there are four main types of problems that are met.

1. Using a pure drug to secure a given amount of solution of a required strength.

2. Using a standard preparation or a "stock solution" to secure a solution of a given strength.

3. Using a given amount of a drug to secure a solution of a required strength.

4. To secure dosage of required strength from tablets of other values (weaker, stronger).

The following problems include illustrations of both metric and apothecaries' systems.

TYPE 1

How much pure drug is required to make up a given amount of a solution of a given strength?

From Powder or Crystal

PROBLEM 1

How much boric acid powder will it take to make up 1 L. of a 4 per cent solution?
Method:

$$x : 1,000 :: 4 : 100$$
$$100 x = 4,000$$
$$x = 40$$

∴ 40 Gm. of boric acid powder is required.

PROBLEM 2

A gastric lavage of 5 per cent sodium bicarbonate has been ordered. Prepare 5 pt. of this solution.
Method:

$$5 \text{ pt.} = 2,500 \text{ cc.}$$
$$x : 2,500 :: 5 : 100$$
$$100 x = 12,500$$
$$x = 125$$

∴ Add 125 Gm. of sodium bicarbonate to 2,500 ml.

PHARMACOLOGY

From Liquid

PROBLEM

How much pure Lysol will be required to make 1 pt. (500 cc.) of a 2½ per cent solution?

Method:

$$2\frac{1}{2}\% = 2.5\%$$
$$x : 500 :: 2.5 : 100$$
$$100 \, x = 1,250.0$$
$$x = 12.5$$

∴ To 12.5 ml. of pure Lysol add sufficient water to make 500 ml.

From Tablets

PROBLEM

How many tablets of bichloride of mercury 0.5 Gm. will be required to make 2 L. of a 1:4,000 solution?

Method:

$$x : 2,000 :: 1 : 4,000$$
$$4,000 \, x = 2,000$$
$$x = \frac{1}{2} \text{ or } 0.5$$

∴ One 0.5 Gm. tablet will be required.

TYPE 2

How much stock solution is required to make up a given amount of solution of a given strength?

Problem

How much KMnO₄ (Potassium Permanganate) 1:20 will be needed to make 12 L. of a 1:5,000 solution?

Method:

$$1:20 = 0.05 \ (5\%)$$
$$0.05 \, x : 12,000 :: 1 : 5,000$$
$$250 \, x = 12,000$$
$$x = 48$$

∴ To 48 ml. of KMnO₄ 1:20 add sufficient water to make 12 L.

Problem

How much of a 5 per cent solution of bichloride of

mercury will have to be used to make up 1,000 ml. (1 L.) of a 1:2,500 solution?

Method:

$$0.05 \ x \ : \ 1,000 \ :: \ 1 \ : \ 2,500$$
$$125 \ x = 1,000$$
$$x = 8$$

∴ Add to 8 ml. of the 5 per cent solution sufficient water to make 1,000 ml.

TYPE 3

How much water will you add to a drug to get a given strength?

Problem

How much water will you add to 1 Gm. bichloride of mercury to get a 1:2,000 solution?

Method:

$$1 \ : \ x \ :: \ 1 \ : \ 2,000$$
$$x = 2,000$$

∴ To 1 Gm. bichloride of mercury add 2,000 ml. of water.

CLASSIFICATION OF DRUGS ACCORDING TO PHYSIOLOGIC OR CHEMICAL ACTION

ABSORBENTS increase the absorption of drugs by tissue.

ANALGESICS alleviate pain without causing loss of consciousness.

ANALEPTICS are drugs that are central nervous system stimulants.

ANESTHETICS produce insensibility to pain.

General anesthetics produce insensibility to pain in all parts of the body. These drugs also produce unconsciousness.

Local anesthetics produce insensibility to pain at the site of application.

ANODYNES are drugs that relieve pain. See Analgesics.

ANTACIDS neutralize acids. They are given usually to neutralize the acid in the stomach.

ANTHELMINTICS destroy or expel worms.

ANTIARTHRITICS relieve arthritis or gout.

PHARMACOLOGY

ANTIBIOTIC (destructive of life) A chemical substance produced by micro-organisms which has the capacity, in dilute solutions, to inhibit the growth of or to destroy bacteria and other micro-organisms: used largely in the treatment of infectious diseases of man, animals and plants.

ANTICONVULSANTS prevent and control convulsive seizures.

ANTIEMETICS check vomiting.

ANTIPYRETICS reduce fever.

ANTISEPTICS inhibit the growth of bacteria.

ANTISIALOGOGUES check the secretion of saliva.

ANTISPASMODICS lessen contractions of muscles, and also lessen convulsions.

AROMATICS stimulate gastric secretion.

ASTRINGENTS contract tissues.

ATARACTICS are tranquilizers.

BITTERS are drugs with a bitter taste, used to increase the appetite.

CARDIAC DEPRESSANTS reduce the heart action, so that the heart beats are slower and weaker.

CARDIAC STIMULANTS increase the activity of the heart, so that the beats are stronger and faster.

CARMINATIVES produce a feeling of comfort in the stomach and relieve the formation or cause the expulsion of gas from the stomach and the intestines.

CATHARTICS cause evacuation of the bowel.

CAUSTICS burn or destroy tissues.

CEREBRAL DEPRESSANTS lessen brain activity. The patient is dull and less active. In large doses they may produce sleep.

CEREBRAL STIMULANTS increase brain activity, making the patient more active, brighter, and more talkative (in large doses such drugs may produce delirium, hallucinations, convulsions, etc.).

CHOLAGOGUES increase the flow of bile.

CONVULSANTS produce convulsions.

COUNTERIRRITANTS act on the skin. They irritate nerves in the skin, thus relieving irritation in deeper or adjacent organs or tissues.

DEMULCENTS are bland soothing liquids, used to coat, protect and lubricate mucous membrane or surface areas of the body.

DEODORANTS destroy unpleasant odors.

DETERGENTS are used to clean wounds or the skin.

DIGESTIVES OR DIGESTANTS aid in the digestion of food.

DISINFECTANTS destroy pathogenic micro-organisms.

DIURETICS increase the excretion of urine.

ECBOLICS stimulate contraction of the uterus and hasten expulsion of its contents, thereby producing abortion or assisting labor.

EMETICS produce vomiting.

EMMENAGOGUES bring about or increase menstruation.

EMOLLIENTS soften and protect the skin and other tissues.

EPISPASTICS produce blisters.

ESCHAROTICS are corrosive substances that destroy the tissue to which they are applied.

EXPECTORANTS increase bronchial secretions and promote expulsion of mucus.

HEMOSTATICS check bleeding.

HORMONES are chemical substances produced in the body which regulate specific activities of tissues, glands or organs.

HYPNOTICS produce sleep.

LAXATIVES produce mild evacuation of the bowel.

MYDRIATICS dilate the pupil of the eye.

MIOTICS contract the pupil of the eye.

NARCOTICS are drugs which produce sleep or stupor. The narcotics also relieve pain (see ANALGESIC; ANODYNE).

OXYTOCICS increase contractions of the uterus. See ECBOLICS.

PARENTERALS are drugs, solutions or suspensions which are prepared and packaged in a sterile manner and are to be used primarily for hypodermic injection.

PROPHYLACTICS ward off disease.

PURGATIVES produce moderately active and frequent evacuation of the bowel.

RESPIRATORY DEPRESSANTS lessen the frequency and depth of breathing.

RESPIRATORY STIMULANTS increase the depth and frequency of breathing.

RUBEFACIENTS redden the skin by dilating the capillaries.

SALINE PURGATIVES are mineral salts that cause evacuation of the bowel.

PHARMACOLOGY

SEDATIVES diminish the activity of an organ or part or all of the body. Usually, they are drugs that reduce nervous excitability.

SOMNIFACIENTS or SOPORIFICS produce sleep.

SPECIFICS are drugs that cure specific diseases, usually by destroying, or combining with, the causative agent.

STEROIDS are substances that have a characteristic chemical structure, such as cholesterol, sex hormones, adrenal cortical hormones and some of the carcinogenic hydrocarbons.

STYPTICS stop bleeding.

TENIACIDES destroy tapeworms.

VERMICIDES destroy worms.

VERMIFUGES expel worms.

HARRISON NARCOTIC ACT

The Harrison Narcotic Act, passed in 1914 and amended several times since, regulates the importation, the sale and the use of narcotic drugs, *viz.*:

1. Opium and its compounds and derivatives
2. Coca and its compounds and derivatives
3. Other compounds found to have addictive properties similar to those of morphine or cocaine.

PROVISIONS OF THE HARRISON ACT

1. Every wholesale dealer, pharmacist, physician, dentist, and other practitioner dispensing or prescribing narcotics must register with the Internal Revenue Service and purchase a special federal tax stamp.

2. Pharmacists:

A. May sell narcotics only on the prescription of persons registered under this law.

B. Must use official forms for purchase, issued by the Internal Revenue Service.

C. A record of each purchase must be kept by the distributor and a duplicate of this record must be kept by the purchaser.

D. Records must be kept for at least 2 years and must be produced for inspection whenever demanded by a revenue official.

3. Physicians and dentists must keep an account of the amount and the disposal of all narcotics.

4. Prescriptions for narcotics cannot be renewed and must show:

    A. Name, address and registry number of the prescribing physician.

    B. Name, age and address of the patient.

    C. Date on which the prescription was written.

5. Violations of any of the provisions of this law are liable to punishment. The penalties have been increased in recent years.

6. It is illegal to possess heroin, except for scientific research.

7. State regulations in regard to narcotics and other "habit-forming" drugs (e.g., barbiturates) may vary from the provisions of the Harrison Act and the stricter of the two or both must be followed.

APPLICATION OF LAW TO HOSPITALS

1. Hospitals must be registered with the Internal Revenue Service, receive a registry number and are subject to the same regulations as physicians.

2. Every order for narcotics must be signed in the order book by the prescribing physician.

3. Accurate records of all narcotics used or discarded must be kept on a special sheet.

    A. Name of patient, amount administered and signature of the nurse must be recorded.

    B. Record must tally in amount with amount received from pharmacy.

APPLICATION OF LAW TO NURSES

Nurses are not registered with the Internal Revenue Service, but act as agents of the physician. They may administer narcotics only under the physician's direct order.

They must not retain narcotics in their possession when they leave a case or when the patient no longer needs them.

They are obligated to return unused narcotics to the

physician prescribing them, or, if this is not possible, to destroy them.

METHODS OF ADMINISTERING DRUGS

Route of administration of a drug varies according to:
1. Effect desired;
2. The manner in which absorption takes place, and
3. The significance of metabolic changes of the drug.

ADMINISTRATION OF DRUGS
FOR LOCAL EFFECT

The drugs are administered to the skin, the mucous membrane or the wounded tissue in the form of irrigations, sprays, painting, instillations, steam inhalations, wet dressings; or they may be administered orally, and, for anesthesia, by infiltration of tissues or injection close to nerves.

ADMINISTRATION OF DRUGS
FOR SYSTEMIC EFFECT

1. Oral route is one of the safest and most convenient methods, although absorption may be slow and uncertain.

A. Absorption is more rapid if drug is in solution and the stomach is empty. (NOTE: Some drugs are more toxic when taken on an empty stomach.)

B. Dilution with ice water improves the taste of the drug and tends to allay local irritation of the gastric mucosa.

C. Irritating drugs, such as iron compounds, should be well diluted and given after meals or with food, through a straw. Some irritating drugs are given as enteric-coated tablets.

2. Rectal route offers a good absorbing surface for many drugs.

A. Dose of drug is usually approximately double that of the oral dose.

B. To prevent expulsion, amount of fluid should be limited to not more than 120 ml.

C. Irritating drugs should be dissolved in some demulcent substance to soothe the rectal mucosa and prevent peristalsis.

3. Subcutaneous or hypodermic injection is given at a 45 degree angle into the loose tissues beneath the skin.

A. There are fewer surface blood vessels on the outer aspect of the upper arm or the thigh.

B. Drug must be nonirritating and administered in small amounts of fluid to avoid irritation and subsequent sloughing of tissue.

C. Area of injection should be massaged gently to aid absorption.

4. Intracutaneous or intradermal injection is introduced between the layers of the skin. It is used for local anesthesia, prophylactic inoculations, diagnostic tests, etc.

5. Intramuscular injection is given at a 90 degree angle through the skin and the subcutaneous tissues into the underlying muscle.

A. Site of injection is usually the upper outer gluteal quadrant, the lateral surface of the thigh, or the deltoid muscle, where there is less danger of involving sensory nerves.

B. Irritating drugs or larger amounts of fluid may be administered.

C. Introduction of drug into blood vessels should be avoided. Plunger should be pulled back after injection to note whether or not there is blood in the syringe.

D. Area should be massaged well to ensure diffusion of drug into adjacent tissues in most instances.

6. Intravenous injections introduce drug directly into blood stream for immediate and certain effect.

A. Tourniquet first applied to distend the vein.

B. After needle is in vein, tourniquet is released and solution injected very slowly and carefully.

C. If repeated injections are necessary, site is changed to avoid injuring or thrombosing the vein.

7. Intrathecal or intraspinal injections introduce drug into the subarachnoid space.

A. Used for spinal anesthesia, antisera, etc.

B. To avoid an increase in intracranial pressure, a like amount of fluid may be withdrawn before injection of drug.

8. Inhalation is effective because of the rich blood

supply and large absorbing surface in the alveoli of the lungs.

A. Used for administration of volatile drugs and gases.

B. Action is rapid, and, when administration is stopped, absorption ceases.

9. Iontophoresis is the percutaneous administration by means of direct electric current, of drugs that ionize.

A. One electrode may be applied to the back and the required current turned on gradually and allowed to remain on for 20 to 30 minutes. The other electrode is connected to the positive or the negative pole, depending on the charge of the therapeutic ion.

B. Positive ions (cations) (e.g., metals, alkaloids) are applied adjacent to a positive electrode.

C. Negative ions (anions, e.g., halides) are applied at a negative electrode.

D. Deep iontophoresis is not possible: as drug is carried away by blood and lymph, drug ion loses charge to electrolytic salts in the body.

OFFICIAL AND PROPRIETARY PREPARATIONS

The importance of standardizing drugs and ensuring their safety and uniform potency is well recognized. This is accomplished by various types of assay and by the use of official books.

An "official drug" is one that has been admitted to the current edition or revision of an official book, viz.:

1. *The United States Pharmacopeia (U.S.P.),* which describes and defines approved therapeutic agents in respect to: (a) source, (b) chemistry, (c) physical properties, (d) tests for identity and purity, (e) methods of assay, (f) methods of packaging and storage, (g) average doses.

2. *The National Formulary (N.F.),* which at present is revised and published simultaneously with the *U.S.P.* It contains similar information about drugs or dosage forms approved by the Committee on National Formulary.

A "proprietary drug" is one that is protected against free competition as to name, product, composition, or processes of manufacture by secrecy, patent or copyright:

Proprietary drugs are apt to be more expensive than the nonproprietary equivalent.

1. When the manufacturer has done a great deal of expensive research in his own laboratories, in return for his investment he is privileged to enjoy exclusive rights on the manufacture and the sale of products.

Part 2.   Drugs to Promote Sleep and Relieve Tension

BARBITURATES

Synthetic preparations of barbituric acid, barbiturates, may be habit forming, and tolerance may be acquired. When long-acting preparations are used, lassitude and depression may persist for 24 to 48 hours.

Accidental poisoning, intensification with alcohol and many other drugs, chronic intoxication and addiction are serious problems. For this reason many states have passed rigid laws for the control of barbiturates.

Actions and Uses

To produce hypnosis: administered after the patient has been prepared for sleep.

As a mild sedative in small doses for nervous conditions such as the nervousness of:

Hyperthyroidism

Hypertension

Menopause, etc.

In large doses to act on the motor cortex of the brain to relieve convulsions or convulsive twitchings.

To potentiate the action of analgesic drugs by synergistic action. However, barbiturates are not analgesic.

Several of the preparations have the power to produce some degree of anesthesia:

1. General anesthesia when given intravenously—Pentothal sodium.
2. Basal anesthesia prior to the administration of a general anesthetic.

PHARMACOLOGY

3. Obstetrical amnesia—used with scopolamine.
Hypnosis in neuropsychiatry: Sodium Amytal, pentobarbital, thiopental (Pentothal).

Side and Toxic Effects

Excitement
Stupor and coma
Slow, shallow respirations
Low blood pressure
Shock and death

Treatment of Overdosage

Respiratory and circulatory stimulants
Open airway at all times

Preparations and Dosage

For long action (6 to 8 hours):
Barbital, 0.3 Gm. in warm milk .
Barbital Sodium (Medinal), 0.3 Gm.
Phenobarbital (Luminal), 60 to 100 mg. by mouth
or by hypodermic.
For action of moderate duration (4 to 6 hours):
Amobarbital (Amytal), 0.1 to 0.2 Gm. by mouth or
by intramuscular or intravenous injection.
Pentobarbital (Nembutal), 0.1 Gm.
Vinbarbital (Delvinal), 30 mg. orally 3 to 4 times
a day for sedation and 100 to 200 mg. as a
hypnotic.
For action of short duration (2 to 4 hours):
Heptabarbital (Medomin), 200 to 400 mg. orally
for sleep; 50 to 100 mg. 2 to 3 times a day for
sedation.
Hexobarbital (Evipal), 2 to 4 ml. intravenously.
Secobarbital (Seconal), 50 to 100 mg.
For ultra-short action as an anesthetic:
Thiopental (Pentothal sodium), 2½ to 5 per cent.

NONBARBITURATE SEDATIVES
AND HYPNOTICS

GLUTETHIMIDE (DORIDEN)

This is a rapid-acting hypnotic, the effect lasting 4

to 8 hours. It lacks the after-depression of barbiturates. It may be used also as a mild sedative.

Dosage and Administration

For hypnosis, 500 mg. orally at bedtime
For sedation, 250 mg. 3 times a day

Side and Toxic Effects

Skin rash
Nausea and vomiting
Essentially the same as for barbiturates
May be fatal in combination with alcohol or other depressants
Has addiction liability
No known treatment for severe intoxication

ETHCHLORVYNOL (PLACIDYL)

This is a mild sedative and hypnotic, which has seemed to be relatively safe.

Dosage and Administration

For hypnosis, 500 mg. orally at bedtime
For sedation, 200 mg. 2 or 3 times a day
Should be given with a glass of milk or light food

Side and Toxic Effects

Headache
Dizziness
Nausea and vomiting
Hypotension
Possibly mental confusion

METHYPRYLON (NOLUDAR)

This drug acts as do short-acting barbiturates, with less depression of the respiratory center.

Dosage and Administration

300 mg. orally at bedtime for sleep
50 to 100 mg. 3 or 4 times a day for sedation

PHARMACOLOGY

Side and Toxic Effects

Nausea and vomiting
Vertigo
Toxicity typical of central nervous system depressant
Possible agranulocytosis
Habituation, tolerance, addiction have been reported

ETHINAMATE (VALMID)

This is a drug with a mild depressant effect for the treatment of simple insomnia. Its action is of short duration and leaves no depressant after-effects. Serious side effects have not been reported. Physical dependence has occurred with large doses used over long periods by chronic alcoholics or emotionally disturbed persons.

Dosage and Administration

500 mg. orally at bedtime.

CHLORAL

One of the oldest and most efficient hypnotics, chloral is considered to be relatively safe unless cardiac impairment is very marked.

Action and Uses

As a sedative
As a hypnotic
Drowsiness usually occurs promptly and is followed quickly by natural sleep.
The patient can be aroused easily.

Preparations and Dosage

Chloral Hydrate, 0.3 to 0.6 Gm. well diluted to prevent gastric irritation.
Chloral Hydrate capsules, 0.5 Gm.

PARALDEHYDE

Paraldehyde is a colorless fluid with a pungent and disagreeable odor and taste.

Action and Uses

An efficient, prompt and relatively safe hypnotic.

Sleep resembles natural sleep, and there are no after-effects.

It is used extensively in cases of delirium and excitement.

It can be used in an emergency for convulsions of drug poisoning.

Contraindications to Its Use

Pulmonary disease, as the drug is excreted largely through the lungs.

Severe cardiac failure when ventilation is poor.

Gastroenteritis or ulceration of the gastrointestinal tract. It is extremely irritating to the gastric mucosa.

Extensive liver damage because much of the drug is destroyed in the liver.

If the patient is ambulatory. The disagreeable odor persists on the breath as long as 24 hours.

If the patient is receiving disulfiram (Antabuse).

Preparations and Dosage

Orally, 4 to 8 ml. on cracked ice or flavored with some syrup, such as orange, cinnamon, etc.

Rectally, 10 to 15 ml. with 1 to 2 parts of olive or cottonseed oil.

Intramuscularly, 1 to 5 ml. Very irritating. Must be injected deep into the muscle and massaged well.

Intravenously, 1 to 2 ml. By this route paraldehyde is extremely toxic, and may even be lethal.

Paraldehyde should not be dispensed from containers that have been opened more than 24 hours.

SCOPOLAMINE (HYOSCINE)

Scopolamine is obtained from hyoscyamus (henbane).

Action and Uses

It has an effect similar to that of atropine, except on the central nervous system. It depresses rather than stimulates the cerebral cortex. Its therapeutic uses are:

To produce hypnosis, especially when patient is restless or agitated. It has a strong synergistic effect with morphine.

With barbiturates to produce "obstetric amnesia."

As a preoperative agent to dry secretions and to exert a quieting effect on patient.

To aid in the withdrawal treatment of morphine or alcohol addiction.

Preparations and Dosage

Scopolamine Hydrobromide, 0.5 mg.

Side and Toxic Effects

Rapid and thready pulse
Rapid fall in blood pressure
Dilated pupils
Dry mouth
Cold perspiration
Coma and collapse

BROMIDES

Action and Uses

Bromides are seldom used today. They are relatively poor sedatives but they are sometimes used to "take the edge off" nervousness. Many proprietary drugs for "nervousness" contain bromides. Since they are cumulative drugs, toxic symptoms often appear.

Preparation and Dosage

Sodium Bromide, 1 Gm.
Potassium Bromide, 1 Gm.
Ammonium Bromide, 1 Gm.
Triple Bromide, effervescent tablets of sodium, ammonium and potassium bromide to be dissolved in ½ glass of water.

Symptoms of "Bromism"

Salty taste in mouth.

Acneiform rash, beginning at hairline. Rash does not always occur and sometimes the diagnosis of bromide intoxication is difficult to make.

Mental depression
Forgetfulness, confusion of ideas
May be excitement and personality changes
Unsteady gait
Constipation

Treatment of Overdosage

Withdrawal of drug usually is sufficient.

Recovery may be more rapid if sodium chloride (salt) is given to quickly replace the bromide ion.

Caffeine may be given if respirations are depressed.

ETHYL ALCOHOL (ETHANOL)

This is a progressive central nervous system depressant derived from the fermentation of sugar.

Action and Uses

Locally

As an astringent for the skin

To cool by evaporation

As a nerve block to cause protracted anesthesia and analgesia in conditions causing intractable pain. (*See* Drugs to Relieve Pain.)

To act as a solvent for iodine and other drugs

To act as an antiseptic and disinfectant

Systemically

To produce sedation by means of central nervous system depression

To stimulate appetite

After exposure to cold temperature, to allow the absorption of heat by vasodilatation. Heat may also escape because of vasodilatation, and alcohol should not be given unless patient is in a warm atmosphere.

To promote secretion of acid gastric juice.

Preparations and Dosage

Ethanol

20 to 25 per cent, locally as an astringent and for sponges.

70 per cent, as an antiseptic.

60 to 90 per cent, for injection as a nerve block.

95 per cent, as a solvent for iodine.

PHARMACOLOGY

Spiritus Frumenti (whiskey), 15 to 30 ml.
Vinum Xerici (sherry), 15 to 30 ml.

Dangers of Continued Use

Gastroenteritis
Avitaminosis due to insufficient intake of food
Cirrhosis of the liver
Delirium tremens and psychoses

TRANQUILIZERS

The mechanisms of action of the tranquilizers are not entirely clear. They depress the central nervous system and produce sedation, but they also act specifically to reduce tension and anxiety. Some agents relieve acute states of confusion and agitation. They often promote a sense of well-being. They may affect appetite, sleep and blood pressure. Some agents block emetic impulses to the vomiting center. The "major tranquilizers" are more effective in treating psychoses than in treating neuroses.

CHLORPROMAZINE (THORAZINE)

Action and Uses

Acts on the central nervous system, the cardiovascular system and the skeltal muscles. It is used primarily to:
Prevent nausea and vomiting
Relax disturbed and agitated patients
Potentiate action of hypnotic drugs
Potentiate the action of analgesic drugs, especially narcotics
Promote a sense of well-being in carcinoma, neurotic and psychotic states

Dosage and Administration

25 to 50 mg. 3 times a day, orally
25 to 50 mg. parenterally

Side and Toxic Effects

Fever
Drowsiness

Convulsions
Postural hypotension
Dizziness
Dryness of mouth
Nasal congestion
Jaundice
Skin rash, which may be severe
Leukopenia or other blood dyscrasias
Parkinsonlike-syndrome

Patients under the influence of alcohol or other CNS depressants should not be given chlorpromazine or related drugs.

PROMAZINE (SPARINE)

This drug resembles chlorpromazine with all the uses and all the toxic effects of chlorpromazine, except jaundice.

Dosage and Administration

Dose is highly individualized.

Orally, 25 mg. or more 3 or 4 times a day. This is the preferred route.

Intramuscular or intravenous injection may be used.

PROCHLORPERAZINE (COMPAZINE)

This compound is related to chlorpromazine and is used in mild anxiety states and the treatment of severe psychiatric disorders. It also helps control nausea and vomiting.

Dosage and Administration

5 to 10 mg. orally or intramuscularly 3 to 4 times a day

Side and Toxic Effects

Dry mouth
Nasal congestion
Drowsiness

Contraindications

CNS depression

PHARMACOLOGY

MEPROBAMATE (EQUANIL, MILTOWN)

Meprobamate adds the effect of relaxing the skeletal muscle to its tranquilizing effect. There is some danger that some patients may become dependent on the drug. In some cases depression is intensified.

Dosage and Administration
400 mg. orally 3 to 4 times a day

Side and Toxic Effects
Headache
Gastric distress
Drowsiness
Hemorrhagic or erythematous skin rashes
Bronchial spasm
Syncope

PERPHENAZINE (TRILAFON)

This drug is related to chlorpromazine and has similar toxic effects.

Dosage and Administration
2 to 4 mg. orally 3 to 4 times a day

MEPAZINE (PACATAL)

Mepazine is similar to, but less potent than chlorpromazine. It produces less drowsiness and sedation.

Dosage and Administration
Orally 25 to 100 mg. a day to relieve anxiety
        50 to 100 mg. a day to control vomiting

Side and Toxic Effects
Visual disturbances
Constipation
Dry mouth
Blood dyscrasis have been reported

PROMETHAZINE (PHENERGAN)

This drug is actually an antihistaminic, but it has a powerful effect in producing drowsiness and sedation. It also controls nausea and may be used to control motion sickness and preoperative nausea. It potentiates the effect of narcotics and barbiturates.

Dosage and Administration

Orally or by rectum 25 to 50 mg. It may be administered intramuscularly or intravenously.

Side and Toxic Effects

Dizziness
Drowsiness

TRIFLUOPERAZINE (STELAZINE)

This drug is related to chlorpromazine and has similar toxic and side effects.

Dosage and Administration

1 to 2 mg. orally twice daily
Intramuscular route may be used.

FLUPHENAZINE (PROLIXIN, PERMITIL)

In action this drug is similar to chlorpromazine.

THIOPROPAZATE (DARTAL)

In action this drug is similar to chlorpromazine.

THIORIDAZINE (MELLARIL)

This drug is similar in action to chlorpromazine but it is not as effective an anti-emetic.

Dosage and Administration

10 to 100 mg. orally 2 or 3 times a day

PHENAGLYCODOL (ULTRAN)

This drug resembles meprobamate in action.

PHARMACOLOGY

Dosage and Administration
300 mg. orally, 3 times a day

CHLORDIAZEPOXIDE (LIBRIUM)

This drug is different chemically but in action it is similar to but more potent than meprobamate. It is a sedative which relieves anxiety and relaxes muscles.

Dosage and Administration
5 to 10 mg. orally 3 or 4 times a day
Intramuscular or intravenous injection may be used.

RESERPINE (SERPASIL; RESERPOID)

This is an alkaloid of Rauwolfia. It was introduced as the first of the tranquilizers and was widely used to control agitated and aggressive psychotic patients. However, it is now used primarily for treatment of mild hypertension.

Dosage and Administration
For hypertension—0.1 to 0.25 mg. daily, in 2 or 3 divided doses, p.o.

Contraindications
Peptic ulcer
Ulcerative colitis

Side and Toxic Effects
Nasal stuffiness
Abdominal cramps
Hypotension
Nausea and vomiting
Drowsiness
Fluid retention

Gain in weight
Dry mouth
Skin rash
Dizziness
Blurred vision
Severe depression

DESERPIDINE (HARMONYL)

This is an alkaloid of Rauwolfia, similar to reserpine.

RESCINNAMINE (MODERIL)

This is also an alkaloid of Rauwolfia similar to reserpine.

Part 3.   Drugs to Treat
Convulsive Disorders

DIPHENYLHYDANTOIN SODIUM
(DILANTIN SODIUM)

Preparations and Dosage

Capsules, 0.1 Gm., up to 4 times a day, as determined by individual patient response. May be used in conjunction with phenobarbital.

Action and Uses

This is a specific drug to control the frequency and severity of grand mal and psychomotor epileptic convulsions.

It is highly selective for the motor cortex of the brain and does not appreciably depress the sensory functions.

It is free of the lethargy-producing and hypnotic effects of the bromides and large doses of phenobarbital.

Side and Toxic Effects

Dizziness and ataxia
Nervousness and tremors
Dermatitis
Hyperplasia of the gums
Nausea and vomiting

ETHOTOIN (PEGANONE)

This drug, like diphenylhydantoin and phenantoin, is used to control grand mal seizures and is considerably less toxic. It may be combined with other drugs if control is not complete.

Side and Toxic Effects (rarely seen)
Numbness
Nausea and vomiting
Headache and depression

Dosage and Administration
2 to 3 Gm. daily in 4 to 6 divided doses

TRIMETHADIONE (TRIDIONE)

Trimethadione is a synthetic drug employed solely for the control of petit mal and psychomotor attacks of epilepsy. Frequently diphenylhydantoin sodium is administered concomitantly, because many persons suffering from petit mal also have grand mal attacks.

Dosage and Administration
Children under 6 years: 150 to 300 mg. 3 times a day
Adult: 900 mg. to 2.1 Gm. daily in 3 or 4 divided doses

Side and Toxic Effects
Skin rash
Headache
Nausea and vomiting
Respiratory depression
Liver damage
Visual impairment
Blood dyscrasias

PHENACEMIDE (PHENURONE)

This is a drug similar to trimethadione used to treat psychomotor and petit mal attacks as well as grand mal seizures. It should be used with great caution. Side effects may be serious.

Side and Toxic Effects
Personality changes which may lead to suicide attempts
Liver damage

Leukopenia
Aplastic anemia
Ataxia

Dosage and Administration

250 to 500 mg., 3 times a day with meals

PHENSUXIMIDE (MILONTIN)

This is an anticonvulsant drug for use in the treatment of petit mal attacks of epilepsy.

Dosage and Administration

0.5 to 1.0 Gm. 2 or 3 times a day regardless of the age of the patient.

Side and Toxic Effects

Seem to be based on individual sensitivity to drug. There may be drowsiness, nausea and dizziness and skin rash; blood and urine studies should be done at frequent intervals.

METHARBITAL (GEMONIL)

Metharbital is a derivative of barbituric acid with the anticonvulsant properties of phenobarbital. It is used to treat grand mal, petit mal and mixed types of convulsive seizures. It exerts less depressing and hypnotic effects than phenobarbital.

Dosage and Administration

50 mg. 3 times a day for children and 100 mg. 3 times a day for adults, given orally.

Side and Toxic Effects

Drowsiness
Irritability
Dizziness
Skin rash
Gastric disturbances

PHARMACOLOGY

MEPHENYTOIN (MESANTOIN)

A synthetic drug, mephenytoin is similar to diphenyl-hydantoin but causes less hyperplasia of the gums.

Dosage and Administration

100 to 400 mg. daily for children and 400 to 600 mg. daily for adults, given orally.

Side and Toxic Effects

Serious blood dyscrasias have occurred following its use.

MEPHOBARBITAL (MEBARAL)

This is a long-acting barbiturate which is used to achieve sedation but also is extensively used to prevent epileptic seizures.

Dosage and Administration

30 to 100 mg. 3 times a day, orally.

Side and Toxic Effects

Same as for other barbiturates.

PRIMIDONE (MYSOLINE)

Primidone is an anticonvulsant drug that is related to the barbiturates. It is active in all forms of epilepsy.

Dosage and Administration

250 mg. by mouth, daily.

It is recommended that frequent blood studies and studies of kidney and liver function be made.

Side and Toxic Effects

Drowsiness and mental dullness
Ataxia
Edema of the eyelids
Painful gums
Fatigue and irritability
Anorexia
Sexual impotence

Part 4. Drugs to Relieve Pain

ANESTHESIA AND ANESTHETIC AGENTS

ANESTHESIA

Anesthesia produces partial or complete loss of sensation, with or without loss of consciousness.

Divisions of Anesthesia

GENERAL. The drug acts on the brain, producing loss of consciousness. It is administered by:

Inhalation—the lungs offer a large absorbing surface in the alveoli and a rich blood supply.

Intravenous route—the drug enters the blood stream immediately.

Rectum—the rectal mucosa offers a good absorbing surface. (*See* Ether *and* Avertin.)

LOCAL OR REGIONAL. The blocking of nerves over a particular area produced by:

Surface application, called topical anesthesia.

Infiltration into superficial and deep tissues.

Injection in or around nerve trunks.

Freezing the area, as with ethyl chloride.

Refrigeration for amputations:

1. Circulation in the limb is first cut off by applying a tourniquet after patient has been given morphine sulfate.
2. The limb is packed with cracked ice and salt or ice bags, avoiding freezing of the tissues.
3. Anesthesia is complete after 1 to 2 hours, and the limb can be kept bloodless and anesthetized for the period of time required.

SPINAL. The drug is introduced into the subarachnoid space of the spinal canal.

Needle usually is inserted between the 3rd and 4th lumbar vertebrae to avoid hitting the spinal cord.

Entire dose may be administered at one time, or fractional amounts may be added as indicated through a polyethylene catheter.

Level or extent of block will vary according to:
1. Specific gravity of solution used (lighter or heavier than spinal fluid).
2. Position of the patient (Trendelenburg position causes fluid to gravitate upward).
3. Amount of solution used and rate and force of injection.

Fall in blood pressure due to paralysis of the sympathetic nerve supply to the abdominal viscera and the great blood vessels of the abdomen and legs—effectively controlled by preliminary injections of ephedrine or other vasopressors.

CAUDAL. The drug is introduced outside the dura mater into the caudal section of the epidural space—anesthesia limited to lower extremities and perineum.

Stages of Anesthesia

See diagram, p. 617 (note that there are 4 stages with the 3rd stage divided into 4 planes).

Administration

It is imperative that anesthetics be administered only by or under the supervision of personnel highly trained in induction techniques and resuscitative measures.

Emergency Measures

There should always be available
1. A means of administering oxygen by inhalation under positive pressure with anesthesia bag and mask.
2. Intravenous fluids

If the above are not available, mouth to mouth respiration should be used.

A tracheal tube may be inserted, if possible.

Respiratory and cardiac stimulants should be on hand for injection:
Ephedrine
Neo-Synephrine
Caffeine
Coramine
Picrotoxin
Elevate the feet, if possible.

STAGES OF ANESTHESIA		RESPIRATION Abdominal / Thoracic	EYE-BALL ACTIVITY	PUPIL SIZE without preliminary medication	REFLEXES Corneal	Conjunctival	Pharyngeal	Cutaneous	Peritoneal	PULSE	BLOOD PRESSURE	EXAMPLES OF OPERATIVE PROCEDURES
I	ANALGESIA		Voluntary	◯	+	+	+	+	+	Fast	Elevated	First Stage of Labor
II	DELIRIUM		++++ +++ ++ +	◯	+	+	+	+	+	Fast	Elevated	None
III SURGICAL	Plane i		Fixed	◯	+	−	+	+ −	+	Normal	Normal	Thoracic Surgery Laminectomy
	Plane ii		Fixed and Converged	◯ ◯	+ −	−	−	−	−	Normal	Normal	Cesarean Thyroid Brain Mastoid Bladder Urethra Fractures Eye Nose Head and Neck Obstetrical Delivery Hernia
	Plane iii				−	−	−	−	−	Normal	Normal	Tonsils Joints Larynx Rectum Most Abdominal Surgery
	Plane iv			◯	−	−	−	−	−	Fast	Falling	Some Abdominal Surgery Internal Podalic Version Breech Extraction
IV	MEDULLARY PARALYSIS			◯	−	−	−	−	−	Fast and Feeble Absent	Falling Shock Level	

Schematic representation of changes in important physical signs at various levels of anesthesia, and the correlation of depth of anesthesia with the control of surgical reflexes and with specific surgical procedures. (Goodman, L. S., and Gilman, Alfred: The Pharmacological Basis of Therapeutics, New York, Macmillan)

PHARMACOLOGY

ANESTHETIC AGENTS

Preparations and Dosage

LOCAL AND/OR TOPICAL

Cocaine, 5 to 20 per cent, for nose and throat operations or for very small areas. Not suitable for extensive operations.

Ethyl Chloride, in the form of a spray for minor operations, to freeze the area.

Piperocaine (Metycaine), ¼ to 1 per cent, for infiltration; 2 per cent, for the eye; 2 to 5 per cent, for nose and throat; 1.5 to 2 per cent for spinal anesthesia.

Dibucaine (Nupercaine), 0.05 to 0.1 per cent, for infiltration; 1:1,500 solution for spinal anesthesia.

Tetracaine (Pontocaine), 5 to 20 mg., for spinal anesthesia; 1 per cent, for the eye; 1 to 2 per cent, for topical anesthesia.

Procaine (Novocain), ¼ to ½ per cent, for infiltration anesthesia; 1 to 2 per cent, for nerve block. It is short acting.

Mepivacaine (Carbocaine), long-acting, relatively nontoxic, for regional or infiltration anesthesia. Injection, 1 to 2 per cent. May also be used for epidural or spinal anesthesia.

Lidocaine (Xylocaine), 1 to 2 per cent for nerve block anesthesia. May also be used for topical anesthesia in 2 to 4 per cent concentrations.

Phenacaine (Holocaine), similar to cocaine, but more potent and more toxic; use restricted to ophthalmologic procedures.

GENERAL

Chloroform seldom is used at the present time because of its toxicity to liver, kidneys and heart.

It must be dropped slowly on the mask to avoid its concentration and consequent cardiac depression during administration.

Cyclopropane, 13 to 20 per cent of the gas with 87 to 80 per cent oxygen is used in the surgical stage or stage 3 of anesthesia. It is stored in an orange colored tank.

---

* Narcotic.

Induction quiet and pleasant

Relaxation good

Recovery rapid

Highly explosive

It is considered a good agent for use in patients in shock.

Ether (diethyl ether) is one of the safest and best agents to produce adequate relaxation. If it is well administered, the patient's pulse, respiration and color remain good throughout administration.

Used to supplement other gases such as nitrous oxide, ethylene, cyclopropane, for relaxation.

Easily administered by the open-drop method by dropping on a mask covered with gauze. Given slowly at first and thoroughly mixed with oxygen under the mask to avoid choking sensations and irritation of the throat. During induction the mask may then be draped with a towel and the vapor allowed to become concentrated, removing towel for maintenance.

Occasionally administered by rectum, mixed with oil. Olive oil is used to avoid irritating effects which may cause necrosis of the rectal mucosa.

Respiratory center first to be affected by overdosage.

Ethyl Chloride is used for short operations or inducing anesthesia prior to administration of ether, which is unpleasant.

Anesthesia is prompt but of short duration.

Toxicity may be compared to that of chloroform.

Ethylene, 80 per cent, with oxygen 20 per cent

Quiet, smooth induction with no excitement period.

Relaxation often adequate.

Chief disadvantage is its explosiveness. Not often used today.

Halothane (Fluothane), like chloroform, is non-explosive. It has a pleasant odor and is 4 times as potent as diethyl ether and up to 2 times as potent as chloroform. It is non-irritating to mucous membranes. Nausea is infrequent.

For induction 2 to 2.5 per cent vapor is necessary and for maintenance 0.5 to 1.5 per cent. It usually is vaporized in a mixture of oxygen and nitrous oxide. It is used as an inhalation anesthetic in a wide variety of surgical procedures. It does not produce deep muscular relaxation.

To avoid respiratory depression, hypotension and cardiac arrhythmias, concentration must be carefully controlled and special equipment for administration is required.

Nitrous Oxide. Always should be used with at least 20 per cent oxygen.

It is stored in a blue tank.

Gives inadequate relaxation unless used in conjunction with other agents or muscle relaxants such as curare or succinylcholine.

Trichloroethylene (Trilene) is a very weak inhalation anesthetic which is not used in most anesthesia machines because it is decomposed by soda lime. It is most popularly self administered during labor in a small vaporizer attached to the patient's wrist.

Vinethene, a smooth and rapid induction, passes rapidly from the level of surgical anesthesia to overdosage without reliable warning signs.

Frequently used for short operations or as an induction to other anesthetic agents.

Thiopental Sodium (Pentothal Sodium), $2\frac{1}{2}$ per cent intravenously is the usual concentration.

Fractional amounts are injected cautiously while the patient counts. When asleep further need for injections depends on returning reflexes.

Respiratory depression may appear suddenly because of the method of injection and its rapidity of action; therefore it is usually used in conjunction with an inhalation anesthetic and oxygen.

BASAL

Tribromethanol (Avertin), 60 to 100 mg. per kilogram of body weight—based on age, weight and general resistance. Maximum single dose for women 6 to 8 Gm.; for men 9 to 10 Gm.

Administered as solution in amylene hydrate, by rectum.

Should not be administered in the presence of liver, kidney or severe cardiac damage, diseases of the rectum or colon, acidosis, shock, severe anemia, or diabetes mellitus.

PREOPERATIVE MEDICATIONS. *See* Narcotics, *See* Scopolamine, *See* Barbiturates, *See* Atropine, *See* Antibiotics.

NARCOTICS

OPIUM

Opium is obtained from the dried juice of the unripe seed capsule of *Papaver somniferum* or its variety, the white poppy. The "Opium Poppy" is native to Asia. The crude opium is dried and powdered to provide powdered opium.

Preparations and Dosage

Opium, because of its action in lessening intestinal peristalsis, is used primarily to produce constipation.

Camphorated Opium Tincture (Paregoric) contains 16 mg. of opium per 4 ml. Dose usually is 4 to 8 ml.

Opium Tincture (Laudanum), 0.6 ml.

MORPHINE

Action and Uses*

Relieves pain and produces sleep by depressing the sensory areas of the brain:

Lessens the ability of the brain to appreciate painful stimuli. It is unexcelled as an analgesic.

Produces a pleasant drowsiness and an exhilarating sense of freedom from worry and anxiety. Morphine is used preoperatively to allay apprehension.

Produces constipation.

Lessens peristalsis of the intestine by increasing the tone of the muscle to such an extent that spasm occurs.

Activity of digestive glands is decreased and secretions are diminished.

* Actions of papaverine (an alkaloid of opium) and nalorphine (Nalline), a derivative of morphine, differ widely. *See* Papaverine and Nalorphine.

Abolishes the reflex for defecation by preventing the sensory stimuli from reaching the brain.

Depresses the respiratory center.

Respirations may be decreased dangerously in opium and morphine overdosage.

Patients with bronchial asthma tend to show marked respiratory depression following the use of morphine.

Dyspnea of cardiac failure greatly relieved, mostly, however, through depression of central sensory perception.

Cough center is dulled, and sometimes the cough reflex is abolished.

Constricts the pupil of the eye, an important sign in either poisoning or detecting addiction.

Increases sweating.

Dosage and Administration

Morphine Sulfate, 8 to 15 mg. Usual dose is 10 to 12 mg. every 4 hours.

It is usually administered subcutaneously but may be given by other routes.

Always count the respirations before administering. Do not give if the respirations are 12 or under. Note toxic symptoms and report them to the doctor.

Side and Toxic Effects

Sleep and stupor

Depressed respirations, may become Cheyne-Stokes

"Pin-point" pupils

Cyanosis

Subnormal temperature

Low blood pressure may occur later with subsequent shock

Treatment

1. Keep patient awake by any means possible, such as walking, slapping him with wet towels, etc. It is easier to maintain the respiratory rate when the patient is awake.

2. If in coma, artificial respiration may be necessary.

3. Gastric lavage or emetics, if the drug has been ingested.

4. Catheterization is helpful, because the drug is eliminated largely in the urine.

5. Respiratory stimulants such as caffeine, nalorphine (Nalline).

6. Oxygen.

7. Maintain fluid and electrolyte balance.

8. Frequent change of position to avoid respiratory complications.

Evidences of Idiosyncrasy

IDIOSYNCRASY OF EFFECT

Nausea and vomiting
Excitement and delirium
Itching of the skin when the effect wears off
Sneezing

IDIOSYNCRASY OF DOSE

Small doses may produce profound effects
Large doses may produce little or no effect

Tolerance, Habituation and Addiction

Tolerance is acquired easily, and increasing amounts of drug are needed to maintain adequate effect.

The liability of habituation and addiction is greater when the patient is psychologically or emotionally unstable.

Withdrawal symptoms of the addict are pronounced
Yawning
Restlessness
Severe abdominal cramps
Nausea, vomiting and diarrhea
Insomnia
Sweating
Violence
Shock and death

Precautions for Use

Elderly persons and children are very sensitive to opiates, and the dosage must be modified carefully.

Should be avoided if the patient has bronchial asthma.

Should never be used solely as a hypnotic when other

hypnotic drugs are effective. However, its use is important as a means of securing rest and allaying apprehension in coronary occlusion and severe cardiac failure.

Should not be used when pain is mild, and milder analgesics will suffice.

It is wise not to allow the patient to know he is receiving morphine.

Should be avoided when sudden severe undiagnosed abdominal pain occurs, as the relief afforded may mask the symptoms and increase the difficulty of diagnosis.

In head injuries there may be increased intracranial pressure with impingement on the respiratory center.

ETHYLMORPHINE HYDROCHLORIDE (DIONIN)

This is a derivative of opium used internally to allay cough and relieve pain, and locally as an analgesic in painful eye conditions. It is an irritant and produces conjunctival edema, inflammation and increased flow of lymph which is soon followed by local anesthesia.

MEPERIDINE HYDROCHLORIDE (DEMEROL)

This is a synthetic drug possessing characteristics of both morphine and atropine. It is often used to replace morphine when such substitution is feasible.

Action and Uses

Depresses the central nervous system.

Relieves pain. In general, analgesia is comparable to that of morphine.

Sedative effect is definite.

Has the antispasmodic properties of atropine and will relieve the pain of smooth muscle spasm.

Does not depress respirations as readily as morphine and, therefore, can be used more safely in bronchial asthma. However, there is evidence that respiration may be depressed.

Does not produce constipation and, therefore, cannot replace opium.

Does not affect the cough center in the medulla, and, thus, cannot replace codeine.

Preparation and Dosage

Demerol Hydrochloride for oral and parenteral administration:

100 mg. is equivilent to 10 mg. of morphine.

Dosage ranges from 50 to 100 mg. every 4 hours, rarely exceeding 150 mg. in a single dose. Drug may be administered orally, but intramuscular injection is more effective.

Side and Toxic Effects

Resemble those of atropine.

Dry mouth

Flushing of the face and neck

Dizziness, particularly if the patient is ambulatory.

Nausea and vomiting, occurring less frequently than with morphine.

Occasional syncope due to fall in blood pressure

Excitement

Muscular incoordination

Habituation and Addiction

Any drug with morphinelike qualities is liable to cause addiction.

Psychic make-up of the individual strongly influences addiction: physical dependence on the drug is encountered frequently in former morphine addicts.

It is subject to the provisions of the Harrison Narcotic Act.

ANILERIDINE (LERITINE)

In action this analgesic is similar to meperidine.

Dosage and Administration

25 to 50 mg. orally, every 4 to 6 hours.

It may also be given parenterally as a phosphate.

DILAUDID

Dilaudid gives the analgesic effect of morphine without its pronounced hypnotic effect. Also, it seems to produce fewer side effects than morphine. Dose is 2 mg.

PANTOPON

Pantopon, a proprietary mixture of all the alkaloids of opium, is suitable for administration either orally or parenterally. Dose is 20 mg.

METHADONE HYDROCHLORIDE (DOLOPHINE)

Methadone hydrochloride is a synthetic analgesic drug resembling morphine. It is deemed to have more analgesic potency than morphine and to show less liability to develop tolerance with repeated doses. Like morphine, it has addictive qualities, but withdrawal symptoms are less severe than those of morphine addiction, and addiction is more easily treated.

Action and Uses

Primarily used for the relief of pain, including pain of smooth muscle spasm, such as renal "colic."

Depresses cough center and can be used to relieve cough.

Is used frequently to treat morphine addiction.

Is not as satisfactory a preanesthetic agent as morphine or meperidine, because there is relatively little sedative effect.

Causes less respiratory depression than morphine.

Dosage and Administration

Methadone Hydrochloride: 5 to 10 mg. orally or parenterally. May be given every 3 to 4 hours.

Side and Toxic Effects

Dry mouth
Nausea and vomiting, occasionally
Dizziness and light-headedness
Mental depression
Constipation
Diaphoresis

METOPON HYDROCHLORIDE

Metopon hydrochloride is a derivative of morphine designed for oral administration. It is reserved primarily for relieving pain of terminal cancer. Its analgesic potency is greater than that of morphine but it has few advantages over morphine except that it is effective when given orally.

Action and Uses

To treat prolonged and intractable pain of terminal cancer.

To treat morphine addiction.

Has little sedative effect and, therefore, is a rather unsatisfactory preanesthetic agent.

Dosage and Administration

Pain is an index to the frequency of administration. Dosage ranges from 3 to 5 mg. orally.

CODEINE

Codeine is a milder analgesic than morphine. It depresses the cough center in the medulla to a greater extent.

Preparations and Dosage

Codeine Phosphate or Sulfate, 15 to 60 mg.

An ingredient of cough syrups in 15-mg. doses.

ALPHAPRODINE HYDROCHLORIDE (NISENTIL)

This is a synthetic narcotic analgesic, related to meperidine hydrochloride. Its analgesic potency is a little better than that of meperidine hydrochloride. Its effects are prompt but of rather short duration (about 2 hours). Tolerance and addiction may occur, and the drug is subject to Federal legislation.

Dosage and Administration

40 to 60 mg. every 2 hours, subcutaneously or orally

Side and Toxic Effects

Essentially the same as morphine. In obstetrics, if used with barbiturates it may cause a marked depression in respiration of mother and fetus.

LEVORPHANOL TARTRATE
(LEVO-DROMORAN TARTRATE)

This is an agent which definitely resembles morphine, although its action is more prolonged. It has a less constipating effect than morphine.

Dosage and Administration

2 to 3 mg. orally or subcutaneously

Side and Toxic Effects

Essentially the same as morphine

NARCOTIC ANTAGONISTS

NALORPHINE HYDROCHLORIDE (NALLINE)

This is a synthetic derivative of morphine which acts to offset the respiratory and other depressant toxic effects of morphine, methadone hydrochloride and meperidine hydrochloride, but not of barbiturate or other respiratory depressants. In morphine addicts, it produces prompt withdrawal symptoms. It is under Federal control.

Dosage and Administration

5 to 10 mg. parenterally. It may be repeated if necessary.

LEVALLORPHAN TARTRATE (LORFAN)

This has been synthesized more recently than nalorphine. It bears the same relationship to levorphanol tartrate as nalorphine hydrochloride does to morphine.

Dosage and Administration

0.5 to 1 mg. parenterally, repeated as necessary.

NON-NARCOTIC ANALGESICS

d-PROPOXYPHENE HYDROCHLORIDE (DARVON)

This is a synthetic analgesic with about the same

potency as codeine for the relief of pain. It is given orally, 32 to 65 mg. capsules every 4 to 6 hours. It does not affect cough in any way.

ANALGESIC ANTIPYRETICS

SALICYLATES

These drugs are derived chiefly from coal tar.

Action and Uses

Heat-regulating center in the central nervous system acts as a "thermostat." When bacterial toxins, infection, etc., have set the "thermostat" at a high level, antipyretic drugs act to "reset" it at a normal level. However, seldom used for antipyresis because:

1. Reduced fever may mask the progress of the disease.

2. Patient may become dehydrated from profuse diaphoresis.

3. In certain enteric fevers, such as typhoid, the temperature may suddenly drop to shock level.

Relieve pain in such conditions as:

    Nonspecific headache

    Neuralgia

    Muscle aches and pains in colds, influenza, etc.

As a specfic drug to treat rheumatic fever, affording dramatic and prompt relief of symptoms.

Symptoms of "Salicylism"

    Ringing in the ears

    Temporary deafness

    Headache

    Blurred vision

    Nausea and vomiting

    Mental confusion

    Skin rash

    Rapid pulse

Large doses may interfere with prothrombin and cause bleeding tendencies.

Overdosage

    Excitement

PHARMACOLOGY

Delirium followed by stupor and coma
Overventilation followed by alkalosis

Preparations and Dosage

Sodium Salicylate, 1 Gm. 4 or 5 times a day in enteric-coated tablets to treat rheumatic fever.

Acetylsalicylic Acid (Aspirin), 0.3 to 0.6 Gm. for simple headache, etc., and 0.9 to 1.2 Gm. 4 times a day as a specific to treat rheumatic fever. May be used in enteric-coated tablets.

OTHER COAL-TAR DERIVATIVES

Acetanilid, 0.2 to 0.5 Gm.*‡
Phenacetin (Acetophenetidin), 0.3 to 0.6 Gm.*
Aminopyrine (Pyramidon), 0.3 to 0.6 Gm.†‡
Antipyrine, 0.3 to 0.6 Gm.‡
Acetaminophen, 0.6 Gm.*

PHENYLBUTAZONE (BUTAZOLIDIN)

This drug has an analgesic effect and is primarily anti-inflammatory. Its action has been effective in rheumatoid arthritis and gout. It is related to aminopyrine. It is considered a dangerous drug. Toxic effects include skin rashes, gastro-intestinal bleeding, agranulocytosis and other blood dyscrasias, hepatitis.

Dosage and Administration

300 to 600 mg. in divided doses with food or milk

ERGOTAMINE TARTRATE AND CAFFEINE (CAFERGOT)

Cafergot is a mixture of ergotamine tartrate 1 mg. and caffeine 100 mg. per tablet, used to relieve migraine

* May change hemoglobin of the blood to methemoglobin: the patient will be cyanotic.
† May cause agranulocytosis.
‡ Because less toxic drugs are available, these compounds are rarely used today.

headache. Caffeine acts synergistically with ergotamine and reduces dosage of ergotamine necessary and also the toxicity of ergotamine. Its effect on headache probably is to constrict the dilated cerebral arteries.

Dosage and Administration

Determined for each patient, but usually 2 tablets at onset of headache and 1 tablet at 30-minute intervals, the total dosage not to exceed 6 tablets.

Contraindications Because of Vasoconstriction Properties

Peripheral vascular disease
Angina pectoris
During pregnancy
Kidney or liver disease

CINCHOPHEN

This drug is rarely used at the present time. It has been largely replaced by colchicine.

COLCHICINE

Colchicine comes from the dried ripe seed of *Colchicum autumnale*. Preparations are administered every 2 to 4 hours until relief is obtained or diarrhea starts, and then the drug is discontinued.

Action and Uses

A specific in gout to control the pain and to prevent or shorten the attack.

Preparation and Dosage

Colchicine Tablets, 0.5 to 1 mg.

SALICYLIC ACID DERIVATIVES

Methyl Salicylate (Wintergreen Oil; Gaultheria Oil), used externally as a liniment.

BENZOCAINE
(ETHYL-p-AMINOBENZOATE; ANESTHESIN)

Benzocaine is a slowly and slightly soluble anesthetic.

Action and Uses

Slow and slight absorption renders drug safe for painful wounds, and for irritated or ulcerated skin and mucous membranes.

Preparation and Dosage

Dusting powder, either pure or diluted
Ointment of 5 per cent
Suppositories

ALCOHOL

Alcohol is used in a strength of 60 to 90 per cent for nerve block in intractable pain.

ANTISPASMODICS

ATROPINE

Atropine is derived from *Atropa belladonna* (deadly nightshade), from *Hyoscyamus* (henbane) or is produced synthetically.

Actions and Uses

To dilate the pupil of the eye and to paralyze the muscles of accommodation to enable examination or refraction. Now largely superseded by faster-acting drugs.

To prevent or, used alternately with a miotic, to break up adhesions between the iris and the lens.

Preoperatively to check bronchial secretions.

To relax smooth muscle spasm.

In peptic ulcer.

To relax pylorospasm and, thus, relieve pain.

Occasionally, as a heart stimulant in heart block such as that produced by severe digitalis poisoning.

Preparations and Dosage

Belladonna Tincture, 0.3 to 1 ml. Usual dose is 0.6 ml.

Belladonna Extract, 15 mg.

Atropine Sulfate, 0.5 to 1 per cent, locally in the eye. Pressure exerted on the inner canthus during instillation to prevent absorption through nasal mucosa.

Atropine Sulfate, 0.4 to 1 mg., orally or subcutaneously.

Side and Toxic Effects

Excessive thirst and dryness of the mouth and the throat

Flushing of the face and the neck

Widely dilated pupils

Rapid and hard pulse

Hurried respiration

Talkativeness; excitement

Later, stupor; rapid, weak pulse, slow and shallow breathing

HOMATROPINE HYDROBROMIDE

Used only for mydriasis (of short duration), in 1 or 2 per cent solution.

HOMATROPINE METHYLBROMIDE (NOVATRIN)

Antispasmodic and inhibitor of excretions.

2.5 to 5 mg. orally, up to 4 times daily, before meals, in disorders of the gastro-intestinal tract.

AMPROTROPINE (SYNTROPAN)

This was an early synthetic substitute for atropine and was used in treatment of spastic colon and other spasmodic states.

50 to 100 mg. orally, 3 or 4 times a day.

ADIPHENINE (TRASENTINE)

Has direct spasmolytic action on gastro-intestinal muscles; effects on the pupil, secretions and cardiovascular system negligible.

75 to 150 mg. 3 times daily before meals, orally; 50 mg., intramuscularly, repeated as necessary.

METHANTHELINE BROMIDE (BANTHINE)

This is a chemical drug that acts much like atropine, but the effects are of longer duration.

Action and Uses

Relieves symptoms of peptic ulcer and favors healing by decreasing gastric motility and inhibiting the excessive secretion of gastric juice. Since the cause of the ulcer still remains, progress of healing must be watched by means of roentgenograms.

Increases the absorption of food in such conditions as ulcerative colitis by slowing intestinal peristalsis.

Dosage and Administration

50 to 100 mg., orally, every 6 hours before meals and at bedtime. This dose later is reduced to 50 mg. 3 times a day and is given as a maintenance dose.

Dosage should be increased during periods of emotional stress and strain.

Side and Toxic Effects

Dryness of mouth

Dilatation of pupils attended by inability to read fine print

Muscle weakness (when large doses are used)

Urinary retention, especially in those with prostatic hypertrophy

PROPANTHELINE BROMIDE (PROBANTHINE)

This is an analogue of methantheline, but it has more potency in reducing gastric secretions. Its side effects are less severe.

Dosage and Administration

15 mg. orally 3 times a day with meals and 15 mg. at bedtime

METHSCOPOLAMINE BROMIDE
(PAMINE BROMIDE)

This is a drug which both relieves spasm of smooth muscle, hypermotility of the stomach and the small intestine, and reduces gastric acidity and the volume of gastric secretion.

Dosage and Administration

Orally 2.5 mg. before meals and 2.5 or 5 mg. at bedtime

Parenterally 0.25 to 1 mg. every 6 to 8 hours

Side and Toxic Effects

Constipation
Blurred vision
Dry skin
Dry mouth
Dizziness

DIPHEMANIL METHYLSULFATE
(PRANTAL METHYLSULFATE)

This drug acts on the heart, the gastric motility and the secretion of the gastric and the sweat glands. It is used most frequently to treat peptic ulcer and for the relief of excessive sweating which aggravates dermatologic conditions.

Dosage and Administration

100 mg. orally every 4 to 6 hours

Side and Toxic Effects

Essentially those of atropine

PAPAVERINE HYDROCHLORIDE

Papaverine hydrochloride is an alkaloid of opium, but differs essentially in its action by the absence of narcotic effect. Toxicity is very low. Habituation and addiction generally do not follow its use. It is subject to regulation under the Harrison Narcotic Act.

PHARMACOLOGY

Action and Uses

Does not affect the central nervous system to any extent and, therefore, does not produce sleep or analgesia.

Chief action is to relax smooth muscle, especially if spasm has occurred. Is of therapeutic value in:

Peripheral and pulmonary arterial embolism. Increases collateral circulation in reflexly constricted blood vessels.

Raynaud's disease or thromboangiitis obliterans.

Bronchial asthma, although epinephrine is considered to be more effective.

Coronary occlusion. Coronary blood flow usually is improved.

Pylorospasm.

Biliary "colic," etc.

Preparations and Dosage

Papaverine Hydrochloride, 60 to 90 mg. orally, and 10 to 60 mg. intramuscularly.

DIOXYLINE PHOSPHATE (PAVERIL PHOSPHATE)

Paveril phosphate is a nonnarcotic antispasmodic used in conditions in which papaverine is indicated.

Action and Uses

Relaxes smooth muscle spasm. Is used to relieve vasospasm accompanying acute myocardial infarction, angina pectoris, peripheral and pulmonary embolism and peripheral vascular disease.

Dosage and Administration

Given orally, 200 mg. 3 or 4 times a day.

Side and Toxic Effects

Primarily nausea and dizziness, but these occur with much less frequency than with papaverine.

TOLAZOLINE (PRISCOLINE)

Action and Uses

A vasodilator that is used in peripheral vascular

diseases to increase the blood supply to the area of vasoconstriction.

Dosage and Administration

25 to 50 mg. by mouth or parenterally every 3 to 4 hours.

Side and Toxic Effects

Flushing
Abdominal pain
Postural hypotension
The drug is contraindicated in peptic ulcer or instances when there is increased secretion of hydrochloric acid.

TETRAETHYLAMMONIUM CHLORIDE; TEAC (ETAMON)

This is a drug that affects the autonomic nervous system and is called a ganglionic blocking agent. It interrupts sympathetic nervous system stimuli associated with vasospasm, which results in vasodilatation and increased blood supply and a drop in arterial blood pressure. It is being replaced by more specific and more effective drugs.

Uses

Therapeutically and diagnostically in:
Buerger's disease
Raynaud's disease
Thrombophlebitis
Causalgia associated with vasomotor abnormalities
Diagnostically, absence of peripheral vasodilatation may indicate organic changes in the vascular supply to the extremities.

Diagnostically in hypertension, to determine to what degree the sympathetic nervous system is involved in hypertension. If the basis for hypertension is nervous constriction, the blood pressure drops. Sometimes this is used in selecting hypertensive patients suitable for sympathectomy.

PHARMACOLOGY

Administration and Dosage

Intravenously, 200 to 500 mg.

Intramuscularly, 1 to 1.2 Gm.

Patient should be kept lying down for at least an hour after administration to prevent postural hypotension.

Side Effects (may be most disagreeable)

Dyspnea

Weakness and fatigue

Giddiness

Circulatory collapse

Temporary loss of ability to void or defecate

Should be used very carefully in elderly patients or those with severe hypertension or poor renal function and should not be used if there has been recent coronary thrombosis.

AZAPETINE (ILIDAR)

This is a drug used in the relief of vasospasm in peripheral vascular diseases.

Dosage and Administration

Given orally 25 mg. 3 times a day first week. If no side reactions occur, then 50 mg. 3 times a day.

Side and Toxic Effects

Dizziness and faintness

Nausea

Postural hypotension

Is contraindicated in coronary occlusion and used with care in asthma and peptic ulcer.

SKELETAL MUSCLE RELAXANTS

CURARE

Curare long was known as an arrow poison used by tribes of South American Indians. Although known since the latter part of the 16th century, it has had no real place in therapy until recently.

Action and Uses

Primary effect is on skeletal muscle, producing relaxation. It is used:

As an adjunct to shock therapy to reduce severity of convulsions in psychiatric conditions.

To treat various conditions of spasticity due to disease of the central nervous system.

In treating tetanus and other convulsive states.

To supplement anesthetic agents that do not provide sufficient relaxation.

To treat various types of "muscle spasm" to break up the cycle of pain and spasm.

To treat the rigidity of Parkinson's disease.

Preparation and Dosage

Intocostrin, 40 to 60 units intravenously: 20 to 30 units may be added slowly.

Tubocurarine Chloride, 40 to 60 units intravenously; dosage varies according to patient.

Side and Toxic Effects

Low blood pressure

Muscular weakness

Respiratory depression due to involvement of the respiratory muscles

Patients with myesthenia gravis are sensitive to the drug.

GALLAMINE TRIETHIODIDE (FLAXEDIL)

This is an agent which is similar to the curare drugs. Its onset of action is rapid, and its effect is of short duration.

Dosage and Administration

50 to 60 mg. intravenously, often with thiopental sodium

Side and Toxic Effects

Tachycardia
Skin rash if patient is sensitive to iodine

SUCCINYLCHOLINE CHLORIDE
(ANECTINE CHLORIDE)

This is an agent that produces relaxation of skeletal muscle similar to that of curare and curarelike drugs. It is used to produce relaxation of muscles in conjunction with anesthesia, short manipulative procedures and electroshock therapy. Its action is shorter than that of curare.

Dosage and Administration

20 to 30 mg. intravenously in one dose or 0.5 to 10 mg. per minute for continuous drip.

Side and Toxic Effects

May produce respiratory depression, and facilities for artificial respiration should be available.

MEPHENESIN (TOLSEROL)

Action and Uses

Mephenesin relaxes voluntary muscles and is used to relieve muscle spasm in spastic and neuromuscular disorders. It provides relief of tremor in such diseases as Parkinson's disease and acute alcoholism. It may be tried in the muscular spasm of cerebral palsy, bursitis and low back conditions. Since it also acts as a depressant on the central nervous system, temporary but definite improvement may occur in psychotic and anxiety states and it may be used as an adjunct to psychotherapy.

Dosage and Administration

Given orally 1 to 3 Gm. 3 to 5 times daily; intravenously, 30 to 150 ml. of a 2 per cent solution. If there is no favorable response in 72 hours, the drug is discontinued.

Side and Toxic Effects

The following side effects, though infrequent, may occur:

Weakness
Dizziness
Hematuria and leukopenia

METHOCARBAMOL (ROBAXIN)

This drug is similar to mephenesin but it is slower in onset of action and has a longer duration of action.

Dosage and Administration

Orally, 1 Gm. 4 times daily; intramuscularly, 0.5 to 1 Gm., may be repeated in 8 hours.

TRIHEXYPHENIDYL HYDROCHLORIDE (ARTANE)

Action and Uses

Acts like atropine and relaxes smooth muscle spasm and, at the same time, relieves spasticity of voluntary muscle, because of its action on both the parasympathetic nervous system and the motor centers of the brain. It is used to relieve the physical symptoms and the mental inertia of Parkinson's disease. It is used also to relieve various types of muscle spasm and to help the patient to achieve muscular co-ordination.

Dosage and Administration

Given orally 1 mg. the 1st day, increasing by 2 mg. at intervals of 3 to 5 days until a dose of 6 to 10 mg. has been achieved; then this dose is given daily.

Side and Toxic Effects

Dryness of mouth
Blurring of vision
Dizziness
Nausea
Nervousness

Part 5.   Drugs to Control Infection

LOCAL ANTI-INFECTIVES

ANTISEPTICS AND DISINFECTANTS

Action and Uses

For antisepsis. Inhibits the growth of pathogenic bacteria.

For disinfection. Destroys pathogenic bacteria by means of:

> *Precipitation and coagulation* of protein of bacterial cell.
>
> *Oxidation* of the bacteria due to the ability of some drugs to release free oxygen.
>
> *Dehydration* of the bacterial cell.
>
> *Disintegration* of the bacteria.

PREPARATIONS AND STRENGTHS

Acriflavine

1:1,000 solution effective against gram positive organisms in dirty wounds.

Effective against the gonococcus.

Alcohol (Ethanol)

A 70 per cent solution is antiseptic.

Has no effect on the tubercle bacillus.

Ammoniated Mercury

5 to 10 per cent to treat fungous and parasitic diseases of the skin.

Chlorine

Antiseptic action probably due to release of nascent oxygen in the presence of moisture.

1:1,000,000 to purify water.

Chlorinated Lime 5 per cent to disinfect excreta.

Dakin's Solution (dilute solution, 0.5%, of sodium hypochlorite) to irrigate wounds.

> Pus and blood may be dissolved and secondary hemorrhage may occur.

Is irritating to skin surfaces, and skin should be well protected with petrolatum gauze.

Chloroazodin (Azochloramid) is similar to sodium hypochlorite.

1:2,000 sometimes applied to mucous membrane of vagina and rectum.

1:3,300 in isotonic saline for packing and irrigating wounds.

1:13,200 as a mucous membrane antiseptic.

Cresol

Soluble in liquid soap. Has a p/c of 3. Sold under the names of Saponated Cresol Solution, Compound Cresol Solution and many trade names.

½ to 1 per cent as a handwash.

3 to 5 per cent to disinfect bed linen, dishes, instruments, etc.

Formalin

A 40 per cent water solution of formaldehyde gas.

10 per cent solution will preserve specimens.

10 per cent solution will deodorize and disinfect excreta.

Gentian Violet

Aqueous and alcohol solutions 2 to 5 per cent are effective against moniliasis and other fungous infections of skin and mucous membrane.

Hexylresorcinol

Solution sold under the trade name of ST37.

1:1,000 dilution as a mucous membrane antiseptic.

Internally as a urinary antiseptic and anthelmintic.

Hydrogen Peroxide

An oxidizing agent of transitory effect.

Iodine

Tincture of Iodine, 2 per cent to disinfect skin.

Is irritating to skin and excess should be removed with alcohol.

Area should not be covered until thoroughly dry.

Preparation should be fresh.

There are several preparations of water-soluble iodine on the market, some combined with detergents.

Mercuric Chloride
(Bichloride of Mercury; Corrosive Sublimate)

Is used rather infrequently.

1:5,000 to disinfect glassware and enamelware: destroys metal and rubber.

1:10,000 to irrigate wounds, for douches, wet dressings and hand disinfectants: it is felt there might be slight danger of absorption through the skin.

Merbromin (Mercurochrome)

A mercury preparation.

2 per cent as a mild skin antiseptic. Its effectiveness is somewhat controversial.

2 to 5 per cent occasionally used to treat bladder infections.

2 per cent aqueous-alcoholic-acetone solution sometimes used by surgeons as a skin disinfectant.

Thimerosal (Merthiolate)

A mercuric preparation.

1:1,000 to 1:30,000 as a skin and mucous membrane antiseptic.

Same strengths to disinfect instruments.

Nitromersol (Metaphen)

A mercury preparation.

1:1,000 to 1:5,000 applied to the skin.

Also used to disinfect instruments.

Oxycyanide of Mercury

1:1,000 to 1:5,000 does not destroy rubber or metal.

Is less toxic than mercuric chloride.

Phenol (Carbolic Acid)

2 to 5 per cent as an antiseptic.

95 per cent as an escharotic to destroy tissue.

In lotions to relieve itching, because of its slight anesthetic properties.

As a standard for comparing the activity of other disinfectants resembling phenol.

Potassium Permanganate

An oxidizing agent.

1:1,000 as a deodorant for offensive wounds.

1:1,000 to 1:10,000 as a gargle, douche or wet dressing.

Mild Silver Protein (Protargin)

Less irritating than silver nitrate.

10 to 25 per cent for mucous membrane antisepsis.

Strong Silver Protein (Protargol)

½ to 1 per cent for instillations.

1:1,000 to 1:2,000 for irrigations.

Scarlet Red

Stimulates the proliferation of epithelial cells in large wound areas.

Silver Nitrate

Molded "lunar caustic" sticks to remove warts and excessive granulation tissue.

½ to 1 per cent as a mucous membrane antiseptic and astringent.

1 to 2 per cent solution dropped in the eye of the newborn to prevent gonorrheal ophthalmitis.

1:5,000 to irrigate the bladder.

Yellow Mercuric Oxide

1 per cent to treat eye infections.

Benzalkonium Chloride (Zephiran Chloride)

Used as aqueous solution or tincture 1:1,000 to 1:5,000. Articles which have been washed must be thoroughly rinsed, as soap deters its action.

Hexachlorophene
(Ingredient of Gamophen, pHisoHex)

An antiseptic related to the phenol compounds.

PHARMACOLOGY

Inhibits the metabolism, particularly of gram-positive organisms which occur naturally or pathogenically on the skin. The drug is incorporated into soaps, liquid preparations, oils, detergent creams and is used preoperatively and postoperatively to reduce bacterial flora on the skin, and for the prevention of such infections as carbuncles, impetigo and seborrheic dermatitis.

2 to 3 per cent solution is used in soaps and creams.

0.5 to 1 per cent solution is used topically.

Residual amounts remaining on the skin reduce bacterial flora and should not be removed with water or other cleansing agents, alcohol or other organic solvents.

Nitrofurazone (Furacin)

Inhibits the enzyme system of bacterial cells and is used topically for the prevention and also the treatment of superficial contaminated wounds, impetigo, burns, ulcerations, etc.

Prolonged use may produce sensitization of the skin.

0.2 per cent in ointments. Area should be covered to maintain contact with the skin.

0.2 per cent solution.

DRUGS TO TREAT SUPPURATING WOUNDS

STREPTOKINASE-STREPTODORNASE (VARIDASE)

Varidase is a combination of enzymes derived from *Streptococcus hemolyticus.*

Action and Uses

Acts by lysing nucleoproteins that make up much of the sediment of thick purulent exudates. Also stimulates a local outpouring of fluid and phagocytes at the site of inflammation. Used to remove clotted blood and fibrinous or purulent accumulations following trauma or inflammation, thus facilitating the action of the anti-infectives.

Dangers in Use

It should not be used if hemorrhage or cellulitis without suppuration is present, as these enzymes might interfere with blood clotting.

It should not be used when there are bronchopleural fistulas, especially those of tuberculosis, as these fistulas may reopen.

Dosage and Administration

It is used as a solution of 100,000 units of streptokinase and 25,000 units of streptodornase in 10 ml. of isotonic saline solution, applied by injection into cavities or topically as wet dressings.

TRYPSIN (TRYPTAR)

This is a purified preparation of animal pancreatic enzyme with proteolytic action. It is used in much the same way as Varidase.

Dosage and Administration

5 mg. as a buccal tablet

5 mg. per ml. for injection

It may also be applied to the surface as a dry powder or as a solution instilled into wound cavities.

Side and Toxic Effects

Urticaria

Pain and induration at site of injection

Fever

It is not used in the presence of liver disease, actively bleeding areas or tuberculous fistulas.

CHYMOTRYPSIN (CHYMAR)

This is another proteolytic enzyme prepared for intramuscular use and also in buccal tablets. It is used for the same purposes as Varidase and trypsin.

BACITRACIN

Bacitracin is an outstanding antibiotic useful against many gram-positive and some gram-negative organisms, especially those strains of organisms resistant to penicillin. It seems to be particularly free from allergic reactions.

Uses

Skin diseases
Eye infections of a pyogenic nature
Surgical infections
Carbuncles, frequently making surgical treatment unnecessary.

Administration

Primarily, it is used locally by means of:
Topical application to the surface of wounds
Injection for local infiltration
Irrigation of infected wounds
Ointment for skin and eye lesions
Its parenteral use is not widespread because of possible kidney dysfunction.

TYROTHRICIN

Tyrothricin is derived from *Bacillus brevis,* a spore-bearing bacillus found in the soil. It is composed of two antibacterial substances—gramicidin and tyrocidine.

Action and Uses

It has antibacterial action and is used to treat indolent ulcers and wound infections, especially those of the latter caused by gram-positive organisms. It exerts no effect unless it can come in direct contact with the organisms and is not effective if infection is deep seated.

Preparations and Dosage

Topically, 0.5 per cent solution or a concentration of 1:2,000.

Is ineffective by mouth and extremely dangerous if used intravenously.

Use is limited entirely to local application.

May be introduced into body cavities if great care is taken that the drug does not enter the blood stream.

SYSTEMIC ANTI-INFECTIVES

SULFONAMIDE DERIVATIVES

The introduction of the sulfonamide compounds to medicine constituted one of the most important advances in chemotherapy. However, many organisms become resistant to sulfonamides, and they have been replaced largely by the use of antibiotics.

Action of Sulfonamide Compounds

The site of action of the drug is in the bacterium itself.

The metabolism of the organism is affected, so that it cannot grow and reproduce.

The natural defenses of the body are able to resist and overcome the infection before it becomes overwhelming.

The drug is considered to be a bacteriostatic agent rather than bactericidal.

Dosage in General

Dosage is governed chiefly by the blood level.

An adequate blood level is considered to be about 7 to 11 mg. of drug in every 100 ml. of blood (7 to 11 mg. per cent).

An initial dose is administered, usually 2 to 4 Gm., to attain an adequate blood level. This is followed by 1 Gm. every 4 to 6 hours, day and night, to maintain the blood level.

In urinary infections 0.5 to 1 Gm. 3 or 4 times a day may be sufficient.

In severe infections, soluble sodium salts may be given intravenously. The dose usually is 2.5 to 5 Gm. followed by oral maintenance doses.

All of the compounds are relatively insoluble, and many physicians prefer to have the tablets crushed to aid absorption.

Therapeutic Uses

Infections caused by gram-positive organisms—streptococci and pneumococci

PHARMACOLOGY

A few gram-negative organisms—meningococci, gonococci and colon bacilli
Prophylaxis against rheumatic fever
Control of carriers of meningococci
Intestinal antisepsis

Precautions for Use

1. Patient's fluid intake, and particularly the urinary output, must be adequate:
   A. Daily fluid intake should be 2,000 to 2,500 ml.
   B. Urinary output must be at least 1,000 ml., and preferably 1,500 ml. per day. Some of the newer compounds have less tendency to cause crystalluria.

2. Blood counts, especially a white blood cell count, must be done at frequent intervals.

3. Frequent determinations of the blood level are necessary.

4. Frequent urinalyses are essential.

5. Drug must be used very carefully if the patient has poor renal function.

Toxic Effects

Elevated temperature ("drug fever")
Skin rash
Nausea and vomiting*
Leukopenia
Anemia
Jaundice
Mental confusion
Oliguria, anuria and hematuria.† Crystals form in the kidney and the ureters, causing mechanical obstruction and irritation

* Occur with the use of sulfanilamide and sulfapyridine but with less frequency with compounds developed later.

† Occur with the use of sulfapyridine, sulfathiazole and sulfadiazine. This danger is obviated somewhat by the administration of an equal amount of sodium bicarbonate with each dose of drug. Crystallization does not occur as readily when the urine is alkaline.

Preparations for Systemic Effect

Sulfadiazine

Sulfamerazine

Sulfamethazine (Diazil)

Sulfamethoxypyridazine (Kynex)—believed to be retained in body fluids more than most sulfonamides; may be administered at 48-hour intervals. The Food and Drug Administration warns that long acting drugs such as Kynex and Madribon not be used unless the short acting dosage is unacceptable.

Sulfadimethoxine (Madribon)—long acting, administered once daily.

Sulfasoxazole (Gantrisin)—is very soluble in urine and is valuable in treating urinary infections

Sulfisomidine (Elkosin)—used to treat urinary infections

Sulfacctamide (Sulamyd)—to treat urinary infections

Preparations for Intestinal Antisepsis

Salicylazosulfapyridine (Asulfidine) seems to have an affinity for connective tissue and is used to treat chronic ulcerative colitis. It has not proved to be superior to other compounds

Sulfaguanidine

Phthalylsulfathiazole (Sulfathalidine)

Succinylsulfathiazole (Sulfasuxidine)

p-Nitrosulfathiazole (Nisulfazole)

DRUGS TO TREAT LEPROSY

Leprosy, also known as Hansen's Disease, is best treated by the sulfone drugs. The initial dose should be small, and, to avoid making the condition somewhat worse, the dose should be increased gradually.

4,4′-DIAMINODIPHENYLSULFONE (DDS, DAPSONE)

This drug is frequently prescribed in the treatment of leprosy. However, it is a British preparation and is not commercially available in the United States. Given orally, 100 mg. twice a week. The dose is then increased weekly by 100 mg. to the maintenance dose of 300 mg. twice a week.

SULFOXONE SODIUM (DIASONE SODIUM)

Very useful in the treatment of leprosy, this drug is given orally in a dosage of 0.3 Gm. the first week, 0.6 Gm. during the next 3 weeks and then 1.0 Gm. per day.

GLUCOSULFONE SODIUM (PROMIN SODIUM)

Given intravenously, 1 Gm. the first day, gradually increasing the dose to 5 Gm. per day over 4 to 6 weeks.

SOLAPSONE (SULFETRONE)

Given parenterally, 1.5 Gm. twice a week.

Side and Toxic Effects of the Sulfones

Nausea and vomiting
Anemia
Dermatitis
Hepatitis
Glandular enlargement
Occasionally, liver damage
Occasionally, psychosis

DRUGS TO TREAT URINARY INFECTIONS

Older drugs have given way largely to newer sulfonamides, such as sulfisoxazole (Gantrisin), and to antibiotics. However, a few may still be used. (*See also* Antibiotics.)

METHENAMINE; HEXAMETHYLENAMINE (HEXAMINE; UROTROPIN)

This drug is a urinary antiseptic widely used at one time, but used less frequently at present.

Action and Uses

Acts only when the urine is acid. Believed to liberate formaldehyde in an acid medium.

Acidifying drugs such as ammonium chloride, sodium

acid phosphate, etc., are administered with the drug.
For uses, *See* Mandelic Acid, *below*.

Preparations and Dosage

Tablets, 0.5 Gm. every 4 hours.

MANDELIC ACID

Mandelic acid is a urinary antiseptic widely used, although sulfonamides and antibiotics have supplanted all urinary antiseptics to some extent.

Action and Uses

Acts on the principle that a highly acid urine is bactericidal. Uses include:
Treatment of pyelitis and cystitis.
Prophylaxis against infection following instrumentation.

Administration

1. Fluids are limited to not more than 1,200 ml. per day to keep the urine acid.
2. Acid salts are necessary only with the administration of sodium mandelate.
3. Renal irritation may occur if administration is continued for more than 12 to 14 days.

Preparations and Dosage

Mandelic Acid Syrups, 4 ml.
Sodium Mandelate, 3 to 4 Gm. 3 times a day. Administered with an acidifying agent.
Calcium Mandelate, 3 to 4 Gm. 3 times a day.
Ammonium Mandelate, 3 to 4 Gm. 3 times a day.
Methenamine Mandelate (Mandelamine), 1 to 1.5 Gm. 4 times a day; maintenance dose, 1 Gm. 3 times a day.

NITROFURANTOIN (FURADANTIN)

Furadantin is effective against a variety of grampositive and gram-negative organisms, but is not effective against viruses or fungi.

PHARMACOLOGY

Action and Uses

Forty per cent of the drug is excreted unchanged in the urine. It is used primarily in bacterial infections of the urinary tract.

Dosage and Administration

100 mg. 4 times a day, preferably given with food or milk.

Side and Toxic Effects

Nausea and vomiting
Skin reactions due to sensitivity occasionally occur

PHENAZOPYRIDINE HYDROCHLORIDE (PYRIDIUM)

This is an azo dye which now is used more for relief of urinary symptoms such as frequency and burning, than for its antiseptic effect. Sensitivity reactions may occur.

Dosage and Administration

100 to 200 mg. 3 times a day before meals.

ANTIBIOTICS

Many of the antibiotics, when given orally, tend to suppress susceptible organisms in the body (the intestinal flora) rapidly, allowing the nonsusceptible ones (yeasts and fungi) to grow and flourish. This may result in troublesome infections, especially around the mouth, in the intestine and around the anus, due to Candida.

PENICILLINS

Penicillin is derived from an extract of the mold *Penicillium notatum*. It is very soluble, easily destroyed and rapidly excreted.

Action and Uses

Antibacterial agent "par excellence" as it is both bacteriostatic and bactericidal for infection caused by:

Staphylococcus
Streptococcus pyogenes
Pneumococcus
Meningococcus
Gonococcus
Gas gangrene bacillus
Organisms that are resistant to sulfonamides.

To treat syphilis.

As prophylaxis against rheumatic fever.

To prevent infection after oral and, perhaps, other types of surgery.

Has proved to be ineffective in gram-negative bacillary disease (viz., typhoid fever, bacillary dysentery and colon bacillus infections), and in the treatment of tuberculosis or malaria.

Preparations and Dosage

Crystalline Penicillin G is used most frequently. It should be stored in the refrigerator when in solution. Dosage varies according to the severity of the infection and the response of the patient.

Intramuscular injection

1. Aqueous solution. 300,000 units every 4 hours or 400,000 units every 6 hours.

2. Procaine Penicillin G, either in oil or aqueous solution 300,000 to 600,000 units or more every 12 to 24 hours.

3. Procaine Penicillin fortified with penicilln G for rapid action 600,000 units or more every 12 hours.

Inhalation by aerosol 50,000 to 300,000 units every 4 hours.

Oral administration requires 3 to 5 times the parenteral dose to ensure adequate absorption; stomach should be empty and antacid should be given.

Local administration (seldom used because of sensitivity hazard).

Troches
Ointment

Side and Toxic Effects

Relatively rare if solution is pure. Sensitivity to the drug may develop. Allergic reactions, which may be serious, occur more frequently with parenteral than with oral administrations. In some cases these may be treated with penicillinase (Neutropen), which is an enzyme that inhibits the action of penicillin. (Penicillinase itself has been reported to cause allergic reactions.)

Symptoms that have been reported are:

Chills and fever
Headache
Urticaria
Anaphylaxis

BENTHAZINE PENICILLIN G (BICILLIN)

Bicillin is a preparation of penicillin that has more prolonged action than penicillin. When given intramuscularly, a single large dose may be effective for 1 to 4 weeks or longer. When given by mouth it is given every 6 to 8 hours. Its absorption from the gastrointestinal tract is not significantly affected by food intake, nor is it destroyed by gastric juices.

Action and Uses

Indications for its use are the same as for penicillin G.

Because it need be infrequently injected, it is especially suitable for administration before oral surgery or tonsillectomy in rheumatic fever patients and in those with congenital heart defects and is used, also, to prevent recurrences of acute rheumatic fever.

Dosage and Administration

600,000 units intramuscularly every 2 weeks in rheumatic fever.

1.2 million units intramuscularly in gonorrhea or syphilis.

Side and Toxic Effects

Same as for penicillin G.

PHENOXYMETHYL PENICILLIN (PEN-VEE)

This is a preparation for oral administration that resists destruction by digestive juices.

Dosage and Administration
125 mg. to 250 mg. (200,000 to 400,000 units) 4 to 6 times a day.

Side and Toxic Effects
Same as for penicillin G.

AMPICILLIN (POLYCILLIN)

This oral medication is used chiefly for gram negative bacteria in urinary infections. It may be used for enteric infections.

Dosage and Administration
500 mg. every 6 hours

SEMISYNTHETIC PENICILLINS

A number of semisynthetic penicillins are available. Among them are:
Methicillin sodium
Potassium phenethicillin
Nafcillin sodium
Sodium cloxacillin
Sodium oxacillin
All are effective against staphylococcal infections.
All except methicillin may be administered orally.

CHLORTETRACYCLINE (AUREOMYCIN)

An important antibiotic derived from *Streptomyces aureofaciens,* chlortetracycline shows a wide range of bacteriostatic activity. It is the first effective antiviral agent.

Action and Uses
Infections caused by organisms amenable to penicillin and sulfadiazine therapy, such as gonococcal, pneumococcal and meningococcal infections. May be used when patient is sensitive to or organism is resistant to penicillin.

PHARMACOLOGY

Ophthalmic conditions
Various types of conjunctivitis and keratitis
Trachoma
Infections due to staphylococcus, pneumococcus and influenza bacillus
Rickettsial diseases
Typhus fever
Rocky Mountain spotted fever
Brucellosis (in conjunction with other agents)
Virus diseases
Primary atypical ("virus") pneumonia
Lymphogranuloma venereum
Psittacosis
Urinary infections caused by colon bacillus or *Aerobacter aerogenes*

Preparations and Dosage

Aureomycin Hydrochloride. 250 mg. 4 times a day with food or milk. Dosage varies with the type of infection treated. The oral route of administration is preferred.

Side and Toxic Effects

Nausea and vomiting
Loose stools
Monilial infections in mouth, intestine or anorectal area.

TETRACYCLINE HYDROCHLORIDE (TETRACYN; ACHROMYCIN)

Tetracycline hydrochloride is an antibiotic related to chlortetracycline. Indications for therapeutic use are essentially the same as for the latter. It has been found to be effective in amebiasis.

Its chief advantage over chlortetracycline is that the sides effects are much milder.

OXYTETRACYCLINE (TERRAMYCIN)

Oxytetracycline is an antibiotic derived from *Streptomyces rimosus* which is both bacteriostatic and bactericidal.

Therapeutic Uses

Infections with staphylococci, streptococci, pneumo-cocci, colon bacillus

Before and after operation to suppress normal bacterial flora of the intestine

Gonorrhea (although penicillin is better)

Syphilis (although penicillin is the drug of choice)

Rickettsial diseases

Viruses which cause pneumonia, lymphogranuloma and trachoma

Brucellosis

Amebiasis

Dosage and Administration

250 to 500 mg. 4 times a day orally or intravenously in severe infections, and occasionally intramuscularly in doses of 100 to 200 mg.

Side and Toxic Effects

Nausea, vomiting and diarrhea. The drug is given with milk to allay nausea or with Lactinex to restore normal bacterial flora and to help to avoid diarrhea.

Skin rash

Drug fever

CHLORAMPHENICOL (CHLOROMYCETIN)

Chloramphenicol is an antibiotic similar to chlortetracycline in its action and range of activity. It is not quite as effective in treating primary atypical pneumonia as the latter, but seems to be as effective in treating other virus infections. It is effective also in treating typhoid fever, although the temperature does not drop for about 5 days in this disease.

Because of the occurrence of serious blood dyscrasias, the use of the drug is reserved primarily for the treatment of typhoid fever and serious infections that are resistant to other agents.

Dosage and Administration

500 mg. orally every 3 to 4 hours (based on 50 mg. per Kg. of body weight daily)

500 mg. to 1 Gm. intramuscularly
0.5 to 1 per cent ophthalmic ointment

Side and Toxic Effects

Skin rash
Nausea and vomiting
Moniliasis
Blood dyscrasias

ERYTHROMYCIN (ILOTYCIN; ERYTHROCIN)

Erythromycin is an antibiotic made from a fungus, *Streptomyces erythreus*, which was found originally in soil from the Philippines and Colorado.

Action and Uses

Inhibits multiplication of bacteria.

Resembles penicillin in activity and is more effective in infections with gram-positive organisms such as staphylococcus, pneumococcus, streptococcus, anthrax bacillus and gas gangrene bacillus.

Dosage and Administration

250 to 500 mg. every 6 hours.

Side and Toxic Effects

Seems to be little danger of toxicity. If diarrhea occurs, it is due to disturbance of gastrointestinal motility rather than to a reduction of intestinal bacterial flora.

OLEANDOMYCIN (MATROMYCIN)

This drug is useful primarily against gram-positive organism. Resistance of organism occurs promptly.

Dosage and Administration

250 to 500 mg. 4 times a day by mouth. Parenteral injection is possible.

NOVOBIOCIN (CATHOMYCIN, ALBAMYCIN)

This is effective chiefly against staphylococci, even when the organism has become resistant to other agents.

However, organisms readily become resistant to novobiocin. Sensitivity reactions may occur.

Dosage and Administration

Orally 250 to 500 mg. 4 times a day. Parenteral administration is possible.

POLYMYXIN B SULFATE (AEROSPORIN)

Polymyxin is an antibiotic derived from a spore-forming bacillus.

Action and Uses

It is used to treat urinary tract infection, meningitis and bacteremia due to *Pseudomonas pyocyaneus, Aerobacter aerogenes, Escherichia coli* and *Hemophilus influenzae.*

Topically for local infections due to gram negative organisms.

Orally for dysentery due to *Shigella shigae.*

Dosage and Administration

300,000 to 500,000 units orally, intramuscularly or intraspinally in meningitis.

Side and Toxic Effects

Dizziness
Weakness
Paresthesia of mouth
Nausea
Diarrhea
Vertigo
Muscular in-co-ordination
Renal damage

COLISTIMETHATE SODIUM (COLY-MYCIN)

Colistimethate is an antibiotic derived from colistin which is produced by a soil grown bacillus.

Action and Uses

It is particularly useful in combating Pseudomonas and other gram negative organisms. It is effective in the treatment of urinary infections, meningitis and peritonitis.

PHARMACOLOGY

Dosage and Administration

2.5 to 5 mg. per Kg. of body weight given intramuscularly.

Side and Toxic Effects

Kidney damage
Vertigo
Pruritus
Tingling sensations in the extremities
Lingual paresthesias
Blood dyscrasias
Visual disturbances
Gastrointestinal upsets

NEOMYCIN SULFATE

Neomycin is an antibiotic from *Streptomyces fradiae*.

Action and Uses

It is active against gram negative and gram positive organisms, but, in general, it is too toxic to give parenterally, and kidney damage may result from its use in this way. It is used orally for intestinal antisepsis as it is absorbed poorly, and it rarely produces systemic toxic effects. It is used locally, also, for eye infections, burns, impetigo and wound infections.

Dosage and Administration

Orally, 1 to 2 Gm. every 6 hours
Topically, 0.5 per cent ointment or solution

Side and Toxic Effects

Damage to kidney
Loss of hearing
Nausea and vomiting
Diarrhea
Numbness of face and extremities
Blurred vision

MIXTURES OF BACITRACIN AND NEOMYCIN (NEOBACIN, BACIMYCIN)

Action and Uses

Used in the treatment of diarrheal diseases and intestinal amebiasis and preoperatively in surgery of the lower bowel to reduce the bacterial count in the intestine.

Dosage and Administration

1 to 3 tablets 4 times a day by mouth.

Side and Toxic Effects

Both bacitracin and neomycin have a toxic effect on the kidney and, therefore, are used very cautiously if given parenterally.

The preparation is little absorbed from the intestine, so there is little toxicity if given by mouth.

NYSTATIN (MYCOSTATIN)

Nystatin was the first antibiotic to destroy fungi and yeasts, except actinomyces. It is useful in treating intestinal moniliasis. It prevents those infections of the intestine and anus that occur sometimes with the oral administration of antibiotics.

Dosage and Administration

1 or 2 tablets of 500,000 units each 3 times a day. If given with oral antibiotics, it should be continued for as long as the antibiotic is used.

Side and Toxic Effects

Nausea and vomiting may occur with large doses.

VASOCONSTRICTORS TO TREAT NASAL CONGESTION

These agents act by constricting blood vessels in the nasal mucosa, facilitating breathing and the drainage of sinuses. Rebound congestion occurs with many of these agents, and their use should not be continued for long periods.

Preparations and Dosage

Ephedrine, 1 per cent
Phenylephrine (Neosynephrine), ¼ to 1 per cent
Naphazoline (Privine HCl), 0.05 per cent

Phenylpropanolamine (Propadrine), 1 per cent topically

Vonedrine, 2.8 per cent; also inhaler

Propylhexedrine (Benzedrex inhaler)

Racephedrine HCl, 1 per cent

Tuaminoheptane (Tuamine), 1 to 2 per cent

DRUGS TO TREAT TUBERCULOSIS

STREPTOMYCIN

Streptomycin is an antibiotic agent derived from *Actinomyces griseus.*

Action and Uses

In the treatment of tuberculosis, it is felt generally that persons with minimal and nonprogressing lesions and those doing well on conservative therapy should not have streptomycin because of its toxicity when administered in large doses over a long period of time. Aminosalicylic acid (PAS) or isoniazid given with streptomycin seem to lessen the tendency of the *M. tuberculosis* organism to become resistant.

Bacterial resistance and toxicity have limited the usefulness of streptomycin to tuberculosis and in combination with penicillin with which it acts synergistically.

Streptomycin is also effective in tularemia and a number of gram negative infections.

Preparations and Dosage

Sufficient dosage must be administered to overcome infection quickly, as resistance of organisms to drug may occur rapidly. Dosage varies with severity of the infection—0.5 to 1 Gm. intramuscularly 4 times a day.

In meningitis, intrathecal injections are necessary. The total dosage should not exceed 25 to 50 mg.

In tuberculosis, combined therapy is used. Usually 1 Gm. of streptomycin is given twice a week with 12 Gm. PAS once a day or with isoniazid.

Dihydrostreptomycin has a greater tendency to cause deafness than streptomycin and is therefore used very little.

Side and Toxic Effects

Tinnitus, vertigo and deafness due to neurotoxic effect on the vestibular portion of the 8th cranial nerve. This damage may be permanent.

Arthralgia and aching of muscles.

Urticaria and fever, possibly due to sensitivity.

AMINOSALICYLIC ACID (PAS)

Aminosalicylic acid is a chemical substance that inhibits the tubercle bacillus. When combined with streptomycin and/or other antituberculosis drugs, it delays resistance of the tubercle bacillus to these drugs.

Dosage and Administration

2 to 4 Gm. 4 or 5 times a day. If given with meals or with 5 to 10 ml. of aluminum hydroxide gel, gastrointestinal symptoms may be allayed.

Side and Toxic Effects

Epigastric distress

Nausea and vomiting

Soft stools and occasional sensitivity reactions

ISONIAZID (ISONICOTINIC ACID HYDRAZIDE)

This is an antibacterial agent effective against human and bovine strains of the tubercle bacillus.

Action and Uses

It is absorbed almost completely from the gastrointestinal tract and readily perfuses spinal fluid and other body tissues. It is of great value in tuberculous meningitis and miliary tuberculosis.

It is used widely in pulmonary tuberculosis.

Results of Therapy

Increased appetite and gain of weight, strength and well-being

Negative sputum

Changes as revealed by roentgenogram are very slow.

PHARMACOLOGY

Dosage and Administration

Since there is evidence of the emergence of resistant strains of organisms, it is used preferably with other agents such as streptomycin and aminosalicylic acid (PAS).

Used concurrently 50 to 100 mg. with 1 Gm. streptomycin twice a week or every 3 days.

50 to 100 mg. may be given with aminosalicylic acid every 12 hours for 7 to 10 days in tuberculous meningitis, then reduced to twice a week.

Side and Toxic Effects

Vertigo and headache
Drowsiness
Twitching of extremities. The drug must be used carefully in those with convulsive disorders.
Difficulty in urination
Constipation

ETHIONAMIDE (TRECATOR)

Similar to isoniazid, this drug is considered to be less effective and more toxic. Its chief use is in the treatment of tuberculosis.

Dosage and Administration

Orally, 250 mg. 2 or 4 times daily. It is best given with other antituberculosis drugs.

CYCLOSERINE (SEROMYCIN)

This is an agent usually reserved for patients who are not progressing well on other forms of antituberculosis drugs.

Dosage and Administration

0.5 to 1 Gm. every 12 hours
It may be used with streptomycin or isoniazid

VIOMYCIN SULFATE (VIOCIN)

For patients who cannot tolerate other antituberculosis drugs, viomycin can be used. However it is toxic and should be avoided in patients with kidney damage.

Dosage and Administration

Intramuscularly by slow injection, 2 doses of 1 Gm., 12 hours apart, every third day.

DRUGS TO TREAT HELMINTH INFESTATIONS

ANTHELMINTICS

Action and Uses

These drugs paralyze the parasite clinging to the intestinal wall, loosening its hold and making possible its expulsion.

Administration in General

1. Fluid fat-free diet 24 to 48 hours before beginning the drug.

2. Saline cathartic early in the morning, before the drug is administered.

3. After saline cathartic has been effective, drug is administered in divided doses 1 to 2 hours apart. Drug is usually in hard gelatin capsules.

4. Saline cathartic and soapsuds enema are given about 2 hours after the last dose of the anthelmintic drug to expel both the parasite and the toxic drug: oil must never be administered with these drugs, as it is readily absorbable and would hasten absorption of the toxic drug.

5. Long rest periods are indicated between treatments.

6. In hookworm infestations, head of worm must be looked for and located.

PREPARATIONS AND DOSAGE

Aspidium Oleoresin (Male Fern)

Total dose not to exceed 5 Gm. A specific to treat tapeworm. May cause:

Headache and dizziness

667

Nausea and vomiting
Diarrhea
Muscular twitching of the extremities
Coma and collapse

Tetrachloroethylene

This is useful in hookworm infestations. It is given in 4 ml. doses in a gelatin capsule. It may cause dizziness, nausea, vomiting, diarrhea, headache and drowsiness.

Hexylresorcinol (Caprokol)

The least toxic of the anthelmintic drugs. Requires fasting only overnight before the drug is administered and for 5 hours afterward. 1 Gm. in divided doses is used to treat hookworm, pinworm, roundworm, dwarf tapeworm and mixed infestations.

Piperazine Salts

These may be used to treat roundworms and pinworms. Dosage is regulated according to body weight:
    250 mg. once a day for infants up to 15 pounds
    250 mg. twice a day up to 30 pounds
    500 mg. twice a day up to 60 pounds
    3.5 Gm. as a single dose for adults and children over
        60 pounds, or 3 Gm. a day for 2 days
For pinworms a single daily dose is given before breakfast for 7 consecutive days.

Dithiazanine Iodide (Delvex)

This has been useful in single or mixed infestations of whipworm, tapeworm, roundworm, hookworm and pinworm.

Dosage and Administration: 100 to 200 mg. 3 times a day for 5 to 21 days depending on type of infestation.

DRUGS TO TREAT AMEBIASIS

CHINIOFON (YATREN; ANAYODIN)

Chiniofon is a 27½ per cent preparation of iodine.

Action and Uses

Kills amebae and cysts in the intestinal wall, and is used to treat amebic dysentery and to control carriers.

Does not affect the amebae that have invaded the liver and, therefore, does not influence the course of amebic liver abscesses.

Preparations and Dosage

Chiniofon Powder, 1 to 5 Gm. by rectum for 7 to 14 days.

Enteric-Coated Tablets, 250 mg.: administered 4 tablets 3 times a day for 8 days, or 2 tablets 4 times a day for 12 days.

DIODOQUIN

Diodoquin is an iodine-containing amebicidal drug, similar to chiniofon and Vioform. It is considered by some authorities to be more effective and is relatively nontoxic.

Action and Uses

Kills amebae and cysts in the intestinal wall and is used to treat amebiasis and to control carriers.

Preparations and Dosage

650 mg. orally 3 times a day for 20 days.

CHLOROQUINE PHOSPHATE
(ARALEN DIPHOSPHATE)

This is an antimalarial drug which also attacks amebae in the liver. It is not recommended for intestinal amebiasis.

Dosage and Administration

Initial dose of 250 mg. 4 times a day or 500 mg. 2 times a day followed by a maintenance dose of 250 mg. twice a day for 2 to 3 weeks.

EMETINE

Emetine is an alkaloid of ipecac. It is a severe proto-plasmic poison, particularly of the heart muscle. The pulse and blood pressure must be taken before each dose of the drug.

Action and Uses

Destroys amebae that have invaded the liver.

Treatment of intestinal amebiasis must be of short duration.

Is ineffective against cysts and, thus, cannot control carriers.

Side and Toxic Effects

Nausea and vomiting

Diarrhea

Cardiac failure

Eventual disintegration of the myocardium and the liver may occur

Preparations and Dosage

Emetine Hydrochloride, 1 mg. per Kg. of body weight, not to exceed 60 mg., intramuscularly, once a day for 5 to 10 days.

CARBARSONE

Action and Uses

Carbarsone, an arsenical derivative, is effective against amebic cysts because it acts against the trophozoites which give rise to cysts. It is used for chronic amebiasis, often with chloroquine or emetine.

Preparations and Dosage

Orally, 250 mg. twice a day for 10 days.

Rectally, as a retention enema, 2 Gm. in 200 ml. of warm 2 per cent bicarbonate solution.

Side and Toxic Effects

Skin rash, diarrhea, abdominal pain.

It should not be administered in liver or kidney disease.

GLYCOBIARSOL (MILIBIS)

Action and Uses

Glycobiarsol is limited in its usefulness to intestinal amebiasis. It contains both arsenic and bismuth.

Dosage and Administration

500 mg. 3 times a day for 7 days

Side and Toxic Effects

Toxicity is less than carbarsone but because of its arsenic content it should not be used in the presence of liver disease.

PAROMOMYCIN (HUMATIN)

Paromomycin is one of the most valuable antibiotics against amebiasis. It is also effective against enteric bacteria such as Shigella, Salmonella, and Escherichia coli. Because of its slow intestinal absorption, toxicity is seldom seen.

Dosage and Administration

Orally, 25 to 50 mg. per Kg. of body weight daily in divided doses with meals, for 5 to 7 days.

See NEOBACIN AND BACIMYCIN
See CHLOROQUINE

DRUGS TO TREAT MALARIA

QUININE

Quinine is an alkaloid of cinchona bark and is a versatile drug.

Action and Uses

A protoplasmic poison especially active against protozoa, it is used to treat clinical symptoms of malaria and as suppressive treatment.

It reduces fever and was formerly used widely as an ingredient of "cold tablets."

PHARMACOLOGY

It reduces auricular fibrillation, although quinidine is better.

Mildly stimulating to the uterine muscle, it sometimes is used with castor oil as an ecbolic.

It thromboses veins by irritant action and is used with urethane (ethyl carbamate) to inject varicose veins.

It is an ingredient of "bitter tonics."

Preparations and Dosage

Quinine Sulfate, orally 1 Gm. for 2 days, then 600 mg. for 5 days.

Quinine Bisulfate, 1 Gm., daily.

Quinine Dihydrochloride, 1 Gm., daily.

Quinine Hydrochloride, 0.2 Gm., intravenously for severe attacks of *falciparum* or the malignant type of malaria.

Quinine Hydrochloride, and urethane (ethyl carbamate), 0.5 ml., intravenously for sclerosing veins.

Totaquine, a mixture of all the alkaloids of cinchona, 0.6 Gm.

Side and Toxic Effects ("Cinchonism")

Headache and dizziness
Tinnitus and deafness
Disturbed vision
Nausea and vomiting
Skin rashes

QUINACRINE HYDROCHLORIDE
(ATABRINE HYDROCHLORIDE)

Quinacrine hydrochloride is a synthetic yellow dye.

Action and Uses

It destroys the asexual form of the malarial parasite, which is the form causing clinical symptoms.

It will not prevent the relapse of the disease in its tertian or quartan forms.

It is more effective than quinine in curing the *falciparum* or malignant form without danger of recurrence.

This drug has been largely replaced by chloroquine.

Preparations and Dosage

Atabrine Dihydrochloride

1. Suppressive treatment: 0.1 Gm. daily for 6 days.

2. To treat clinical attack: 200 mg. with 1 Gm. of sodium bicarbonate every 6 hours for 5 doses. Then 100 mg. 3 times a day for 6 days.

Side and Toxic Effects

It causes the skin and the urine to become yellow. This is not serious and usually disappears in 3 to 4 weeks.

Headache may occur.

Gastrointestinal symptoms may occur.

CHLOROQUINE PHOSPHATE
(ARALEN PHOSPHATE)

Chloroquine phosphate is a chemical antimalarial drug developed during the course of World War II.

Action and Uses

A single weekly dose adequately suppresses symptoms.

It is more potent and more rapid in clearing the blood of parasites than quinacrine hydrochloride (Atabrine).

It cures attacks of malaria caused by *P. falciparum* but not those caused by *P. vivax*.

It provides longer periods of remission between relapses in *P. vivax* infestations.

To treat amebiasis in the intestinal type and when there is liver involvement. Avoids the toxicity of emetine.

Preparations and Dosage

Chloroquine phosphate

1. Suppressive treatment: 500 mg. once a week.

2. To treat clinical attack: 1 Gm. and an additional dose of 500 mg. after 6 or 8 hours. 500 mg. is repeated on 2 successive mornings.

PHARMACOLOGY

Side and Toxic Effects

Side effects, usually of a mild and transitory nature, are:

> Headache and visual disturbances
> Pruritus
> Nausea and vomiting

AMODIAQUINE HYDROCHLORIDE (CAMOQUIN)

Action and Uses

Amodiaquine is as effective an anti-malarial drug as chloroquine and it also has a low toxicity. It has been known to cure infection caused by *Plasmodium falciparum*. It does not prevent the infection by *P. vivax* but will treat effectively acute attacks. It is helpful in suppressing endemic malaria.

Preparations and Dosage

Orally, 400 to 600 mg. in a single dose for acute attacks of malaria. For suppression, 400 to 600 mg. every two weeks.

Side and Toxic Effects

Gastrointestinal disturbances, spasticity and convulsions, but these are rarely seen.

PYRIMETHAMINE (DARAPRIM)

Action and Uses

Pyrimethamine is an anti-malarial drug whose value lies in its suppressive action. By interfering with the formation of sporozoites in the mosquito, it prevents the transmission of malaria. Its use has often resulted in the cure of falciparum infections.

Preparations and Dosage

Suppressive dose: 25 mg. each week, orally.

Side and Toxic Effects

These are rare although anemia and leukopenia may occur.

DRUGS TO TREAT SCHISTOSOMIASIS AND FILARIASIS

ANTIMONY

Action and Uses

In the form of tartar emetic as an expectorant.

For the treatment of diseases acquired primarily in the tropics.

Schistosomiasis
Kala-azar and other leishmanial diseases
Lymphogranuloma venereum
Filariasis

Most of the preparations may cause severe vomiting.

PREPARATIONS AND DOSAGE

Antimony Potassium Tartrate (Tartar Emetic)

3 mg., as a nauseant expectorant. Seldom used.

40 mg. in a 0.5 per cent solution, intravenously, as an initial dose, increasing each dose every 2 days for a total of 140 mg. in 14 to 18 doses.

Stibophen (Fuadin)

A total of 2.5 Gm. in 15 days. Administered intramuscularly on alternate days. A course of iron therapy is recommended after treatment of schistosomiasis.

Ethylstibamine (Neostibosan)

Initially 200 mg., intramuscularly or intravenously. This may be increased to 300 mg. for a total of 3.5 to 5 Gm. over a 4 week period.

Stibamine Glucoside (Neostam)

0.1 Gm. per 100 lb. body weight, intramuscularly or intravenously, in freshly prepared 4 per cent solution. It is given on alternate days for a total of 3 Gm.

Suramin Sodium

To prevent infection, 1 Gm. is given intravenously twice a week for 3 months. For treatment 1 to 2 Gm., intravenously, are given every week for a total of 5 to 10 mg. The solution should be made fresh each time the drug is administered.

Part 6.   Drugs to Treat Cardiac Disorders

DIGITALIS

Digitalis comes from the leaves of *Digitalis purpurea* or purple foxglove and the *Digitalis lanata* or white foxglove.

Action and Uses

1. To treat cardiac arrhythmias, such as atrial (auricular) fibrillation.

A. Prolongs the refractory period of the heart, thus preventing the conduction of extrasystoles while the heart is at rest.

B. Affects the conduction system itself and retards the conduction of extrasystoles.

2. In congestive heart failure.

A. Directly stimulates the heart muscle, increasing its tone and contractility.

B. Heart beats more effectively.

3. Indirectly produces diuresis by improving general circulation.

Side and Toxic Effects

Side reactions usually are due to cumulative action.

Anorexia, nausea and vomiting

Diarrhea

Slowing of the pulse (pulse below 60)

Extrasystoles manifested by coupling rhythm

Headache

Disturbed vision sometimes occurs

Dosage and Administration

Digitalization to saturate the tissues and relieve symptoms.

For the average patient weighing about 140 to 150

pounds, 1 to 1.5 Gm. of digitalis leaf or 1 to 1.5 mg. of digitoxin or 2 to 4 mg. of digoxin over a 24 to 48 hour period.

Digitalization period may be prolonged.

Maintenance dose of 0.1 to 0.2 Gm. of digitalis leaf or 0.1 to 0.2 mg. of digitoxin or 0.5 mg. of digoxin daily to replace amount excreted daily and to maintain saturation of tissues and prevent a recurrence of symptoms.

PREPARATIONS

Whole Leaf Preparations for Oral Administration

Prepared in ½ or 1 U.S.P. Digitalis units

TABLETS OR PILLS of 50 to 100 mg.

CAPSULES of 50 to 100 mg.

DIGITALIS TINCTURE. 1 ml. containing 0.1 Gm. Seldom used today.

SUPPOSITORIES for rectal administration

Proprietary Preparations of Purified Glycosides

Many can be administered parenterally.

DIGITOXIN (Digitaline-Nativelle), 0.1 to 0.2 mg. This is an important glycoside of digitalis.

1. Absorption from the gastrointestinal tract is almost complete, and oral administration is considered as therapeutically beneficial as parenteral administration.

2. The entire digitalization dose, 1.2 to 1.5 mg., can be administered at once, an impossibility with digitalis leaf.

3. Toxic effects are somewhat less than with digitalis leaf, although cumulative effects are the same.

4. Nausea and vomiting occur less frequently.

GITALIN, 0.25 to 1 mg. daily.

LANATOSIDE C (CEDILANID)

A drug that has been widely used. Lanatoside C is obtained from the leaves of *Digitalis lanata,* which contain more glycosides than the leaves of *Digitalis purpurea.* It is not generally considered more advantageous than digitoxin, which can be administered orally.

PHARMACOLOGY

Action and Uses

The action is the same as digitalis, but has certain advantages over digitalis.

1. The margin of safety between the therapeutic dose and the toxic dose is much greater.

2. Nausea and vomiting occur less frequently.

3. The critically ill patient can be digitalized immediately by giving a single digitalization dose intravenously.

Preparations and Dosage

TABLETS of 0.5 mg. for oral administration.

AMPULES of solution for intravenous administration. Digitalization may be accomplished by:

Administering the digitalization dose of 8 mg. in divided doses.

Administering the digitalization dose of 8 mg. in a single dose.

A daily oral maintenance dose of 0.5 to 1 mg. must follow.

DIGOXIN (LANOXIN)

Digoxin is a glycoside obtained from the leaves of the *Digitalis lanata* or white foxglove.

Action and Uses

Action and toxicity are the same as those of digitalis. However, because it is purified active principle, it is of value for rapid digitalization. Saturation of tissues is achieved in a few hours when given orally and in a few minutes when given intravenously.

Dosage and Administration

If patient has had no drugs of the digitalis group within 2 weeks, rapid digitalization may be accomplished with 0.75 to 1.0 mg. of drug.

Maintenance often is carried out with either digitalis or digitoxin. The maintenance dose of digoxin is 0.25 to 0.75 mg.

ACETYLDIGITOXIN (ACYLANID)

A glycoside derived from *Digitalis lanata,* acetyl-digitoxin is said to have a more rapid rate of dissipation than digitoxin. Toxicity is manifested by nausea and vomiting before cardiac irregularities occur.

Dosage and Administration

Given orally. *For rapid* digitalization 1.2 to 2 mg. within 24 hours is given. *For slow* digitalization 1 mg. daily for 2 to 6 days. *For maintenance,* 0.1 to 0.2 mg. daily.

SQUILL

Squill is derived from a bulb *Urginea martima.*

Action and Uses

Its action is essentially that of digitalis, but it is felt to be less persistent. It is seldom used as a substitute for digitalis, although it may be used when patient cannot tolerate digitalis. (*See* Digitalis, *above.*)

Preparations and Dosage

Frensh squill is poorly absorbed; therefore, its glycosides are used more frequently.

SCILLAREN, 1.6 mg. 3 times a day by mouth until compensation is regained, then 0.8 mg. daily.

SCILLAREN B given intravenously for immediate effect. Not more than 0.5 mg. is administered within 24 hours.

URGININ, 3 mg. in divided doses, then a maintenance dose of 0.5 to 1 mg. daily.

STROPHANTHIN AND OUABAIN

These are glycosides of the *Strophanthus kombé* and the *Strophanthus gratus* and are seldom used at present.

Action and Uses

Their action is identical with that of digitalis: poorly absorbed from the gastrointestinal tract and, therefore, used intravenously for emergency digitalization. Seldom used at present.

PHARMACOLOGY

Preparations and Dosage

STROPHANTHIN, 0.5 mg., intravenously, in a single dose, making sure the patient has not had digitalis within 2 weeks.

OUABAIN (Crystallized Strophanthin). The same as strophanthin.

QUINIDINE

Quinidine is an alkaloid of cinchona bark and a powerful cardiac depressant.

Action and Uses

It is used to abolish atrial fibrillation of the paroxysmal type or of short duration.

Lessen excitability of atria

Reduces rate of conductivity of atria

Increases the refractory period or "rest period" of the heart

Since it is a protoplasmic poison, it is not used to treat atrial fibrillation of long-standing cardiac decompensation, unless all other measures have failed, or unless the patient has been well digitalized.

It has antimalarial action, and is used occasionally when the patient shows an intolerance to quinine.

Preparations and Dosage

Quinidine Sulfate, 0.2 to 0.4 Gm. every 4 hours. If no effect occurs in 2 or 3 days, the drug may be discontinued. The effect may last for several months. Usually, a test dose is administered first to determine any sensitivity to the drug.

Side and Toxic Effects

Nausea and vomiting

Headache and faintness

Tinnitus

Palpitation

Flushing

Convulsions

Embolism—clot of stagnant blood in atrium might become dislodged when atrium contracts.

Contraindications to Use

Marked cardiac insufficiency of long-standing
Arteriosclerosis
Organic heart lesions
History of emboli

PROCAINAMIDE (PRONESTYL)

This amide of procaine was developed following the discovery that procaine given intravenously (usually a dangerous procedure) abolished ventricular fibrillation resulting from cyclopropane anesthesia.

Action and Uses

Used primarily to treat ventricular arrhythmias, but also used to treat atrial fibrillation, the drug apparently depresses the irritability of the ventricles and the atria.

Dosage and Administration

Given orally, or intramuscularly, 1 Gm. every 6 hours. May be given intravenously in an emergency in doses of 0.2 to 1 Gm. very slowly.

Side and Toxic Effects

Low blood pressure producing shock if given intravenously
Nausea and vomiting
Agranulocytosis

OXYGEN

Commercially available pure (99%) oxygen is a gas obtained from liquefied air; it is marketed in steel cylinders. These cylinders must be equipped with reducing valves before use to control the flow of the oxygen, which is under high pressure.

Action and Uses

Oxygen is used in cases of oxygen want, such as:
PNEUMONIA, when there is diminished absorbing surface in the lung.

PHARMACOLOGY

CARDIAC FAILURE, when faulty circulation causes improper oxygenation of blood.

CORONARY OCCLUSION, when anoxia of the heart muscle causes severe pain, necrosis of the heart muscle and subsequent cardiac failure.

HINDRANCE TO RESPIRATION, such as that caused by asthma, pulmonary edema, etc.

CARBON MONOXIDE POISONING

To mix with and dilute anesthetic and other gases.

Dosage and Administration

See pp. 107-111: Technics for the dosage and administration of oxygen by

Nasal catheter

Mask

Pressure Mask

Tent

METHACHOLINE CHLORIDE
(MECHOLYL CHLORIDE)

This drug is a synthetic choline ester of greater stability than the acetylcholine of the body, but with the same stimulating effect on the parasympathetic system.

Action and Uses

Subcutaneously, to treat intractable paroxysmal tachycardia when other measures to end the attack have failed. Stimulates vagus nerve, produces bradycardia.

Occasionally by mouth or by iontophoresis, to treat chronic ulcers, scleroderma and diseases of vascular spasm, such as Raynaud's disease.

Stimulates peristalsis, but this effect is of no therapeutic value.

To treat urinary bladder retention in atonic bladder.

Contraindications to Its Use

Should not be used intravenously because of the danger of cardiac arrest.

Should not be administered if patient has bronchial asthma, coronary artery disease or any severe illness.

Preparations, Administration and Dosage

MECHOLYL CHLORIDE, 10 to 15 mg., subcutaneously.

If a second dose is necessary, 10 to 20 minutes should elapse before it is administered. A dose of 30 mg. is seldom exceeded.

Site of injection should not be massaged.

Atropine, 0.6 mg., should be in readiness in case of extreme bradycardia or other untoward effect.

Patient should be in a recumbent position and should be warned of unpleasant side effects, such as:

Syncope

Dyspnea

Marked intestinal peristalsis leading to involuntary defecation.

For conditions other than paroxysmal tachycardia: orally, 200 to 500 mg. 2 to 3 times a day.

MECHOLYL BROMIDE, 0.2 to 0.6 Gm. 2 or 3 times a day, used by mouth.

Part 7.   Drugs to Treat Edema

AMMONIUM CHLORIDE

Action and Uses

Ammonium ion is converted to urea in the liver, liberating the chloride ion, which is acid. Sodium combines with the chloride ion to neutralize it, and sodium is excreted as sodium chloride. Water is excreted with the sodium.

In 3 or 4 days, the kidney starts manufacturing ammonia to compensate for loss of sodium, and ammonium chloride becomes ineffective.

As a saline expectorant in doses of 0.3 Gm., ammonium chloride is repeated at frequent intervals.

It is used as an agent to acidify urine.

Dosage and Administration

1 to 1.5 Gm. 4 times a day. To avoid irritation it should be well diluted or administered in enteric-coated tablets. It is especially useful when administered for

several days prior to the administration of a mercurial diuretic and seems to potentiate the action of a mercurial.

SALINE DIURETICS

Action and Uses

The possible concentration of electrolytes in the kidney is limited. Drugs that cause this limit to be exceeded cannot be excreted unless diluted by water drawn from the tissues of the body.

Preparations and Dosage

HYPERTONIC GLUCOSE (Dextrose), 50 ml. of 25 to 50 per cent.

UREA, 8 Gm. 4 times a day, is more palatable when administered in a full glass of water with lemon juice and sugar.

XANTHINE DIURETICS

Sometimes these are referred to as stimulating diuretics. They are obtained from the coffee bean, tea leaves and the seeds of *Theobroma cacao* (cocoa). The kola nut also contains caffeine.

Action and Uses

They produce diuresis, especially when edema is due to faulty circulation.

Improve general circulation

Increase circulation of the kidney by dilating kidney blood vessels

Increase permeability of the glomeruli by altering the epithelium of the blood vessels and Bowman's capsule.

Because of the availability of more potent and dependable diuretics, the xanthines are used largely only as adjuncts to other diuretics.

Preparations and Dosage

THEOPHYLLINE, 0.2 Gm. 3 times a day:

The most active and effective, but effect is not sustained.

May cause gastric and renal irritation

THEOBROMINE, 0.3 to 0.6 Gm.:

Is not as active as theophylline, but its action is of longer duration

Is not irritating to the kidney

CAFFEINE. (*See* Caffeine.)

MERCURY COMPOUNDS

Action and Uses

Antiseptic and disinfectant. (*See* Antiseptics and Disinfectants.)

As an irritant diuretic: Interferes with enzyme systems that are responsible for the reabsorption of chloride and reduces the ability of the kidney tubules to reabsorb sodium and, hence, water.

Side and Toxic Effects

See Mercury *under* Poisons: Symptoms and Treatment.

PREPARATIONS AND DOSAGE

Diuretics should be given early in the morning so as not to interfere with the patient's rest. Mercurial diuretics are contraindicated in acute nephritis and generally should not be repeated for 4 to 5 days.

MERALLURIDE (Mercuhydrin Sodium), 0.5 to 1.5 ml. intramuscularly.

MERCUROPHYLLINE (Mercupurin), 0.5 to 1.0 ml., intravenously or intramuscularly.

MERSALYL (Salyrgan) with Theophylline, 2 ml., intravenously or intramuscularly.

CHLORMERODRIN (Neohydrin). A mercurial diuretic with the same action and uses as other mercurials. It has the great advantage of being effective orally, and in some instances parenteral injections of other mercurials are unnecessary. Given orally, 18 to 72 mg.

MERCAPTOMERIN SODIUM (Thiomerin Sodium). An effective mercurial diuretic that is given subcutaneously. It is less irritating than other parenterally administered mercurials. Give 0.5 to 1 ml., making sure the injection is made beneath the subcutaneous fat and that the site of injection is changed frequently.

MERCUMATILIN SODIUM (Cumertilin), 1 to 2 ml., intramuscularly or intravenously.

MERETHOXYLLINE PROCAINE (Dicurin Procaine), 2 ml. intramuscularly.

THIAZIDES AND RELATED COMPOUNDS

CHLOROTHIAZIDE (DIURIL)

Action and Uses

The action of chlorothiazide is not well understood. In large doses it acts as a carbonic anhydrase inhibitor, but this does not seem to be its chief action. It apparently acts on the kidney tubule in such a way that sodium and chloride ions are not reabsorbed readily and urine output is increased. Potassium is excreted also, which may necessitate the administration of potassium chloride.

Chlorothiazide not only relieves edema but also lowers blood pressure in hypertension, probably due to depletion of the body's excess of salt. It should be used with caution in the management of toxemias of pregnancy.

Preparations, Dosage and Administration

Chlorothiazide 0.5 to 1.0 Gm. orally once or twice a day.

Hydrochlorothiazide (Esidrix) 25 to 50 mg. 1 to 2 times a day.

Bendroflumethiazide (Naturatin), initial dose 5 to 20 mg., daily maintenance dose 2.5 to 5 mg. daily.

Benzthiazide (NaClex), initial dose 50 to 200 mg. daily, maintenance dosage reduced gradually to 25 to 50 mg. once or twice a day.

Methyclothiazide (Enduron) 2.5 to 10 mg. daily.

Polythiazide (Renese) 1 to 4 mg. daily.

Trichlormethiazide (Naqua), initial dose 2 to 4 mg. daily, maintenance 2 mg. daily.

Chlorthalidone (Hygroton) 50 to 200 mg. 3 times a week.

Quinethazone (Hydromox) 50 to 100 mg.

Side and Toxic Effects

Weakness
Gastric distress
Joint pains which resemble those of gout
Skin rash
Electrolyte imbalance

SPIRONOLACTONE (ALDACTONE)

Action and Uses

Spironolactone causes diuresis by antagonizing the action of aldosterone, an adrenocortical hormone that regulates retention of sodium, thereby increasing the loss of sodium and water in the distal tubule. It lessens the excretion of potassium and ammonium. It reduces edema in congestive heart failure, hepatic cirrhosis with ascites, and the nephrotic syndrome.

Side and Toxic Effects

Drowsiness
Ataxia
Stupor
Skin rash

Dosage and Administration

25 mg. 4 times a day.

ACETAZOLAMIDE (DIAMOX)

Diamox is a derivative of sulfonamides and is used orally as a diuretic.

Action and Uses

Like sulfonamides, it inhibits the enzyme system, especially carbonic anhydrase, in the kidney, which is responsible for the formation of carbonic acid from carbon dioxide and water. When this process is slowed up, the urine cannot become acid and much sodium is passed out as sodium bicarbonate.

The drug is used primarily to reduce ocular tension in glaucoma.

Dosage

200 to 500 mg. in one dose, by mouth. Must be used on intermittent schedule; is not effective on continuous administration.

Side and Toxic Effects

Gastric discomfort
Fatigue
Drowsiness
Paresthesias of the face and the extremities

CARBACRYLAMINE RESINS (CARBO-RESINS)

Ion-exchange resins long have been used widely in industry to remove unwanted substances. They are used now in medicine to remove ingested sodium and potassium through the intestinal tract.

Action and Uses

They act chemically by giving up hydrogen ions and taking on other ions, principally sodium ions, and excreting them in the feces. Used to control edema in cardiac failure, cirrhosis of the liver, kidney conditions when excretion of sodium is low, and to enhance the action of mercurial diuretics.

Danger in Use

As the increased excretion of sodium reduces the amount of sodium available, care must be taken to maintain the acid-base balance or acidosis may occur. There should be 1.5 Gm. of sodium given in the diet. If the diet is suspended or reduced, the drug should be discontinued or given in smaller dosage.

Potassium deficiency may occur unless potassium is given or is incorporated in the resin, as potassium is removed before sodium.

Dosage and Administration

Each gram of the ion-exchange resins will remove 23 mg. of sodium. Given orally about 16 Gm. as a flavored powder in water or fruit juice 3 times a day, although dosage is adjusted to patient's needs. Body weight is the best indication for control of dosage.

See also AMINOPHYLLINE
See also CAFFEINE

Part 8.   Drugs to Treat Hypertension

NITRITES

Action and Uses

Chief action is to relax smooth muscle of blood vessels. Vasodilatation is followed by a fall in blood pressure.

1. Used primarily to relieve or prevent attacks of angina pectoris.
   - A. Rapid-acting nitrites, such as amyl nitrite or nitroglycerin, offer immediate relief of attack.
   - B. Longer acting nitrites, such as sodium nitrite, erythrityl tetranitrate, mannitol hexanitrate etc., are best for relieving the severity and reducing the frequency of attacks.
2. Nitroglycerin is employed sometimes to distinguish between an attack of acute angina pectoris, which is relieved promptly by nitrites, and the pain of coronary thrombosis, which is not influenced by nitrites.
3. None of the preparations is of long enough duration to be effective, except symptomatically, in treating hypertension.

Occasionally used to relax bronchial muscle and relieve asthma.

Sometimes affords relief in ureteral spasm or "colic."

PREPARATIONS AND DOSAGE

AMYL NITRITE, 0.2 ml., by inhalation. Ampule is

crushed and its contents inhaled. Action of about 7 minutes' duration.

GLYCERYL TRINITRATE (NITROGLYCERIN), 0.3 to 0.6 mg. tablets sublingually. Action is of about 20 minutes' duration.

PENTAERYTHRITOL TETRANITRATE (PERITRATE), 10 to 20 mg. 3 to 4 times a day to prevent anginal attacks or to decrease their severity.

Side and Toxic Effects

Dizziness and faintness
Headache and feeling of fullness in the head
Flushing of the face and neck
Increased heart rate
Cyanosis due to the formation of methemoglobin
Convulsions
Unconsciousness
Tolerance to preparations often is acquired.

HYDRALAZINE HYDROCHLORIDE (APRESOLINE)

Hydralazine hydrochloride is a hypotensive agent.

Action and Uses

It inhibits the action of pressor substances that cause hypertension and is used in cases that persist after sympathectomy, essential hypertension, hypertension of acute nephritis and toxemias of pregnancy.

Dosage and Administration

10 to 20 mg., 3 or 4 times a day. Blood pressure is taken frequently. It may be combined with other hypotensive agents.

Side and Toxic Effects

Fever
Tachycardia
Dizziness and faintness
Weakness
Nausea and vomiting
Nasal congestion
Psychoses

A dangerous drug and should not be used in coronary disease, incipient or existing cerebral accident or renal damage.

HEXAMETHONIUM CHLORIDE
(METHIUM CHLORIDE)

Hexamethonium chloride is a ganglionic blocking agent.

Action and Uses

It inhibits nerve impulses transmitted through both sympathetic and parasympathetic ganglia. Its blocking effect on sympathetic stimuli causes lowering of blood pressure. It is used primarily for the management of hypertension. At present other ganglionic blocking agents are replacing it.

Dosage and Administration

Give 125 to 250 mg. orally or 50 mg. subcutaneously. It may be repeated in 6 hours if necessary.

Side and Toxic Effects

Loss of ocular accommodation
Decrease in gastrointestinal motility
Alteration of bladder function
Nausea and vomiting
Used carefully in arteriosclerosis, old age, coronary disease and renal damage

RAUWOLFIA SERPENTINA (RAUDIXIN)
AND RAUWOLFIA ALKALOIDS

Although more than 20 alkaloids have been isolated, the entire root of the plant is still used. However, reserpine, one of the alkaloids, is used most commonly.

Action and Uses

The mechanism of action that results in reduction of blood pressure is not well understood. It is used in essential hypertension—alone if the hypertension is mild, and combined with other drugs if the condition is severe.

PHARMACOLOGY

It is given also with other drugs to reduce the dosage of other hypotensive agents. It is used also in psychiatry for a calming effect.

Preparations, Dosage and Administration

Rauwolfia (Raudixin), 50 to 300 mg. a day orally in divided doses.

Reserpine (Serpasil), 0.1 to 0.25 mg. daily in 2 or 3 divided doses orally or parenterally.

Alseroxylon (Rauwiloid), 2 to 4 mg. daily orally.

Rescinnamine (Moderil), 0.5 mg. twice daily orally, for 2 weeks, then 0.25 mg. daily.

Side and Toxic Effects

Drowsiness
Loose stools
Slow pulse
Increased secretion of gastric juice
"Stuffy" nose
Bizarre dreams
Long term use of dosages higher than 0.25 mg. may have more serious reactions:
Perforation of ulcers
Gastrointestinal hemorrhage
Severe depression (and suicidal attempts)

PENTOLINIUM TARTRATE (ANSOLYSEN)

Action and Uses

This is a ganglionic blocking agent. It is used in the management of moderately severe, severe and malignant hypertension, but it is not recommended for mild forms. It is of great potency, and its action seems to be quite predictable.

Dosage and Administration

Often given with rauwolfia serpentina (Raudixin) or reserpine (Serpasil).

Given by mouth 20 mg. 3 times a day the first week, and increasing 20 mg. each week, until minimum effective dosage is reached (average, 20 to 200 mg. every 8 hours).

Side and Toxic Effects

Postural hypotension
Constipation
Dryness of mouth
Cycloplegia

Contraindications

Pyloric stenosis
Myocardial infarction
Severe coronary insufficiency
Cerebral arteriosclerosis

MECAMYLAMINE HYDROCHLORIDE (INVERSINE)

This is a potent ganglionic blocking agent similar to hexamethonium, but with more prolonged action. It is used for the same purposes as other ganglionic blocking agents. Like all ganglionic blocking agents, use requires careful supervision and regular observation. Contraindications are the same as for other ganglionic blocking agents.

Dosage and Administration

2.5 mg. 2 times a day by mouth. This is increased at intervals of not less than 2 days until desired effect is obtained; average maintenance dose is a total of 25 mg. a day.

Side and Toxic Effects

Constipation
Dry mouth
Nausea and vomiting
Postural hypotension

CHLORISONDAMINE CHLORIDE (ECOLID)

This is a ganglionic blocking agent similar to others. It is less predictable in action than mecamylamine hydrochloride but is more potent than pentolinium tartrate or hexamethonium. It is used for more severe types of hypertension.

Dosage and Administration

Orally, 10 mg. in morning and evening, increasing until 200 mg. daily is reached, if patient needs it.

Parenterally, 1 to 10 mg. in a single dose.

Side and Toxic Effects

Same as other ganglionic blocking agents

VERATRUM VIRIDE ALKALOIDS
ALKAVERVIR (VERILOID)

Veratrum viride alkaloids are hypotensive agents.

Action and Uses

They decrease blood pressure by dilating the arterioles, which is accompanied by constriction of the venous beds. They are used primarily for hypertensive crises, eclampsia, acute nephritis and toxemias of pregnancy. Uses are limited. Dosage is variable.

Toxic Effects

Epigastric burning
Nausea and vomiting
Salivation
Low blood pressure and collapse
Heart block

Part 9.   Drugs Used to Treat Hypotension and Cardiac Collapse

LEVARTERENOL BITARTRATE
(/-NOREPINEPHRINE; LEVOPHED)

Action and Uses

A powerful vasoconstrictor, levarterenol bitartrate raises blood pressure without increasing cardiac output (unlike epinephrine in this respect). It is used to maintain blood pressure in surgery, hemorrhage and vaso-motor depression.

Dosage and Administration

2 to 4 micrograms per minute in saline isotonic with 5 per cent dextrose, or in 5 per cent dextrose in distilled water, intravenously.

Blood pressure should be taken every 2 minutes until desired level of blood pressure is reached, then checked very frequently until administration is discontinued.

If it extravasates into the subcutaneous tissue, slough-ing may occur.

Side and Toxic Effects

Rash
Headache
Pain in chest
Nausea and vomiting
Extreme pallor
Photophobia
Bradycardia, which is abolished by atropine
Is not used during cyclopropane anesthesia as the danger of ventricular fibrillation is increased.

METARAMINOL BITARTRATE
(ARAMINE BITARTRATE)

Metaraminol bitartrate is used like levarterenol bi-tartrate to raise blood pressure in acute hypotensive states. Its action is more gradual in onset but is more prolonged than that of levarterenol.

Dosage and Administration

2 to 10 mg. subcutaneously, intramuscularly or by intravenous infusion. Intravenous injection should be used only in extreme emergencies and with great care.

Side and Toxic Effects

These seldom occur with therapeutic doses. However, as the drug is a vasopressor, care needs to be taken in its use. To avoid cumulative effect due to prolonged action, at least 10 minutes should elapse before dosage is increased.

ISOPROTERENOL HYDROCHLORIDE
(ISUPREL; ALUDRINE)

This is an agent which is related to epinephrine and levarterenol. It is used to increase the ventricular rate in heart block and to prevent cardiac arrest. Since it relaxes bronchial muscle, also, it is a powerful drug for the treatment of bronchial asthma.

Dosage and Administration

10 to 15 mg. sublingually 3 to 4 times a day
0.5 ml. of a 1:200 solution by nebulizer

Side and Toxic Effects

Palpitation
Anginal pain
Headache
Nausea and vomiting
Nervousness and excitement
Precordial pain
Low blood pressure

EPINEPHRINE (ADRENALIN)

Epinephrine is a hormone secreted by the medulla of the adrenal gland. It is obtained by extraction from adrenal glands and is also produced synthetically.

Action and Uses

A vasoconstrictor, it is used:

To raise blood pressure temporarily. Action is of short duration, and increase in blood pressure is probably due to increased cardiac output, which may be unwise in cardiac disorders.

To shrink mucous membrane of the nasal passages.

To control superficial capillary hemorrhage.

To localize a local anesthetic agent such as Novocain.

To relieve urticaria, anaphylactic shock or the nitritoid crisis of arsphenamine reaction.

Relaxes constricted bronchial muscle and relieves asthma.

Releases glycogen from the liver and is used occasionally to raise blood sugar in insulin shock.

In extreme emergencies is used intracardially or intravenously for its direct stimulation of the heart.

Preparations and Dosage

EPINEPHRINE HYDROCHLORIDE (ADRENALIN)

1:100 in a spray or nebulizer to treat asthma.

1:500 in oil, 0.2 to 0.5 ml., intramuscularly. Forms a depot for the slow release and absorption of adrenalin, giving it more sustained action.

1:1,000 solution, 0.3 to 1.0 ml. for hypodermic injection.

SUPRARENALIN, 1:10,000 ampules of 1 ml.

SUPRARENIN BITARTRATE, 1:1,000 in ampules of 1 ml.

Side and Toxic Effects

Insomnia
Nervousness and anxiety
Tremors
Headache
Tachycardia

PHENYLEPHRINE HYDROCHLORIDE
(NEO-SYNEPHRINE HYDROCHLORIDE)

Phenylephrine hydrochloride is a synthetic drug with properties similar to epinephrine and ephedrine.

Action and Uses

A vasoconstrictor, it is used

1. To shrink mucous membrane of nasal passages.

2. With a local anesthetic agent to retard absorption and prolong its action.

3. With spinal anesthetic to combat the fall of blood pressure.

4. When collapse occurs because of failure of the peripheral blood vessels, rather than a decrease of circulating blood volume.

In ophthalmology

1. As a mydriatic for fundus examination.

2. With cycloplegic drugs to prevent or free adhesions between the iris and the lens.

PHARMACOLOGY

Preparations and Dosage

NEO-SYNEPHRINE HYDROCHLORIDE

Orally 10 to 25 mg.

Subcutaneously 0.2 to 1 per cent solution

½ to 1 per cent solution for nasal congestion or sinusitis.

0.1 to 1.0 ml. of 1 per cent solution for systemic effect.

In ophthalmology:

1 or 2 drops of 1 per cent solution for mydriasis.

1 drop of 10 per cent solution as a vasoconstrictor. Should be preceded by Holocaine or Pontocaine to reduce irritation of the drug.

EPHEDRINE

Ephedrine comes from the twigs of a Chinese shrub (ma huang). It is also prepared synthetically. Symptoms of anxiety sometimes follow its use.

Action and Uses

A vasoconstrictor, it is used:

1. To shrink mucous membrane of the nasal mucosa.

2. To raise blood pressure in collapse. Action is more sustained than that of epinephrine.

3. Administered with spinal anesthesia to maintain blood pressure.

4. To relieve hay fever and urticaria.

Relaxes constricted bronchial muscle and affords relief in bronchial asthma.

Preparations and Dosage

EPHEDRINE SULFATE OR HYDROCHLORIDE, 1 to 3 per cent, in oil or saline.

Saline felt to be the preferred medium.

Oily preparations discouraged. If improperly administered, oil may enter the lung and lipoid pneumonia may result.

EPHEDRINE SULFATE OR HYDROCHLORIDE, 25 to 50 mg., by mouth, intramuscularly or intravenously.

MEPHENTERMINE SULFATE (WYAMINE)

Mephentermine sulfate increases blood pressure by improving cardiac contractions. It exerts pressor action and is therefore a nasal decongestant when applied topically and a vasoconstrictor when given parenterally. It is used to combat high blood pressure and certain cardiac arrhythmias.

Dosage and Administration

Orally, 12.5 to 25 mg. 2 or 3 times daily

Intravenously or intramuscularly, 15 to 30 mg.

Topically, 0.5 per cent concentration, 2 to 3 drops every 4 hours for nasal congestion.

METHOXAMINE HYDROCHLORIDE (VASOXYL)

The action of methoxamine hydrochloride is very similar to that of other drugs that constrict the blood vessels.

Dosage and Administration

Intramuscularly, 10 to 15 mg. At least 15 minutes should elapse before second dose.

Intravenously, 5 to 10 mg. (for emergency use only)

Topically, 1 to 3 drops, 2 to 4 times daily.

See also WHOLE BLOOD
See also BLOOD SUBSTITUTES *and*
PLASMA EXPANDERS
See also ATROPINE

Part 10. Drugs to Treat Depressive States

RESPIRATORY DEPRESSION

NALORPHINE HYDROCHLORIDE (NALLINE HYDROCHLORIDE)

Nalorphine hydrochloride is a derivative of morphine, but has quite different properties. It is not used as an analgesic because of undesirable side effects. It antagonizes the effects of morphine and its derivatives.

PHARMACOLOGY

Action and Uses

To prevent respiratory depression when large doses of morphine are needed. Given about 30 minutes before dose of morphine or any of its derivatives.

To reverse respiratory depression, hypotension and neurologic changes due to narcotic poisoning.

Will produce abstinence symptoms in addicts.

Has no effect in respiratory depression due to barbiturates or anesthesia.

Dosage and Administration

Given parenterally 5 to 10 mg., repeated in 10 to 15 minutes if necessary. A dose of 40 mg. may be safely used in severe poisoning.

It is subject to the provisions of the Harrison Narcotic Act.

LEVALLORPHAN TARTRATE (LORFAN)

(See NARCOTIC ANTAGONISTS for more information, p. 628)

CAFFEINE

Caffeine is one of the oldest and best known stimulants. The average cup of coffee contains 60 to 120 mg. of caffeine.

Action and Uses

Principal stimulating effect is on the cerebral cortex, resulting in clearer and more rapid thought.

Often effective to relieve headache, possibly due to cerebral vascular constriction.

Occasionally used to relieve fatigue and drowsiness.

As an emergency measure in respiratory failure, especially that of narcotic poisoning.

As a heart stimulant, as adjunct in treatment of circulatory collapse. Acts directly on the heart muscle: in cardiac disease it is deemed unwise to use caffeine as a stimulant as the nervous system and the processes of the body are stimulated and the patient needs rest.

As a diuretic* when edema is due to faulty circulation. Other types of diuretics are used more frequently, at present.

Preparations and Dosage

1. Caffeine, U.S.P. 0.2 Gm.
2. Caffeine, citrated, N.F., 60 to 300 mg. for oral and parenteral use.
3. Caffeine Sodium Benzoate, U.S.P., 0.2 to 0.5 Gm. subcutaneously or intramuscularly.
4. An ingredient of various headache remedies.

Side and Toxic Effects

Insomnia and restlessness
Anxiety
Palpitation
Dizziness
Nausea

NIKETHAMIDE (CORAMINE)

Nikethamide is a synthetic preparation.

Action and Uses

It is used most widely as an emergency respiratory and circulatory stimulant. The main site of action is on the central nervous system.

Preparations and Dosage

1 to 3 ml. of 25 per cent solution. Usually administered parenterally.

PENTYLENETETRAZOL (METRAZOL)

Action and Uses

As an emergency stimulant in respiratory and circulatory collapse.

* If tolerance has been built up by the continued use of caffeine-containing beverages, the therapeutic result may be disappointing.

PHARMACOLOGY

As a sustaining agent and restorative in chronic cardiac and circulatory disorders.

In convulsive doses in psychiatric institutions to treat mental disorders. Causes severe convulsions, and vertebral fractures have been reported following its use. Has been replaced by electroshock therapy.

Preparations and Dosage

Orally, 0.1 to 0.5 Gm. several times daily.

Intramuscularly, intravenously or subcutaneously 0.1 to 0.5 Gm. of 10 per cent solution.

PICROTOXIN

Picrotoxin is obtained from the berries, commonly called "fish berries," of the East Indian plant *Anamirta cocculus*.

Action and Uses

A powerful central nervous system stimulant, picrotoxin is used to treat poisoning by central nervous system depressants, specifically barbiturates. Many physicians prefer to use physiologic measures.

Dosage and Administration

The amount of drug administered depends on the severity of the poisoning.

1. Aim of treatment is to keep patient in a restless and active state, stopping short of muscular twitching, to avoid possibility of convulsions.

2. Patient needs careful watching.

Given intravenously only, usually at rate of 1 ml. containing 1 mg. of drug per minute; 6 mg. may be given initially with an addition of 3 mg. at 15 minute intervals until 15-mg. dose has been administered or until desired effect is obtained.

1. Stimulation usually measured by increased muscle tone and reflex activity.

2. Dosage level adequate at return of corneal and pupillary reflexes.

3. *No attempt should be made to restore consciousness with picrotoxin.*

4. Barbiturate preparation for cutaneous injection should be at hand to use as antidote for possible overdose of picrotoxin.

Side and Toxic Effects

Salivation and vomiting
Elevated blood pressure
Slowing of the heart rate
Convulsions
Respiratory failure leading to death

CARBON DIOXIDE

Action and Uses

To stimulate the respiratory center in the medulla and to increase the rate and depth of respirations.

1. In asphyxia, if respiration has not ceased.
2. When respiratory failure is due to poisoning.
3. During anesthesia to combat respiratory depression that might occur from anesthetic agent or from hyperventilation.
4. After anesthesia, to aid in eliminating anesthetic gases.
5. To prevent postoperative pneumonia or atelectasis.

To treat hiccoughs, although the exact action is not known. Perhaps it stimulates the respiratory center and makes the diaphragm contract more rhythmically.

Preparations and Dosage

By mask, or funnel in an emergency, inhaled in 5 to 10 per cent carbon dioxide and 95 to 90 per cent oxygen mixture for 3 to 5 minutes.

Side and Toxic Effects

When administered in too high a concentration or over too long a period of time, toxic symptoms may appear.

Hyperpnea and dyspnea
Vomiting
Disorientation
Elevated blood pressure
Convulsions

CIRCULATORY DEPRESSION

AMMONIA

Action and Uses

In liniments as a rubifacient and counterirritant.

As an antacid.

As a carminative because of its volatility.

As a temporary and emergency respiratory and circulatory stimulant. Produces reflex stimulation by irritating the mucous membrane of the respiratory and the gastrointestinal tracts.

Dosage and Administration

Smelling Salts, containing ammounium carbonate and lavender.

Aromatic Spirits of Ammonia, containing ammonium carbonate in aromatic oils, 2 ml. well diluted.

See DRUGS TO TREAT HYPOTENSION
(VASOCONSTRICTORS)

> EPINEPHRINE
>
> NOREPINEPHRINE
>
> EPHEDRINE
>
> NEO-SYNEPHRINE
>
> *See also* CAFFEINE

ALCOHOLISM

DISULFIRAM (TETRAETHYLTHIURAM DISULFIDE; ANTABUSE)

Disulfiram is a drug to treat alcoholism only when the patient has a real desire to stop drinking. It is important for him to know what he is getting and the violent effect the drug will have on him if he drinks.

Action and Uses

Acts to increase the oxidation of alcohol to acetaldehyde. The high concentration of acetaldehyde in the

704

body probably gives rise to the unpleasant symptoms—extreme flushing, increased pulse and respiration, dizziness, nausea and vomiting, and throbbing headache. It is used as an adjunct to psychiatric treatment of chronic alcoholism.

Dosage and Administration

After at least 12 hours of abstinence from alcohol, or when all signs of alcohol intoxication have disappeared, 500 mg. every day taken orally for 2 to 3 weeks; then a daily maintenance dose of 125 to 500 mg.

Side and Toxic Effects

It is not dangerous in the absence of alcohol. It is a dangerous drug when combined with alcohol as noted above and ingestion of even small amounts of alcohol have caused death. Reaction to alcohol will continue for about a week after a single large dose of the drug.

Patients on disulfiram should not be given medications that contain alcohol (spirits; tinctures; many elixirs and cough "syrups," etc.). Rubbing alcohol must not be used.

LETHARGY AND DEPRESSION

AMPHETAMINE SULFATE (BENZEDRINE)

Amphetamine sulfate is a synthetic preparation.

Action and Uses

A powerful vasoconstrictor, and, when used locally, shrinks the mucous membrane of nasal passages, facilitating breathing and the drainage of sinuses.

When used systemically, its chief effect is on the cerebral cortex. It has a stimulating effect on the brain and is used to treat:

Narcolepsy
Postencephalitis lethargy and other sequelæ
Mild depressive psychotic states
Alcoholism, as an adjunct to treatment
Subcutaneously as a respiratory stimulant.
To control appetite in obesity.

PHARMACOLOGY

Dangers of Use

When used indiscriminately as a "pick-me-up" to abolish fatigue and drowsiness, the initial stimulation is sometimes followed by collapse.

Produces euphoria and habituation.

Contraindicated in cardiovascular disease, especially when hypertension is present.

Dosage and Administration

Amphetamine Sulfate, 5 to 10 mg. twice daily, preferably administered in the morning or early afternoon and not at bedtime. Subcutaneously 10 mg. in 1 to 2 ml. distilled water.

Side and Toxic Effects

Anxiety and restlessness
Insomnia
Dizziness
Palpitation

DEXTRO-AMPHETAMINE (DEXEDRINE) AND METHAMPHETAMINE HYDROCHLORIDE (DESOXYN HYDROCHLORIDE)

These are similar to amphetamine sulfate (Benzedrine); the three compounds differ primarily in degree of activity.

Action and Uses

Same as for amphetamine sulfate, except that vasoconstrictor effect is milder and central nervous stimulation is greater.

As an adjunct to the treatment of obesity by:

1. Decrease in appetite by decreasing gastrointestinal motility.

2. Creation of a feeling of satisfaction and well-being which allays "nervous nibbling."

3. Increase in will power to stick to diet.

Dosage and Administration

5 mg. every 4 to 6 hours.

Side and Toxic Effects

Same as for amphetamine sulfate.

DEXTRO-AMPHETAMINE SULFATE AND AMOBARBITAL (DEXAMYL)

Action and Uses

The combination of drugs acts to provide an elevation of mood and a sense of well-being and, at the same time, exerts a calming effect and relieves anxiety. The amobarbital offsets the stimulating effect of the Dexedrine Sulfate and the Dexedrine Sulfate offsets the depressant effect of amobarbital.

Dosage and Administration

Tablets containing dextroamphetamine 5 mg. and amobarbital 32 mg.: 1 tablet 2 or 3 times a day, at breakfast time, lunch and dinner. Timed release capsules, double or triple the strength of the tablet: 1 capsule on arising.

Contraindications

Essentially the same as for amphetamine.

METHYLPHENIDATE HYDROCHLORIDE (RITALIN)

This drug apparently acts as a stimulant to the higher brain centers, the cerebral cortex included. Mental acuity and alertness is increased in depressed, regressed, and inactive patients.

Dosage and Administration

Orally or parenterally, 5 to 20 mg. 2 to 3 times a day. The 3rd dose, if administered, is given early to avoid insomnia.

Side and Toxic Effects

Nervousness and insomnia
Dizziness
Palpitation
Anorexia

Part 11. Parenterals

SODIUM CHLORIDE

Isotonic, normal or physiologic saline solution has the same osmotic pressure as blood serum and body fluids have and is not injurious to cells. It is of 0.85 to 0.9 per cent concentration.

A hypertonic solution has higher osmotic pressure than does serum or body fluids.

A hypotonic solution has lower osmotic pressure than does blood serum or body fluids.

Action and Uses

To replace fluids and electrolytes (sodium and chloride) lost by diarrhea, vomiting, excessive diaphoresis or hemorrhage.

To maintain fluid and electrolyte balance when the patient can take nothing by mouth.

As irrigations for wounds and mucous membranes. Isotonic solution is much less irritating to abraded and irritated surfaces than plain water.

In an emergency, to restore circulating volume in the blood vessels and to raise blood pressure. (*See* Blood Substitutes, *below.*)

As a vehicle for parenterally administered drugs.

Preparations and Dosage

SODIUM CHLORIDE, 0.85 to 0.9 per cent by hypodermoclysis or infusion. Usually given 500 to 1,500 ml. or more. The flow rate varies according to doctor's orders.

SODIUM CHLORIDE, 0.85 per cent with dextrose, 5 per cent.

HYPOTONIC SALINE, 0.45 per cent, used for daily maintenance.

HYPERTONIC SALINE, 3 per cent and 5 percent, for severe salt depletion.

SOLUTIONS FOR ELECTROLYTE THERAPY

RINGER'S INJECTION (and Solution), containing sodium, calcium and potassium as chlorides.

LACTATED RINGER'S INJECTION, containing sodium lactate.

SODIUM LACTATE ONE-SIXTH MOLAR, to treat acidosis and to alkalinize urine. Used alone or combined with Ringer's Solution.

SODIUM BICARBONATE 5 PER CENT. Preferred to sodium lactate solution in metabolic acidosis.

BUTLER'S MULTIPLE ELECTROLYTE SOLUTION, contains sodium, potassium, magnesium, chloride, carbonate and phosphate.

HYALURONIDASE (ALIDASE; WYDASE)

Hyaluronidase is an enzyme isolated from bacterial cultures or animal tissues.

Action and Uses

It hydrolyzes hyaluronic acid, which is a component of the "ground substance" of tissues that acts as a barrier to the free spread of fluid. Thus, when this enzyme is injected into the body, it helps spread fluid faster and aids in its more rapid absorption. It is used to:

Facilitate the absorption of hypodermoclysis solutions

Aid in the diffusion of certain drugs

Help diffuse local anesthetic agents

Aid in absorption of accumulated fluids, such as those resulting from injury to a joint

Prevent and treat urinary calculi

Dangers in Use

Sensitivity may occur

If used in infections, the infection may spread

Dosage and Administration

150 turbidity-reducing units per 1 ml. of isotonic saline, given by injection.

WHOLE BLOOD

Action and Uses

To restore circulating volume and to raise blood pressure when shock occurs.

To supply red blood cells, hemoglobin and platelets in anemia or blood dyscrasias.

Preparations and Administration

Whole blood, with sodium citrate added to prevent clotting, often is administered as an indirect transfusion in amounts of 500 ml., although larger amounts may be given in severe hemorrhage or anemias.

Transfusion Dangers

1. Transmission of disease: to prevent such occurrence donors must be screened, by
   A. Taking of blood Wassermann
   B. Inquiring into history of malaria, allergies, jaundice, etc.
   C. Careful sterilization of needles and syringes to avoid transmission of infectious hepatitis
2. Transfusion "reaction," manifested by:
   A. Chills
   B. Fever
   C. Urticaria
3. Mismatched blood—rarely occurs, because of careful typing and cross-matching, consideration of Rh factor, etc.—leading to:
   A. Agglutination of cells
      a. Backache, an ominous sign
      b. Dyspnea
      c. Rapid pulse
      d. Collapse
   B. Hemolysis of blood cells

SODIUM CITRATE

10 ml. of 2½ to 4 per cent per 100 ml. of blood may be used as an anticoagulant for plasma and for blood for fractionation. Anticoagulant Acid Citrate Dextrose Solution is used for storage of whole blood.

BLOOD SUBSTITUTES

Preparations, Dosage and Administration

ISOTONIC SALINE or GLUCOSE to replace circulating fluid and raise blood pressure in an emergency is administered intravenously at a high rate of flow. The effect is temporary.

PLASMA or SERUM, 500 ml., although any amount needed can be safely administered.

Replaces circulating volume
Supplies protein

SERUM ALBUMIN in nephrosis promotes diuresis.

Advantages of Plasma Over Whole Blood

No need to find a compatible donor
Large quantities can be stored for immediate use
Time saved because typing tests are not necessary
Can be transported easily
Relatively free of reactions

PLASMA EXPANDERS

DEXTRAN

Dextran is a plasma expander.

Action and Uses

When properly diluted, it is approximately equivalent, osmotically, to serum albumin. It is used to increase plasma volume and maintain blood pressure in the emergency treatment of hemorrhage and shock. It is not a substitute for whole blood or plasma and will not restore blood proteins. A few persons show sensitivity to it.

Dosage and Administration

Given intravenously as a 6 per cent solution in isotonic saline in 500 ml. amounts.

GELATIN
(SPECIAL INTRAVENOUS SOLUTION)

Action and Uses

Gelatin is a specially prepared colloidal solution used in an emergency as a substitute for whole blood and plasma when it is not available.

It maintains blood pressure in shock.

It remains in the circulation for about 24 to 48 hours. Since it is excreted by the kidneys, it should be used very carefully when there is evidence of kidney damage.

Gelatin solution may interfere with blood grouping and cross matching, so these procedures should be done before gelatin is administered.

Dosage and Administration

Given about 500 ml. at 30 ml. per minute. Solution should be warmed to about 50°C. before using, as it gels at lower temperature.

PLASMA PROTEIN FRACTION-HUMAN
(PLASMANATE)

Plasma Protein Fraction (Human) is similar to serum albumin in its action and uses. It expands plasma volume and is useful in combating shock, hemorrhage, hypoproteinemia, and in supplying the patient unable to take protein by mouth.

Dosage and Administration

Intravenously, 1,000 ml. containing 50 Gm. of protein, at a rate not to exceed 5 to 8 ml. per minute.

SOLUTIONS FOR NUTRITION

DEXTROSE

Dextrose is used in a 5 to 10 per cent solution intravenously to supply carbohydrate and calories.

FRUCTOSE (LEVULOSE)

Fructose is used for the same purposes as dextrose;

it is metabolized and converted to liver glycogen more rapidly.

Given intravenously in 10 per cent solution.

INVERT SUGAR

Invert sugar is used in the same way as dextrose; it is utilized more rapidly, and can be administered more rapidly without causing glycosuria.

Given intravenously in 5 to 10 per cent solution.

AMINO ACIDS

The amino acids often are referred to as the "building stones of protein."

Hypoproteinemia leads to:
    Alterations in water balance
    Lowered resistance to infection
    Retardation of wound healing

Action and Uses

1. To supply nitrogen necessary to produce hemoglobin and to build the stroma of red blood cells when anemia has occurred.

2. To restore the nitrogen balance of the body and to raise the blood proteins to normal level in:

    A. Surgery

    B. Extensive wounds and burns, in which the oozing of serum has caused excessive loss of proteins.

    C. Gastrointestinal diseases, when dietary restrictions are necessary or when there is difficulty in absorption.

    D. Kidney diseases in which albuminuria causes extensive loss of protein.

Preparations and Dosage

PROTEIN HYDROLYSATES.

Amigen, 50 to 100 Gm. per 1,000 ml. of solution by hypodermoclysis or intravenous infusion.

Parenamine

These preparations may be administered orally by dissolving them in milk, water or fruit juice. They are somewhat unpleasant by this route.

COTTONSEED OIL EMULSION (LIPOMUL)

This is an emulsion of cottonseed oil to be administered intravenously to patients who cannot achieve sufficient caloric intake by mouth. Fat yields 9 calories per gram as opposed to 4 calories per gram of other nutritional components. However, side effects of this type of parenteral administration may be severe.

Dosage and Administration

Cottonseed oil is not mixed with any other parenteral fluid. The intravenous drip must be kept at an extremely slow rate. 250 or 500 ml. of a 15 per cent emulsion may be administered daily for not more than 14 infusions.

Side and Toxic Effects

Back and chest pain
Difficult respirations
Urticaria
Chills and fever
Nausea and vomiting
Abdominal pain
Headache and dizziness
Bleeding from the gastrointestinal tract

Part 12.   Drugs to Treat Blood Dyscrasias

ANEMIAS

IRON

Iron is used chiefly in the form of ferrous salts.

Action and Uses

1. Very small portions of ingested iron are absorbed in the intestine, chiefly the duodenum, and are deposited in the blood-forming organs.

A. Some of this "reserve iron" is used in forming hemoglobin, which enters the red blood cells.

B. Excretion of absorbed iron is minimal.

C. Variations in the amount of iron stored by the normal adult does not affect levels of hemoglobin and red blood cells.

2. Used to restore hemoglobin concentration and red blood cell count in anemias due to:

A. Nutritional iron deficiency

B. Blood loss from massive or slow hemorrhage

C. Chlorosis

Side and Toxic Effects

Gastric distress unless given with or immediately after food

Abdominal cramps

Diarrhea or constipation

Hemosiderosis

Hemochromatosis

Preparations and Dosage

FERROCHOLINATE (CHEL-IRON), orally 330 to 660 mg. 3 times a day.

REDUCED IRON in capsules, 0.5 Gm. (Seldom used at present)

FERROUS SULFATE, 0.3 to 0.6 Gm. orally.

IRON AND AMMONIUM CITRATE, 1 Gm. well diluted and through a straw to protect the teeth from stain.

FERROUS FUMARATE, 200 mg. 3 times a day.

IRON-DEXTRAN COMPLEX (Imferon), used only when oral iron is contraindicated. 50 to 250 mg. intramuscularly, deep into gluteal muscle with long needle after subcutaneous tissue has been displaced laterally. (To be used only in severe iron deficiency anemia. Patient should be watched for anaphylactic reaction.)

LIVER EXTRACT

Until recent years liver extract was used as the only specific drug available in the treatment of pernicious anemia. Today cyanocobalamin has largely replaced it for this purpose, but liver extract is still used for its cyanocobalamin activity to increase the number of red blood cells produced in the bone marrow. Liver Extract is administered deep into the muscle.

CYANOCOBALAMIN (VITAMIN B-12)

Cyanocobalamin in 1948 was discovered to be the antianemic principle in liver extracts. Since that time, it has become increasingly important in the treatment of pernicious anemia. Today it is the drug of choice.

Action and Uses

Its action is that of the antianemic principle of the liver.

1. Stimulates production of red blood corpuscles.
2. Effectively treats pernicious anemia (with or without neurologic symptoms).
3. Useful in treating tropical and non-tropical sprue.
4. Useful in treating nutritional macrocytic anemia due to vitamin B-12 deficiency.

Dosage and Administration

Since it cannot be absorbed if there is a lack of "intrinsic factor" (still not identified) in the gastric juice, and since this lack is characteristic of pernicious anemia, it is not practical to give the drug orally. Dosage schedule in severe pernicious anemia is 15 mcg. to 30 mcg. 2 or 3 times a week until remission occurs, then a maintenance dose of 15 mcg. every other week.

FOLIC ACID

Folic acid is a component of vitamin B complex that can be chemically synthesized. It is generally used in combination with liver therapy or vitamin B_{12}. Folic acid should never be used alone in the treatment of pernicious anemia because it is ineffective in the control of the neurologic symptoms. It has no effect on any anemia except the macrocytic type.

Action and Uses

To treat anemia of:

Pernicious anemia, in conjunction with liver extract or vitamin B_{12}

Sprue

Pellagra

To treat nutritional macrocytic anemia

To treat macrocytic anemia of pregnancy

It is relatively free of side effects in any dosage.

Preparations and Dosage

10 mg., orally or intramuscularly. Oral administration is considered as effective as parenteral administration.

See also WHOLE BLOOD

LEUKEMIAS

SODIUM RADIOPHOSPHATE
(SODIUM PHOSPHATE P 32; PHOSPHOTOPE)

This radioactive substance now is readily available and relatively inexpensive because of widespread construction of atomic reactors. It is similar in effect to external radiation, but not necessarily considered superior to it. Radiation sickness and the toxic effects of antineoplastic drugs are avoided by its use. Its effect is only palliative.

Action and Uses

It concentrates in long bones and in bone marrow and slows the rate of blood cell formation.

In polycythemia vera, a single intravenous dose of 2.5 to 5 millicuries may provide a longer period of remission than can be obtained with drug or x-ray therapy. A 2nd or 3rd dose may be necessary at intervals of 8 to 12 weeks. The effects of the drug are not noted for about 6 weeks.

In chronic myelogenous leukemia, doses of 1 to 2 millicuries intravenously are given weekly for 4 to 8 weeks to suppress white blood cell formation but avoid too great suppression of red cells. The drug does not reduce the size of the spleen as rapidly as radiation therapy and, therefore, may not provide as prompt relief of pressure symptoms.

Side and Toxic Effects

Leukopenia

Anemia

Hemorrhagic tendencies due to destruction of platelets

NOTE: As with all radioactive substances, extreme care should be observed in handling, which requires special training and experience.

URETHAN (ETHYL CARBAMATE)

Action and Uses

Urethan acts possibly by interfering with the metabolism of nucleic acid needed for cell division and thus inhibits leukemic cells. However, it is not considered the best agent for treating leukemia.

Dosage and Administration

Given orally 2 to 4 Gm. in enteric-coated tablets.

Side and Toxic Effects

Nausea and vomiting

Dizziness

Drowsiness

Leukopenia and anemia

Possibly hepatitis

SODIUM AMINOPTERIN

Sodium aminopterin blocks folic acid needed to produce white blood cells and inhibits division of leukemic cells in acute leukemia. However, use of the drug is often followed by serious toxic effects and its use is limited to the treatment of acute leukemia in children.

Dosage and Administration

0.25 to 0.5 mg. orally 3 to 6 times a week until remission occurs.

Side and Toxic Effects

Ulceration of tongue and mucous membranes
Nausea
Diarrhea
Loss of hair
Persistent hemorrhage requiring transfusion

METHOTREXATE

This is similar in action to sodium aminopterin and is used to treat acute leukemia. It is a very toxic compound.

Dosage and Administration

0.12 mg. per kilogram of body weight orally or parenterally for children and 5 mg. 3 to 6 times a week for adults.

Side and Toxic Effects

The same as for sodium aminopterin

MERCAPTOPURINE (PURINETHOL)

This is a synthetic and potent drug that interferes with the formation of nucleic acids. It has produced periods of remission in acute leukemias and in some cases of chronic myelogenous leukemia. It is of no value in chronic lymphatic leukemia.

Dosage and Administration

Initial, daily, oral dose is 2.5 mg./Kg. of body weight. However, the amount of drug that can be tolerated differs from patient to patient.

Side and Toxic Effects

Leukopenia
Thrombocytopenia and bleeding
Nausea and vomiting
Anorexia

PHARMACOLOGY

BUSULFAN (MYLERAN)

This is a powerful synthetic drug to treat chronic myelogenous leukemia. The hemoglobin rises, the white blood count decreases, the immature myeloid cells decrease, the size of the spleen decreases and the patient seems improved subjectively. It resembles nitrogen mustard in its action.

Dosage and Administration

2 to 6 mg. daily by mouth until improvement occurs. Whether maintenance dosage is continued is determined by the condition of the patient. Complete blood count must be done at least once a week.

MECHLORETHAMINE HYDROCHLORIDE (MUSTARGEN HYDROCHLORIDE) (NITROGEN MUSTARD)

Nitrogen mustard is related to the mustard gas used in gas warfare in World War I.

Action and Uses

It is especially toxic to rapidly growing cells, although skin, blood vessels and other tissues are involved.

It has shown good results in treating Hodgkin's disease, lymphosarcoma, and certain chronic leukemias, but is not intended to be used as a substitute for radiation therapy.

It has been disappointing in acute leukemias.

Preparations and Dosage

Solution must be freshly prepared in saline.

It is administered intravenously and must not be allowed to come in contact with the skin or to extravasate into the tissues.

Course of treatment is 0.1 mg./Kg. of body weight daily for 4 days. Treatment may be repeated in 1 month.

Side and Toxic Effects

Nausea and vomiting occur rapidly
Severe diarrhea

Dehydration and prostration due to loss of water and electrolytes

Anemia and leukopenia due to damage of the hema topoietic system.

TRIETHYLENEMELAMINE (TEM)

This drug is similar in action and use to the nitrogen mustards. It is given orally. Less nausea and vomiting seem to result from its use.

Dosage and Administration

2.5 mg. with 2 Gm. sodium bicarbonate on 2 successive mornings, then, if there is no anorexia, an additional dose of 2.5 mg. Treatment may then be continued after 3 to 5 days or stopped.

Side and Toxic Effects

Same as mechlorethamine hydrochloride except for nausea and vomiting. Cumulative toxicity is greater.

CHLORAMBUCIL (LEUKERAN)

This is a derivative of nitrogen mustard which may be of value in treating chronic lymphatic leukemia and Hodgkin's disease.

Dosage and Administration

Orally, 0.1 to 0.2 mg./Kg. of body weight for 3 to 6 weeks.

Side and Toxic Effects

Gastric distress
Depression of bone marrow

TRIETHYLENETHIOPHOSPHORAMIDE (THIO-TEPA)

This drug is used in the same way as nitrogen mustard and chlorambucil. It is not effective in acute leukemias. It is used primarily when radiation therapy is not effective. It may depress the bone marrow unduly.

Dosage and Administration

0.2 mg./Kg. of body weight intramuscularly or intravenously for 3 to 5 days. Dose must be carefully individualized.

CYCLOPHOSPHAMIDE (CYTOXAN)

Cyclophosphamide is a nitrogen mustard derivative but is not irritating. It has been used with good results in Hodgkin's disease, lymphomas, and chronic lymphocytic leukemia.

Dosage and Administration

Intravenously, 2 to 3 mg./Kg. of body weight for 6 to 8 days.

Orally, the maintenance dose is 50 to 200 mg. daily.

Side and Toxic Effects

Gastro-intestinal disturbances
Anemia and leukopenia
Thrombocytopenia
Alopecia (temporary)

Part 13.   Drugs to Treat Thrombophlebitis

ANTICOAGULANTS

HEPARIN SODIUM

Heparin sodium is a purified anticoagulant substance obtained from animal lung and liver.

Action and Uses

Heparin sodium is believed to prevent the conversion of prothrombin to thrombin and, thus, prolong the clotting time of blood. Action is immediate. Sometimes, it is administered simultaneously with Dicumarol and is withdrawn as soon as the effect of Dicumarol takes place

(24 to 48 hours). Uses are the same as Dicumarol. (*See* Dicumarol, *below.*)

Preparations and Dosage

Dosage varies and is regulated according to the coagulation time of the blood, frequently 10,000 to 12,000 units every 8 hours intramuscularly or by deep subcutaneous injection.

Continuous intravenous drip of 10,000 to 20,000 units in 1,000 ml. of 5 per cent dextrose or normal saline solution.

Dangers and Disadvantages of Use

Difficult to administer. It is administered by intravenous drip or by deep intramuscular injection, which is painful.

Is very expensive.

Difficult to maintain a constant clotting time, as it raises clotting time rapidly and must be watched carefully.

Dangerous hemorrhages may occur, which may be terminated by the administration of protamine.

PROTAMINE SULFATE

Protamine sulfate is a heparin antagonist and neutralizes the anti-coagulant effect of protamine. It is used to treat bleeding tendencies resulting from heparin administration.

Dosage and Administration

An amount equal to the amount of heparin over a 3 to 4 hour period, given intravenously, the dose not exceeding 50 mg. at one time.

BISHYDROXYCOUMARIN (DICUMAROL)

Dicumarol is an anticoagulant substance originally derived from spoiled clover but now made synthetically.

Action and Uses

Dicumarol is believed to retard prothrombin formation by the liver and, thus, prolong clotting time of the blood.

PHARMACOLOGY

It is used therapeutically:

To prevent postoperative thrombosis when thrombosis seems liable to occur.

To treat thrombophlebitis and embolism.

In coronary occlusion to lessen incidence of complications.

Pulmonary embolism.

Preparations and Dosage

DICUMAROL, 0.2 to 0.3 Gm. by mouth. Its effect is not seen for 24 to 48 hours.

1. When drug has been administered for 2 days, a prothrombin time of the blood is determined: if prothrombin time is satisfactory, 0.2 Gm. is administered daily. Prothrombin time then is done frequently and should be kept between 13 and 15 seconds.

2. Should never be administered unless a frequent prothrombin time can be determined.

Contraindications to Use

1. If the patient shows any bleeding tendencies: Hemorrhage may occur with the use of the drug, but is controlled easily by transfusion and large doses of vitamin K.

2. Marked liver or kidney impairment.

PHENINDIONE (DANILONE; HEDULIN)

This is an agent which is similar in action to bishydroxycoumarin but acts more promptly and is effective in smaller doses. It has produced agranulocytosis.

Dosage and Administration

100 to 150 mg. orally twice a day.

DIPHENADIONE (DIPAXIN)

Diphenadione reduces prothrombin in the blood and delays coagulation of the blood. It is prompt in action and its action is prolonged. Depression of blood elements may occur.

Dosage and Administration

20 to 30 mg. by mouth initially, followed by 10 to 15 mg. thereafter, depending on the prothrombin time.

WARFARIN SODIUM (COUMADIN)

This is used in the same manner as other anticoagulants and has the same dangerous potentialities.

Action and Uses

Its action is essentially the same as that of Dicumarol, but it has faster and more prolonged action. It takes effect in 12 to 24 hours and its effect lasts 3 to 5 days.

Dosage and Administration

40 to 50 mg. initially by mouth or parenterally, followed by 5 to 10 mg., depending on the prothrombin time.

Toxic Effects

Same as Dicumarol

ETHYL BISCOUMACETATE (TROMEXAN)

This drug is an anticoagulant related to Dicumarol.

Action and Uses

Its action is essentially the same as that of Dicumarol, except that the effect is seen much more rapidly. It is active in 24 hours, but its action is of shorter duration.

Dosage and Administration

Given orally 1.5 Gm. as an initial dose and 0.6 to 0.9 Gm. every day subsequently, depending on the prothrombin time. (*See* Dicumarol.)

Toxic Effects

Same as Dicumarol

ACENOCOUMAROL (SINTROM)

Acenocoumarol is an anticoagulant which lies between bishydroxycoumarin and ethyl biscoumacetate in the speed of its action. Its use and the precautions for its use are similar to other coumarin type drugs.

Dosage and Administration

Orally, 16 to 28 mg. on the 1st day, 8 to 16 mg. on the 2nd day and a maintenance dose of 2 to 10 mg. daily, depending on the prothrombin time.

Part 14. Drugs to Treat Bleeding Tendencies

MENADIONE

Menadione is an official synthetic vitamin K preparation. It is essential to the synthesis of prothrombin by the liver.

Action and Uses

1. Maintains a normal prothrombin time of the blood, and is used:

A. Preoperatively when biliary obstruction is present and hemorrhage is apt to occur at operation or postoperatively.

B. Preoperative prophylaxis for jaundiced patients.

C. To prevent postpartum hemorrhage when the prothrombin time is lengthened.

2. Useful only when hemorrhagic conditions are not due to injury of the liver cells themselves.

3. Absorption is directly related to the presence of bile in the intestine. Vitamin K is a fat-soluble vitamin.

4. To treat hemorrhagic tendencies when there has been an overdosage of bishydroxycoumarin and related drugs.

Preparations and Dosage

MENADIONE, 1 to 2 mg. daily by mouth or subcutaneously. Must be administered with bile salts.

MENADIONE SODIUM BISULFITE (HYKINONE) is a water soluble preparation which can be given orally without bile salts; 0.5 to 2 mg. daily parenterally.

MENADIOL SODIUM DIPHOSPHATE (SYNKAYVITE), orally or parenterally without bile salts, 5 mg.

PHYTONADIONE (MEPHYTON, KONAKION, VITAMIN K_1), 1 to 25 mg. orally; 5 mg. as an emulsion diluted in sterile water parenterally.

See also CALCIUM

ASCORBIC ACID

Ascorbic acid is used widely in bleeding from the gums, anemia, gum infection, etc. However, unless these bleeding tendencies are due to ascorbic acid deficiency, it is not of much value. It is used rationally to treat scurvy and its manifestations.

Preparations and Dosage

100 to 150 mg. by mouth or parenterally daily.

Part 15. Drugs to Treat Common Gastrointestinal Disorders

NAUSEA AND VOMITING

DIMENHYDRINATE (DRAMAMINE)

This is a drug that is related to the antihistamines and to diphenhydramine (Benadryl Hydrochloride).

Action and Uses

Its mechanism of action is not well understood. It causes slight sedation. The drug is used primarily for the prevention of motion sickness. It is most useful in controlling motion sickness of travel by boat, train or car and, to a lesser extent, by airplane. It has been found also to be useful in controlling both the vertigo and the nausea of Menière's syndrome, the labyrinth dysfunction of other conditions, and the nausea of radiation, hypertension, pregnancy, drug administration, etc.

Dosage and Administration

For the prevention of motion sickness, 50 mg. orally 30 minutes before departure, and repeated every 4 hours during the journey.

For the control of nausea in other conditions, 50 to 100 mg. every 4 hours.

Side and Toxic Effects

Like the antihistamines, this drug produces drowsiness. There may be danger to the blood-forming organs if administration is prolonged.

MECLIZINE HYDROCHLORIDE
(BONAMINE HYDROCHLORIDE)

This drug is related to the antihistamines and is used to control motion sickness. Its effect is quite prolonged. Slight drowsiness seems to be the only side effect.

Dosage and Administration

25 to 50 mg. orally.

CYCLIZINE (MAREZINE HYDROCHLORIDE)

This is an antihistaminic drug used to control nausea and vomiting during pregnancy, motion sickness, inner ear surgery and vertigo. Side effects of drowsiness seem to be very minimal, but dry mouth and blurred vision may occur.

Dosage and Administration

Essentially the same as dimenhydrinate.

PYRIDOXINE HYDROCHLORIDE (VITAMIN B$_6$)

Pyridoxine hydrochloride is a drug that, except nutritionally, has limited value in medicine. It is used primarily to control the nausea and vomiting of pregnancy and of radiation sickness.

Dosage and Administration

5 mg. orally, or 25 to 50 mg. intramuscularly or intravenously.

TRIMETHOBENZAMIDE HYDROCHLORIDE (TIGAN)

Trimethobenzamide, a new antiemetic, shows promise of being very helpful in controlling nausea and vomiting in the postoperative period, in pregnancy, motion sickness, and intoxication from drugs. Effects appear 20 to 40 minutes after administration.

Dosage and Administration

Orally or intramuscularly, 100 to 300 mg. 1 to 4 times a day.

CONSTIPATION

CATHARTICS

Action

1. Irritate nerve endings in the intestine and, thus, increase motor activity.
2. Increase bulk by means of:
    A. Adding indigestible bulk
    B. Preventing absorption of water by using such preparations as hydrocarbons, viz., mineral oil
    C. Drawing fluid from the tissues to the intestine by using saline cathartics
3. Lubricate and facilitate the passage of feces by using bland oils.

Indications for Use

Drug or food poisoning
After anthelmintics
To relieve cerebral or other types of edema by using saline cathartics
Enforced inactivity of bed rest

PHARMACOLOGY

Contraindications to Use

Appendicitis, or any undiagnosed abdominal pain
Typhoid fever, or any ulcerative condition of the intestine
Intestinal obstruction of paralytic ileus
Diverticulitis, or other inflammatory condition of the intestine
During late pregnancy

Preparations and Dosage

LAXATIVES

Albolene (Mineral Oil; Liquid Paraffin; Liquid Petrolatum), 15 to 30 ml.

Agar-agar, 4 to 15 Gm.

Bisacodyl (Dulcolax), 10 to 15 mg. Through action on nerve endings in the mucosa of the colon, this contact laxative stimulates peristalsis.

Milk of Magnesia (Magnesium Hydroxide), 15 to 30 ml.

PURGATIVES

Alophen Pills, 1 pill.

Cascara Sagrada Pills, 0.3 to 0.6 Gm.

Cascara Fluidextract, 2 to 4 ml.

Castor Oil (Oleum Ricini), 15 to 30 ml. Methods of administration:

1. Castor Oil "cocktail" of equal amounts of oil, Lactopeptone Elixir and a few drops of peppermint oil.
2. Mixed with orange or dilute lemon juice and sodium bicarbonate and taken through a straw while effervescing.
3. Oil preceded and followed by sucking a piece of ice.
4. Prepared with orange or dilute lemon juice—a layer of fruit juice, a layer of oil and a layer of fruit juice.

Phenolphthalein, 60 mg. An ingredient of many proprietary cathartics.

Saline Cathartics

1. Magnesium Citrate, 150 to 250 ml.
2. Magnesium Sulfate (Epsom Salts), 15 to 30 Gm.
3. Sodium Sulfate (Glauber's Salts), 15 Gm.

4. Sodium Phosphate, 4 to 8 Gm.
5. Potassium and Sodium Tartrate (Rochelle Salts). The contents of the white and blue papers are mixed and administered during effervescence.

FECAL SOFTENING AGENT

Dioctyl Sodium Sulfosuccinate (Doxinate, Colace). This is an agent which lowers the surface tension in the intestinal tract and permits water to mix with fecal material. It may be used to treat or to prevent constipation, although it has no action on intestinal peristalsis. Dosage is 10 to 20 mg. orally for infants and children, and 10 to 60 mg. for adults.

DRUG OR FOOD POISONING

EMETICS

Emetics were used widely at one time, but they are employed less frequently now since the advent of the stomach tube.

Action and Uses
1. Produce vomiting by means of:
   A. Gastric irritation
   B. Stimulation of the vomiting center in the medulla
2. Primary uses:
   A. After poisoning by food or drugs
   B. In acute alcoholism

Preparations and Dosage
APOMORPHINE, 5 mg. used very occasionally—in acute alcoholism:

A morphine derivative, it is somewhat depressant, although it lacks the main depressant effect of morphine.

It is felt that if the patient is too intoxicated to stand unaided, he is too depressed to be a safe subject for the drug.

COPPER SULFATE, 1 to 2 Gm. Used infrequently.

IPECAC, 0.5 Gm.

MUSTARD, 4 Gm. in a glass of water.

SODIUM CHLORIDE (salt), 4 Gm. in a glass of tepid water.

ZINC SULFATE, 0.6 to 1.0 Gm.

DIARRHEA

BISMUTH

Bismuth compounds are used as insoluble compounds. The oral administration of soluble compounds leads to irritation.

Preparations are used to allay nausea and vomiting due to gastric irritation, and to check diarrhea, because of astringent and protective qualities.

Preparations and Dosage

To treat diarrhea and peptic ulcer:

BISMUTH SUBCARBONATE, 1 Gm.

BISMUTH SUBNITRATE, 1 Gm., used less frequently than subcarbonate: nitrate radical changed to nitrite in the intestine and may give rise to nitrite poisoning.

KAOLIN

Kaolin is a substance not absorbed from the gastro-intestinal tract and used as a physical adsorbent to absorb toxins, moisture, etc. It is used to treat diarrhea.

Preparations, Dosage and Administration

Kaolin, 50 to 60 Gm. of powder mixed with water.

Kaopectate (kaolin with pectin), 15 to 30 ml.

Pectin is an emulsifying agent with limited use in treating diarrhea.

See also OPIUM
See also ANTIBIOTICS
See also SULFONAMIDES

DISTENTION

CARMINATIVES

Composed of volatile or mildly aromatic substances, carminatives give their best effect if they are administered in hot water.

Preparations and Dosage

AROMATIC SPIRITS OF AMMONIA, 2 ml.
GINGER FLUIDEXTRACT, 2 ml.
PEPPERMINT OIL, 8 to 10 drops of Peppermint Water, 4 ml.
RHUBARB AND SODA, 4 to 8 ml.

See also PROSTIGMINE

ENZYME DEFICIENCY

DIGESTANTS

Digestants are drugs that promote the process of digestion in the gastrointestinal tract, although their use in medicine is limited.

Action and Uses

As replacement therapy in deficiency states.
1. Deficiency of hydrochloric acid in the stomach.
2. Deficiency of enzymes of:
   Stomach
   Pancreas
3. Deficiency of bile.

Preparations and Dosage

BILE SALTS
   Ox Bile Extract (Fels Bovis), 0.5 Gm.
   Dehydrocholic Acid (Decholin), 250 to 500 ml.
DILUTE HYDROCHLORIC ACID 10 per cent, 1 to 2 ml. in a glass of water. Patient uses a glass tube to protect the teeth.
GLUTAMIC ACID HYDROCHLORIDE *(Acidulin),* 300 mg.
PANCREATIN, 0.5 Gm. Protected from the action of gastric juice by enteric coating.

PEPTIC ULCER

ANTACIDS

Action and Uses

To neutralize excessive acidity of the stomach by means of:

1. Chemical reaction to form neutral salts.
2. Physical adsorption. Molecules of acid adhere to the surface of an antacid of a colloidal nature and become inactive.

Preparations and Dosage

SYSTEMIC ANTACIDS, which are soluble and absorbable and, therefore, are capable of changing the pH of the blood and producing alkalosis.

Sodium Bicarbonate, 2 to 4 Gm.

NONSYSTEMIC ANTACIDS, which are relatively insoluble and nonabsorbable and are incapable of changing the pH of the blood.

Calcium Carbonate, 1 Gm. Is very constipating.

Magnesium Oxide, 0.3 to 1.0 Gm. Is laxative, and is used often as an adjunct to constipating substances.

Magnesium Trisilicate, 2 to 4 Gm. Has the advantage of adsorptive properties.

Aluminum Hydroxide Gel (Amphogel; Creamalin, etc.), 15 to 30 ml. Exerts a demulcent, astringent and antacid effect. Is sometimes administered by nasal drip. Also available in tablets.

Aluminum Phosphate Gel, 15 to 30 ml.

POLYAMINEMETHYLENE RESIN (RESINAT)

This is a synthetic acid-binding resin.

Action and Uses

It acts by withdrawing acids from solution and binding them, then excreting them through the intestinal tract. It is used as an adjunct to the treatment of peptic ulcer to relieve symptoms.

Dosage and Administration

Given 0.5 to 1.0 Gm. orally every 2 hours.

Side and Toxic Effects

Nausea and vomiting may occur unless the taste of the resin is disguised.

Part 16.   Drugs to Treat Vitamin Deficiencies

VITAMIN PREPARATIONS

The availability of expensive vitamin compounds and extensive advertising have led to a great deal of abuse of these preparations.

Action and Uses

They are valuable as replacement therapy in nutritional deficiencies of vitamins due to:

Inadequate diet

Difficulties in absorption

There is felt to be no rationale for the use of vitamins for symptoms resembling, but not caused by, deficiencies.

Preparations and Dosage

For deficiencies treated by vitamin preparations, *See* Summary of Vitamins *under* Diet.

Vitamin A. Oleovitamin A, 7.5 mg.

Vitamin B

Vitamin B Complex. Dosage is variable.

Thiamine Chloride (Vitamin B_1), 1 to 15 mg. orally daily (may cause diarrhea).

Riboflavin (Vitamin B_2 or G), 5 to 10 mg. orally.

Nicotinic Acid and *Nicotinamide* (Niacin; Niacin Amide), 25 to 50 mg. May cause transient but unpleasant flushing.

Pyridoxine to treat the nausea and vomiting of x-ray and radium sickness. 5 to 100 mg. daily.

Folic Acid. See Folic Acid, *under* Drugs to Treat Blood Dyscrasias.

Vitamin B_{12}. Is specific in the treatment of pernicious anemia. Pernicious anemia is caused by a deficiency of "intrinsic factor," an as yet unidentified substance that facilitates gastric absorption of B_{12}. Large amounts of B_{12} are believed to keep the posterior column of the spinal cord normal. Cyanocobalamin 1 microgram per day. Dose is variable.

VITAMIN C

Ascorbic Acid, 50 to 100 mg.

VITIMIN D. Most preparations named contain A and D.*

Cod Liver Oil (Oleum Morrhuae), 8 to 10 ml. Calciferol, 125 micrograms to 5 mg.

Drisdol (Vitamin D_2), 2 to 20 drops for infants. Does not contain Vitamin A.

Halibut Liver Oil, 0.1 to 0.5 ml.

Viosterol (Ergosterol). Does not contain Vitamin A.

Oleum Percomorphum, 10 to 15 drops.

VITAMIN E (alpha-tocopherol). Its usefulness in man has not been established. Experimentation continues but it apparently has no value in the treatment of sterility and habitual abortion. Many claims for therapy in common diseases have been made but none substantiated.

VITAMIN K. *See* Menadione *under* Drugs to Treat Bleeding Tendencies.

Part 17. Drugs to Treat Bronchial Asthma

THEOPHYLLINE ETHYLENEDIAMINE (AMINOPHYLLINE)

This is a synthetic drug.

Action and Uses

Has diuretic action and, like other xanthine derivatives, is particularly useful when edema is due to congestive heart failure.

Dilates coronary blood vessels and sometimes is used

*A high calcium level and calcification of tissues may occur from overdosage.

to treat coronary artery disease by increasing the blood supply to the heart, but its position is not definitely established.

Relaxes constricted bronchial muscle and is used widely to treat bronchial asthma.

1. Is not generally as effective as epinephrine.
2. Is especially useful if the patient has become "epinephrine-fast."
3. Often administered intravenously or intramuscularly to relieve a severe attack.

Preparations and Dosage

AMINOPHYLLINE TABLETS, 200 mg. 3 times a day.

AMPULES of 250 and 500 mg. for intravenous and intramuscular injection.

SUPPOSITORIES of 250 and 500 mg.

See also EPINEPHRINE
See also DEMEROL HYDROCHLORIDE
See also ANTIHISTAMINICS

Part 18.   Drugs to Treat Endocrine Disorders

HYPOTHYROIDISM

THYROID EXTRACT

Thyroid extract is obtained from the dried animal gland and assayed according to its iodine content.

Action and Uses

1. Acts by virtue of the thyroxin contained in the gland.
2. Used as replacement therapy in deficiency of the gland:

A. Myxedema and cretinism

B. Low metabolic rate, seemingly unassociated with deficiency of gland

C. In menstrual disorders if due to glandular deficiency

PHARMACOLOGY

D. Sometimes in obesity, to increase the amount of foodstuffs burned, although dietary control is better and safer.

Preparations and Dosage

THYROID TABLETS, U.S.P., 30 to 60 mg. or more. Some authorities advocate chewing the tablet to promote better absorption.

THYROXIN, the hormone of the gland, 0.05 to 0.5 mg.

SODIUM LEVOTHYROXINE (Synthroid), 0.05 to 0.1 mg. orally daily.

SODIUM LIOTHYRONINE (Cytomel), 5 to 25 mcg. (micrograms) daily.

Side and Toxic Effects

Nervousness and tremors
Headache
Palpitation
Loss of weight
Sweating

PARATHYROID EXTRACT (PARATHORMONE; PAROIDIN)

This is an animal extract containing parathyroid hormone.

Action and Uses

To replace the active principle of the parathyroid gland in hypoparathyroidism.

1. Relieves the symptoms of tetany by controlling the excitability of nervous and muscular tissue.

2. Restores and maintains normal balance of calcium and phosphorus in the blood serum.

A. Causes a rise in blood calcium in about 4 hours, lasting about 18 to 20 hours.

B. Blood calcium level must be watched carefully since overdosage can have serious consequences.

Preparations and Dosage

25 to 40 U.S.P. units intramuscularly every 12 hours for 5 or 6 days.

A calcium salt is administered simultaneously. If administration is continued for more than 10 days, parathyroid extract loses its effect.

CALCIUM

Action and Uses

As an antacid. *See* Antacids *under* Drugs to Treat Gastrointestinal Disorders.

To aid in the formation of bones and teeth.

To regulate the activity of nerve and muscle and relieve the symptoms of tetany.

To increase the coagulability of the blood.

To treat urticaria and angioneurotic edema.

Preparations and Dosage

CALCIUM LACTATE, 5 Gm.

CALCIUM GLUCONATE, 5 Gm. orally, 1 Gm. intramuscularly or intravenously.

DIHYDROTACHYSTEROL (HYTAKEROL)

This is a preparation with effects similar to those of parathyroid hormone and vitamin D. However, it is expensive and is used only when hypoparathyroidism cannot be controlled adequately with calcium and vitamin D.

Action and Uses

Used to control tetany of hypoparathyroidism by means of:

Influencing excretion of phosphorus

Mobilizing calcium from the bones

Aiding the absorption of calcium from the intestine.

Preparations and Dosage

Capsule, 0.625 mg. per 0.5 ml.

Solution, 6.25 mg. per 5 ml.

An initial dose of 3 to 10 ml., then a maintenance dose of 1 to 7 ml. daily.

Level of blood phosphorus and calcium is watched carefully.

PHARMACOLOGY

Side and Toxic Effects

Polyuria
Excessive thirst
Dizziness and tinnitus
Nausea and abdominal cramps
Demineralization of bone

HYPERTHYROIDISM

THIOURACILS

Thiouracils are synthetic drugs.

Action and Uses

1. Action is not known exactly, but it is thought to inhibit the production of thyroxin by the thyroid gland.

2. Used preoperatively to lower the basal metabolic rate in hyperthyroidism.

A. Supplemented by sedatives, rest and dietary and vitamin therapy. A remission of symptoms occurs and the patient is clinically improved.

B. The basal metabolic rate can be maintained at a lowered level and operation delayed for a longer period of time than when iodides are used.

Preparations and Dosage

PROPYLTHIOURACIL, which is less toxic than thiouracil, is the drug of choice. 50 to 100 mg. orally daily.

METHYLTHIOURACIL (Methiacil, Thimecil), 200 mg. daily.

IOTHIOURACIL SODIUM (Itrumil Sodium), 150 to 300 mg. daily.

Side and Toxic Effects

Headache and dizziness are most common
Skin rash similar to that of iodides
"Drug fever"
Serious complications of agranulocytosis and renal involvement

METHIMAZOLE (TAPAZOLE)

Methimazole is a synthetic antithyroid drug.

Action and Uses

Blocks the synthesis of thyroxin by preventing the thyroid gland from taking up iodine. It is more potent and faster acting than propylthiouracil. Its effect is seen in 2 to 6 weeks and is used for the long-term treatment of hyperthyroidism. When the drug has been used for a year, the percentage of cure is high in the younger age group.

Dosage and Administration

Given 5 to 10 mg. orally daily.

Side and Toxic Effects

1. *Agranulocytosis*. The patient is warned to report a sore throat immediately
2. *Skin rash* similar to an iodide rash may occur
3. *Hyperplasia* of the thyroid gland. Iodine sometimes is given at the end of treatment to overcome this.

IODIDES

Action and Uses

In hyperthyroidism, to prevent the rapid release of the hormone into the blood stream.

To supply iodine and prevent simple goiter.

Preoperatively in hyperthyroidism to depress metabolism and irritability of the thyroid gland.

As a saline expectorant in bronchitis.

Preparations and Dosage

SODIUM IODIDE, 0.3 ml.* In syphilis, 2 to 5 Gm.

POTASSIUM IODIDE, same dose as sodium iodide.*

LUGOL'S SOLUTION, 0.5 ml. 1 to 3 times a day for 7 to 10 days for preoperative treatment.*

* Iodides are irritant to the gastric mucosa and should be administered in milk or should be well diluted in water.

PHARMACOLOGY

Symptoms of "Iodism"

Sneezing and coryza
Conjunctivitis
Frontal headache
Skin rash

SODIUM IODIDE I 131
(RADIOACTIVE IODINE)

A radioactive isotope, it is used in the treatment of hyperthyroidism and cancer of the thyroid. The substance is taken up into the thyroid gland and acts as local x-ray radiation, causing the gland to shrink. It is used when recurrence occurs after surgery.

It is used most frequently to test the function of the thyroid gland.

Dosage and Administration

1 to 100 microcuries as a test dose (not during pregnancy as the effect on the fetus is not known). 1 to 100 millicuries by mouth.

Toxic Effects

Usually not used in women of child-bearing age, due to the possibility that sterility may occur.

DIABETES MELLITUS

INSULIN

Insulin is an aqueous solution of an active principle of the pancreas. It affects the metabolism of carbohydrates and is a specific drug to treat diabetes mellitus.

Action and Uses

Temporarily restores the ability of the body to utilize carbohydrates.

Causes the storage of glycogen in the liver.

In diabetes mellitus, insulin maintains the blood sugar at a normal level, ketone bodies do not appear in the urine and diabetic acidosis is avoided.

Occasionally used to increase appetite in malnutrition.

Employed in schizophrenia to produce shock, but its use is attended by danger.

Preparations, Dosage and Administration

1. Dosage is variable and must be determined for each individual patient.

    A. Aim is to give sufficient amount of insulin to enable the patient to utilize an adequate diet.

    B. Should be administered in large enough doses to prevent glycosuria and excessive hyperglycemia.

2. Insulin is destroyed in the digestive tract and, therefore, cannot be given orally but must be used subcutaneously.

STANDARD INSULIN. 1 ml. contains 20, 40, 80 or 100 units.

    1. Administered 30 minutes before meals.

    2. Has a very rapid effect. Effect lasts 6 to 8 hours.

    3. If no insulin reaction has occurred in 6 hours it is unlikely that any will occur.

CRYSTALLINE INSULIN for those allergic to regular insulin.

PROTAMINE ZINC INSULIN. 1 ml. contains either 40 or 80 units.

    1. Introduced primarily for the diabetic patient who cannot be controlled without many injections of standard insulin.

    2. Is administered once a day and shows reduction of blood sugar in 3 to 6 hours. Maximum effect appears in 16 to 24 hours.

        A. Effect may be prolonged for 24 to 36 hours or longer, resulting in overlapping of insulin action.

        B. Insulin shock can occur at any time, and frequently occurs at night.

    3. Does not take care of the immediate rise in blood sugar after meals, necessitating one injection of standard insulin before breakfast.

    4. Is in suspension and must be agitated before use.

GLOBIN INSULIN, sometimes called an "intermediate" insulin. 1 cc. contains 80 units.

PHARMACOLOGY

1. Is administered once a day ½ hour before breakfast, as it has rapid action.

2. Has an activity of longer duration than standard, but shorter than protamine insulin.

   A. Shows maximum effect in 8 to 16 hours.

   B. Rate of insulin release almost negligible after 24 hours.

3. Supplementary injections of standard insulin are frequently unnecessary.

ISOPHANE INSULIN (NPH Insulin). A modified insulin that contains more insulin, because it is prepared from insulin crystals, rather than amorphous, and has less protamine than protamine zinc insulin.

1. It has intermediate action between the short action of standard insulin and the long action of protamine zinc insulin.

2. Action usually begins within 2 hours after injection, its peak is reached in 10 to 20 hours and its effect lasts 28 to 30 hours.

3. It is possible to mix standard insulin with NPH insulin for rapid effect. Like protamine zinc insulin, it must be rotated gently to mix it.

LENTE INSULIN. This is the purest form of modified insulin as it contains no foreign protein and cannot produce local sensitivity reactions. Its activity is comparable to that of isophane insulin.

Symptoms of Hyperinsulinism

Cold clammy skin
Pallor
Nervousness
Hunger
Disorientation
Collapse

HYPOGLYCEMIC AGENTS OTHER THAN INSULIN

SULFONYLUREAS

These are agents which may be given orally to reduce blood sugar and to treat mild diabetes either with or without insulin as a supplement. They are thought to act principally by stimulating the pancreas to secrete insulin. In severe diabetes, the islets may have lost their ability to secrete insulin.

Preparations and Dosage

TOLBUTAMIDE (Orinase), given orally in an initial dose of 0.5 Gm. twice daily. This is gradually changed to a maintenance dose of 0.5 to 2 Gm. in divided doses.

CHLORPROPAMIDE (Diabinese), initial oral dose 100 to 250 mg., daily maintenance dose 100 to 500 mg.

PHENFORMIN HYDROCHLORIDE (DBI), daily dose of 50 to 150 mg. given with breakfast and the evening meal.

Side and Toxic Effects (incidence is low)

Nausea and vomiting
Dermatitis due to sensitivity
Weakness
Tinnitus
Headache
Leukopenia
Possible furthering of liver damage, if present

MENOPAUSE AND RELATED DISORDERS

ESTROGENS

Therapy with follicular hormones is widely used, and all the preparations mentioned, except progesterone, are follicular.

Action and Uses

1. Follicular hormone is used:

A. To relieve symptoms of the menopause due to the cessation of ovarian functioning, necessitating a readjustment of hormonal balance.

B. To treat gonorrheal vaginitis in children and senile vaginitis by changing the vaginal mucosa to the adult type, thus increasing its bactericidal acid secretions.

C. To treat menorrhagia and metrorrhagia if bleeding is due to hormone deficiency.

PHARMACOLOGY

    D. To treat prostatic cancer in the male.

    E. To treat cancer of the breast.

  2. Luteal hormone, progesterone, reduces uterine motility and is used:

    A. Occasionally, to treat habitual abortion.

    B. To treat dysmenorrhea, but its value is questionable.

Preparations, Dosage and Administration

FOLLICULAR HORMONES

    Estriol (Theelol), 60 to 120 mg. orally, 1 to 4 times daily

    Estrone (Theelin), 1 to 5 mg. parenterally

    Estradiol (Progynon), 0.25 mg. orally or parenterally

    Ethinyl Estradiol (Estinyl), 20 to 50 mcg., 1 to 3 times a day

    Diethylstilbestrol (Stilbestrol), a synthetic preparation, 0.5 to 1 mg. daily, orally. May cause nausea and vomiting, epigastric pain or malaise.

    Estrogenic substances (Premarin), 1.25 mg. daily, orally

    Dienestrol (Restrol, Synostrol), 0.1 to 1.5 mg. daily, orally or parenterally

    Chlorotrianisene (Tace), 12 to 24 mg. daily by mouth

    Hexestrol, 2 to 3 mg. orally daily

    Methallenestril (Vallestril), 6 to 9 mg. orally daily

All these preparations are used in large doses for palliation of breast and prostatic cancer.

LUTEAL HORMONE

    Progestrone (Progestin), 25 mg. intramuscularly

    Ethisterone (Pranone), 25 mg. orally 4 times a day

    Norethindrone (Norlutin), 10 to 20 mg. orally

    Hydroxyprogesterone (Delalutin), 125 to 250 mg. intramuscularly every 4 weeks

    Medroxyprogesterone Acetate (Provera), 2.5 to 10 mg. for 5 to 10 days in amenorrhea.

Side and Toxic Effects

Nausea and vomiting

Diarrhea

Skin rash

HYPOGONADISM

ANDROGENS

Action and Uses

They are used as replacement therapy in testicular failure or loss of testes.

They are used experimentally in the treatment of functional bleeding and to relieve symptoms of the menopause. If therapy is extended over a long period of time, there is danger of producing permanent virilism in the female.

They are used to treat cancer of the breast.

Preparations and Dosage

TESTOSTERONE PROPIONATE (Oreton, Andronate) in oil, intramuscularly.

METHYLTESTOSTERONE, a synthetic preparation for oral use. 5 to 10 mg. daily, sublingually or buccally.

NORETHANDROLONE (Nilevar), 30 to 50 mg. daily.

FLUOXYMESTERONE (Halotestin), 4 to 10 mg. orally daily.

TESTOSTERONE CYPIONATE, 50 to 100 mg. every 7 to 14 days, intramuscularly.

TESTOSTERONE ENANTHATE (Delatestryl), 100 to 400 mg. intramuscularly at intervals of 2 to 4 weeks.

METHANDROSTENOLONE (Dianabol), orally 5 to 10 mg. daily, for not more than 6 weeks.

NANDROLONE PHENPROPIONATE (Durabolin), intramuscularly, 25 mg. once a week.

OXYMETHOLONE (Anadrol), orally, 5 to 10 mg. daily for not more than 6 weeks at a time.

STANOLONE (Neodrol), intramuscularly, 100 mg. daily.

STANOZOLOL (Winstrol), orally, 2 mg. 3 times a day.

Side and Toxic Effects

General: Heart failure due to retention of electrolytes and water
Nausea and vomiting

Female: Hirsutism
Deepening of voice
General masculinization

DEFICIENCIES OF ADRENAL CORTEX

ADRENAL CORTEX HORMONES

Adrenal cortex hormones are natural hormones derived from the cortex of the adrenal gland. They are available also in synthetic preparations that are cheaper.

Action and Uses

As a specific for adrenal insufficiency to correct the defect in electrolyte metabolism. It may be supplemented by the administration of enteric-coated salt tablets.

Preparations and Dosage

Dosage varies according to the condition of the patient. Too rapid a gain in weight is an indication of overdosage and subsequent retention of too much sodium, resulting in edema:

Desoxycorticosterone Acetate ("Doca"), 1 to 2 mg. intramuscularly daily, or by pellet implantation 75 or 125 mg., under the skin every few weeks.

Fludrocortisone (Florinef), orally 0.25 to 1 mg. daily.

See also *Cortisone* and *Hydrocortisone*.

ACTH (ACTHAR, CORTICOTROPIN)

ACTH is a hormone secreted by the anterior pituitary gland which stimulates the adrenal cortex to release cortisone and hydrocortisone.

Action and Uses

These substances have anti-inflammatory and anti-pyretic effect. They do not cure disease but enable the body to endure the stress of disease and provide periods of remission, or enable the body to endure disease until it is cured. They are used primarily in:

Rheumatoid arthritis

Acute rheumatic fever and pancarditis

Disseminated lupus

Allergic manifestations such as bronchial asthma, penicillin reaction, poison ivy, etc.

Gout

Eye and skin diseases
ACTH is ineffective in Addison's disease.

Dosage and Administration

ACTH is given intramuscularly, 40 to 100 units daily in 4 divided doses, or by intravenous drip, 5 to 20 units administered over an 8-hour period.

Side and Toxic Effects

Edema, elevated blood pressure and cardiac failure due to salt retention
Wasting of tissue due to nitrogen imbalance
Glycosuria
Failure of wound healing due to anti-inflammatory action of drug which does not allow the formation of fibrous tissue
Spread of tuberculosis due to breaking down of fibrous tissue
Poor antibody formation in disease
Hirsutism, virilism and voice changes due to effect of drug on secondary sex characteristics
Mental changes
Thrombophlebitis
Peptic ulcer may occur

GLUCO-CORTICOIDS

These are hormones of the adrenal cortex which regulate carbohydrate, fat and protein metabolism. Hydrocortisone and cortisone also have an effect on water and electrolytic balance. They protect against stress, and have anti-inflammatory action. Their effects and side and toxic effects are essentially those discussed under ACTH. Sudden withdrawal may result in adrenal insufficiency.

Preparations, Dosage and Administration

CORTISONE ACETATE (Cortone Acetate) may be given parenterally, orally or topically. 80 to 100 mg. daily may be administered orally or parenterally. 1.5 to 2.5 per cent may be used topically.

PHARMACOLOGY

HYDROCORTISONE (Cortef, Cortril, Hydrocortone) seems to have greater anti-inflammatory action than cortisone and is effective in smaller doses in rheumatoid arthritis and other conditions. May be administered orally or parenterally in 10 to 20 mg. doses 3 to 4 times a day for not more than 2 weeks; then dose is gradually reduced. It may be injected directly into the synovia or the joint.

HYDROCORTISONE SODIUM SUCCINATE (Solu-Cortef) is given parenterally in the same dosages as Cortef.

PREDNISONE (Meticorten, Deltasone, Deltra) is an extremely potent compound and is used in as small doses as possible. It is given orally 30 to 50 mg. initially, then reduced by 5 to 10 mg. every 4 to 5 days until the threshold maintenance dose is obtained.

PREDNISOLONE (Delta Cortef, Meticortelone, Sterane) is an analogue of hydrocortisone which is less irritating to tissues and is perhaps better for intrasynovial injection. Dosage is the same as for prednisone.

METHYLPREDNISOLONE (Medrol) is administered orally 5 to 10 mg. 4 times a day, initially. In chronic conditions initial dosage is lower. Its anti-inflammatory effect is somewhat greater than prednisolone, and it seems to cause less water retention.

FLUDROCORTISONE ACETATE (Alflorone Acetate, F-Cortef Acetate, Florinef Acetate) is an analogue of hydrocortisone, effective in smaller doses. It is administered orally 0.1 to 0.3 mg. daily. Topically, it is used in 0.05 to 0.25 per cent.

DEXAMETHASONE (Decadron) is similar to hydrocortisone in actions and uses. It appears to cause less water retention. It may be given orally, 1.5 to 3 mg. initially, in divided doses, and decreased gradually to minimum satisfactory for maintenance. Topically as an aerosol, the dosage varies with the severity of the condition.

TRIAMCINOLONE (Aristocort, Kenacort) is a potent compound with greater anti-inflammatory action. It is given orally 2 to 5 mg. 3 to 4 times a day.

TRIAMCINOLONE ACETONIDE (Kenalog) is used topically in 0.01 to 0.1 per cent preparations for various dermatoses.

Part 19.   Drugs to Treat and Prevent Postpartum Hemorrhage

PITUITARY EXTRACT (POSTERIOR)

Action and Uses

Stimulates contraction of the uterus and has the same uses as ergot. (*See* Ergot, *below.*)

Stimulates intestinal peristalsis and is used to relieve postoperative ileus and distention or that induced by toxic febrile conditions.

Enables the tubules of the kidney to reabsorb water and is used as an antidiuretic in diabetes insipidus.

Preparations and Dosage

SOLUTION OF POSTERIOR PITUITARY OR PITUITARY EXTRACT, 1 ml. subcutaneously, intramuscularly or on cotton pledgets inserted in the nostrils.

ACTIVE PRINCIPLES

Pitocin, 0.3 to 1.0 ml., intramuscularly, for obstetric use.

Pitressin, 0.3 to 1.0 ml., intramuscularly or nasally, as an antidiuretic.

Pitressin, intramuscularly, for relief of distention.

ERGOT AND ITS DERIVATIVES

Ergot is derived from a fungus growing on rye, *Claviceps purpurea.*

Action and Uses

Stimulates the contraction of the uterus and is used:

1. During and after the third stage of labor and if hemorrhage occurs before delivery of the placenta.

2. To control postpartum hemorrhage.

3. To hasten normal retraction of the uterus.

4. Occasionally, to control uterine bleeding in menorrhagia and metrorrhagia.

PHARMACOLOGY

Preparations and Dosage

ERGOT FLUIDEXTRACT, 2 ml. (seldom used)

ACTIVE PRINCIPLES; less toxic and more widely used.

Ergonovine Maleate (Ergotrate) 0.2 to 0.4 mg. 2 to 3 times a day, orally or parenterally.

Methylergonovine Maleate (Methergine), synthetic, given 0.2 mg., 3 to 4 times a day, orally or parenterally.

Ergotamine Tartrate (Gynergen), 0.5 mg., intramuscularly. Used empirically to relieve certain cases of migraine headache, although its action is not well understood. Probably it relaxes dilated blood vessels in head.

Methysergide Maleate (Sansert), orally, 4 to 6 mg. daily. Its action is still being studied.

Side and Toxic Effects

Cramplike pains in the abdomen

Nausea, vomiting and diarrhea

Dry gangrene of the extremities due to continued contraction of the blood vessels

Abortion or fetal asphyxiation may occur if drug is used prematurely

Part 20.   Drugs to Treat Myasthenia Gravis

NEOSTIGMINE (PROSTIGMIN)

Action and Uses

1. Stimulates intestinal peristalis and is widely used to relieve distention and ileus.
   - A. Peristaltic action occurs rapidly.
   - B. Rectal tube facilitates expulsion of gas.
   - C. Small low enema sometimes necessary to aid action of drug.

2. Stimulates contraction of the bladder and is used frequently to prevent or treat atony of the bladder. Repeated catheterization with subsequent risk of infection may be avoided.

3. Stimulates contraction of skeletal muscle and is used orally as a specific drug to treat myasthenia gravis.

Preparations and Dosage

NEOSTIGMINE BROMIDE (Prostigmin Bromide), 15 mg. 3 times a day for oral administration. Much more may be needed.

NEOSTIGMINE METHYLSULFATE (Prostigmin Methylsulfate), 0.5 mg. intramuscularly. May be used to treat distention of the intestine.

PYRIDOSTIGMINE BROMIDE (Mestinon), 60 to 360 mg. a day. Valuable in treating myasthenia gravis because of its more prolonged action. The patient may still be able to swallow in the morning to take his dose orally and thus avoid a morning intramuscular injection.

Side and Toxic Effects

Nausea and vomiting
Abdominal cramps
Diarrhea
Profuse salivation
Muscle twitchings
Pulmonary edema due to increase in pulmonary secretions

EDROPHONIUM CHLORIDE (TENSILON CHLORIDE)

This is an antagonist of skeletal muscle relaxants such as curare.

It is especially useful in diagnosis and evaluation of treatment in myasthenia gravis, although the action of the drug is too short to treat the disease to any extent. It can be used for repeated tests on the same day and within a short time of each other. It is used also to overcome the effects of curare when its action is no longer necessary, or when respiratory depression has occurred.

Dosage and Administration

Given intravenously 10 to 30 mg.

Side and Toxic Effects

Increased salivation
Tachycardia
Flushing
Nervousness and fright

See also EPHEDRINE

Part 21. Drugs to Treat Urinary Retention

BETHANECHOL CHLORIDE (URECHOLINE CHLORIDE)

Action and Uses

Constricts smooth muscle and is used to treat gastric retention after vagotomy, postoperative urinary retention and postoperative abdominal distention.

Dosage and Administration

Given orally 10 to 30 mg. 3 or 4 times a day. Occasionally given subcutaneously (2.5 to 5 mg.). It should never be given intramuscularly or intravenously.

Side and Toxic Effects

Headache
Abdominal discomfort
Sweating
Bronchial constriction
Low blood pressure

See also NEOSTIGMINE
See also METHACHOLINE

Part 22. Drugs to Treat Arthritis

GOLD

Action and Uses

1. Has shown beneficial results in the treatment of lupus erythematosus; this is believed by some authorities to be its only valid use.
2. Used to treat rheumatoid arthritis.
   A. Results not entirely convincing. Spontaneous remission of the disease presents difficulties in evaluating treatment.
   B. Severe systemic reactions occur.

Preparations and Dosage

GOLD SODIUM THIOMALATE (Myochrysine), 25 to 50 mg. intramuscularly weekly until 700 mg. to 1 Gm. total is reached.

AUROTHIOGLUCOSE (Solganol), 25 to 50 mg. intramuscularly weekly until a total of 1 Gm. is reached.

AUROTHIOGLYCANIDE (Lauron), 25 mg. intramuscularly, increasing 25 mg. weekly for 22 weeks, but not to exceed 150 mg. in a single dose.

Side and Toxic Effects

Elevated temperature
Vomiting and diarrhea
Albuminuria
Stomatitis
Severe exfoliative dermatitis
Hepatitis
Shock
Aplastic anemia and agranulocytosis have occurred. Its use is contraindicated in kidney, liver or other severe organic diseases.

INDOMETHACIN (INDOCIN)

Action and Uses

This synthetic drug effects anti-inflammatory, analgesic and anti-pyretic action in rheumatoid arthritis.

Dosage and Administration

Indomethacin is given orally, 25 mg. 2 or 3 times a day.

Side and Toxic Effects

Peptic ulcer
Dizziness, light headedness
Nausea and vomiting
Diarrhea
Abdominal pain

See also ACTH AND CORTISONE

See also SALICYLATES

Part 23.   Drugs to Treat Heavy Metal Poisoning

DIMERCAPROL (BAL)

Dimercaprol (BAL—British Anti-Lewisite) is an interesting development of World War II.

Action and Uses

An antidote to gold, mercury or arsenic poisoning and used chiefly for:

Acute toxicity resulting from the gold treatment of rheumatoid arthritis

Bichloride of mercury and other types of heavy metal poisoning

Preparations and Dosage

A 10 per cent solution in oil is given intramuscularly. It is administered 3 mg. per kilogram of body weight every 4 hours the first 2 days, 4 injections the third day, 2 injections daily for a further 10 days, or until recovery occurs.

Side and Toxic Effects (usually transient)

Malaise
Nausea and vomiting
Salivation and lacrimation
Paresthesia
Sense of warmth
Pain in head, abdomen and extremities

CALCIUM DISODIUM EDETATE (CALCIUM DISODIUM VERSENATE)

Action and Uses

Calcium disodium edetate treats lead poisoning by combining with the heavy metal ions and forming a stable, non-ionized, water-soluble complex or chelate.

Dosage and Administration

5 ml. of the drug is added to 250 to 500 ml. of sterile 5 per cent dextrose or isotonic saline solution and given by slow intravenous drip over a period of 1 hour.

In mild cases of lead poisoning the drug may be given orally, 4 Gm. a day in divided doses.

Part 24. Drugs Relating to Allergy

ALLERGENIC PREPARATIONS

These agents are extracts of solutions of the various substances to which patients may become sensitive.

Action and Uses

1. To diagnose various allergic phenomena. Some extracts or solutions produce a reaction.

    A. When applied to the skin or mucous membrane, sensitivity can be determined by the "patch test."

    B. When introduced internally, sensitivity may be determined by the "scratch test" and by intradermal injection.

2. For prophylaxis of hay fever and asthma arising from allergy.

3. To "desensitize" in conditions due to hypersensitivity.

4. To treat perennial asthma and rhinitis if the offending substances can be determined.

    A. Is not satisfactory if the offending substance is food.

    B. Treatment administered by subcutaneous inoculation.

Preparations and Dosage

No uniform dosage can be stated.

Preparations include protein extracts of bacteria, foods, animal epidermis, fur, hair and dander, pollens of plants and grasses, fungi and Rhus extracts of poison ivy, oak and sumac.

PHARMACOLOGY

ANTIHISTAMINICS

These drugs are powerful histamine antagonists and relieve the symptoms of allergy but in no way affect the underlying cause of allergy. They probably act by preventing histamine from being taken up by and combining with the cell. Hypnotic, sedative and narcotic drugs should be used carefully during their administration as the most common side effect is drowsiness. Persons should also be cautioned against driving a car or working around machinery while they are using any of these preparations.

Therapeutic Uses

Rhinitis
Hay fever
Pruritus and urticaria
Contact dermatitis
Drug sensitization
Bronchial asthma

Preparations and Dosage

These are just a few of the many preparations.

DIPHENHYDRAMINE HYDROCHLORIDE (Benadryl Hydrochloride), 50 mg. 4 times a day until symptoms are relieved.

TRIPELENNAMINE HYDROCHLORIDE (Pyribenzamine Hydrochloride), 50 mg. 1 or 2 times a day until symptoms are relieved.

ANTAZOLINE PHOSPHATE (Antistine Phosphate), 1 or 2 drops in each eye of 0.5 per cent solution.

PROMETHAZINE HYDROCHLORIDE (Phenergan Hydrochloride), 25 to 50 mg. up to 4 times a day.

DOXYLAMINE SUCCINATE (Decapryn Succinate), 12.5 to 25 mg. up to 4 times a day.

CHLORCYCLIZINE HYDROCHLORIDE (Perazil), 50 mg. 2 or or 3 times a day.

CHLORPHENIRAMINE (Chlor-Trimeton Maleate). An antihistamine drug with the same action as other antihistamines but with a very low incidence of side effects and given in very small doses, 2 to 4 mg. up to 4 times a day.

BROMPHENIRAMINE MALEATE (Dimetane), 4 mg. 4 times a day.

DEXCHLORPHENIRAMINE MALEATE (Polaramine), 2 mg. 3 or 4 times a day.

DIMETHINDENE MALEATE (Forhistal), 1 mg. 3 times daily.

PHENIRAMINE MALEATE (Trimeton), 25 mg. 3 times daily.

TRIMEPRAZINE TARTRATE (Temaril), 2.5 mg. 4 times daily.

Side and Toxic Effects

Drowsiness
Nausea
Headache and disturbance of vision
Dryness of mouth

Part 25. Drugs Used in Dermatologic Conditions

EMOLLIENTS

These are oily substances that are used to soothe and soften the skin. Substances used may be glycerine, cottonseed oil, ointments containing benzoated lard, lanolin, petroleum jelly, cold cream, cocoa butter and zinc ointment.

ANTISEPTIC AGENTS

These may be used in various skin infections and infestations. Their use should be preceded by thorough cleansing of the skin.

Preparations might include as ointments or as wet dressings:

Bacitracin
Iodochlorhydroxyquin (Vioform)
Neomycin
Tyrothricin
Ammoniated Mercury 5 per cent
Nitrofurazone (Furacin) 1:50,000

ANTIFUNGAL AGENTS

These agents include:
Salicylanilide (Salinidol)
Propionate Compound (Propion Gel) 5 per cent
Diamthazole Dihydrochloride (Asterol) 5 per cent
Coparaffinate (Iso-Par) 17 per cent
Gentian Violet 1 per cent
Griseofulvin given orally 1 Gm. daily

KERATOLYTICS

These agents are used for removal of warts, corns, fungus growths, etc.
Salicylic Acid, ointment, 2 to 10 per cent.

Part 26.   Drugs Used in Conditions of the Eye

These drugs usually are employed in the form of drops because of rapid absorption through the conjunctiva and the cornea. Always use very weak solutions.

The drug should be fresh and the dropper sterile.

Solutions

IRRIGATIONS: Normal saline (0.85 per cent)

ANESTHETICS

Cocaine—2 to 4 per cent. For operations on lids and eyeballs. Dilates pupil.

Phenacaine Hydrochloride (Holocaine)—1 per cent (or ointment, 1 to 2%). For foreign bodies, taking tension, treatments, etc.

Tetracaine Hydrochloride (Pontocaine)—0.5 to 1 per cent. Will not dilate pupil.

Procaine Hydrochloride—1 to 2 per cent, by injection. For lid anesthesia or facial nerve block.

ANTISEPTICS

Zinc sulfate—0.25 per cent for conjunctivitis, 1 or 2 drops 3 or 4 times a day.

PHARMACOLOGY

Ointments of neomycin, bacitracin, polymyxin and oxytetracycline. Penicillins are seldom used topically today, to avoid sensitization.

HEMOSTATIC

Epinephrine—1:1,000.

MYDRIATIC

Dilates the pupil $\begin{cases} \text{Paredrine, 1 per cent} \\ \text{Phenylephrine Hydrochloride} \\ \quad \text{solution 10 per cent} \end{cases}$

CYCLOPLEGIC: Paralyzes the ciliary muscle. Dilates pupil.

Atropine—1 per cent. For refraction in children, for intra-ocular inflammation, and after intra-ocular operations. Lasts 7 to 14 days.

Homatropine—2 per cent. For fundus examination. For refractions after 12 years of age. Lasts 24 hours.

Hyoscine (Scopolamine)—0.2 per cent. Used when sensitivity to atropine occurs. For refractions between 8 and 12 years old. Lasts 3 days.

Hydroxyamphetamine (Paredrine)—0.5 to 1 per cent. Lasts 6 days.

MIOTIC: Contracts the pupil.

Carbachol—0.75 to 1.5 per cent. For glaucoma.

Pilocarpine—0.5 to 4 per cent. For glaucoma.

Physostigmine (Eserine)—0.2 to 0.5 per cent. For glaucoma and after homatropine.

Isoflurophate (Floropryl)—ointment 0.025 per cent, solution 0.1 per cent.

FLUORESCEIN: 2 per cent bicarbonate solution. To stain wounds of cornea and conjunctiva (for diagnosis).

Many of the above preparations are used in ointment form when prolonged action is desired.

Steroids are used to treat inflammatory conditions of the eye.

See also ANTIBIOTIC OINTMENTS
See also CORTISONE OINTMENT

Part 27.   Diagnostic Preparations

ACTION AND USES

Certain substances are radiopaque and are used to outline various systems of the body for x-ray examination.

Dyes that are excreted readily are used to test the function of certain organs; the amount of excretion is determined by colorimeter.

Some drugs stimulate glandular secretion for diagnostic purposes.

Occasionally, stains are used to locate lesions.

PREPARATIONS AND DOSAGE

Barium Sulfate

150 to 300 Gm. in 400 ml. of water or milk to outline the stomach or as an enema to outline the intestinal tract.

Sulfobromophthalein

2 to 5 mg. per kilogram of body weight, intravenously to test liver function.

In 30 minutes a blood sample is drawn, and the dye content of serum is determined.

In the normal subject, at least 90 per cent of the dye should have been excreted at the end of 1 hour.

Iodopyracet (Diodrast)

An iodized oil; 20 ml. of solution is given intravenously to outline the urinary tract. The patient has previously followed a routine of fasting and dehydration.

Sodium p-Aminohippurate

50 ml. of 20 per cent solution of sodium *p*-aminohippurate is given intravenously to determine the functional capacity of the tubules in excretion.

Contraindicated when there is evidence of liver damage, nephritis or uremia.

Sodium Acetrizoate (Thixokon, Urokon)

This is used as a contrast medium; for intravenous pyelogram, 25 ml. of a 30 per cent solution intravenously is the usual dose.

Sodium Diatrizoate (Hypaque)

This is also an agent used for intravenous excretory urography. It is given intravenously. 30 ml. of a 50 per cent solution is the usual dose.

Meglumine Diatrizoate (Renografin, Gastrografin)

This is another agent for intravenous excretory urography. 20 ml. of a 76 per cent solution is injected very slowly over 3 to 5 minutes into the antecubital vein.

For roentgenography of the gastrointestinal tract, the oral dose is 30 to 90 ml. of a 76 per cent solution. The solution may be diluted.

Histamine Phosphate

0.3 mg. subcutaneously to test the ability of the stomach to secrete hydrochloric acid.

May cause transient flushing, headache, sweating, drowsiness, allergic manifestations and dizziness. Severe reactions likely in patients with bronchial disease.

Has also been used as a test for pheochromocytoma. Should not be used with aged patients or those with hypertension.

Betazole Hydrochloride (Histalog) has fewer side effects and may be used. Usual dose 50 mg. subcutaneously.

Sodium Diprotrizoate (Miokon)

This is used for intravenous excretory urography. The dose is 20 to 30 ml. of a 50 per cent solution given intravenously, slowly over 3 to 4 minutes. It is best to give a "test dose" of 1 ml. intravenously to note any untoward reactions.

Azuresin (Diagnex Blue)

This is an agent containing a resin and a dye. Patient has fasted and bladder must be empty. After oral administration of 2 Gm. of the granules the blue dye is displaced by hydrogen ions, is absorbed and then excreted in the urine. The determination of the amount of dye in the urine after 2 hours indicates the amount of free hydrochloric acid in the stomach. Intubation is unnecessary.

Two tablets of caffeine sodium benzoate to stimulate gastric secretion are given 1 hour prior to the administration of the resin.

Mannitol

This is an alcohol which is filtered at the glomeruli but is little absorbed by the tubules. It is used to test glomerular filtration and is given intravenously in a 25 per cent solution.

Iophendylate (Pantopaque)

This agent is used for myelography. It provides good visualization of the spinal cord. 6 to 12 ml. may be slowly injected intrathecally into the subarachnoid space by lumbar puncture.

Iodized Oil (Lipiodol)

An iodized vegetable oil, used to outline the bronchial tree.

Locates bronchial and pulmonary lesions.

Is considered a surgical procedure, and substance is carefully introduced by tracheal catheter, immediately before the roentgenogram is taken.

Phenolsulfonphthalein (Phenol Red)

1 ml. (6 mg.) intravenously or intramuscularly to determine kidney function.

Patient drinks 200 ml. of water.

First urine specimen is discarded, then specimens taken at the end of 15 minutes, 1 hour and 2 hours.

In the normal subject, 65 to 85 per cent of the dye should appear in the urine at the end of 2 hours.

Gallbladder Dyes

Several agents have been introduced as contrast media for visualization of the gallbladder by x-ray.

PREPARATIONS AND DOSAGE

Iodoalphionic Acid (Priodax), given orally, 3 Gm. with several glasses of water after a light fat-free meal in late afternoon. Nothing should be taken by mouth until after the examination the next morning.

Iopanoic Acid (Telepaque) given orally 3 Gm. 10 hours before examination after a fat-free meal.

Iophenoxic Acid (Teridax) given orally 3 Gm. after a fat-free evening meal, 10 hours before examination.

Appendix

Tables of Measurement

METRIC TABLE OF WEIGHTS

1000	Gm.	=	1 kilogram
100	"	=	1 hectogram
10	"	=	1 decagram
1.0	"	=	unit of weight
0.1	"	=	1 decigram
0.01	"	=	1 centigram
0.001	"	=	1 milligram
0.000001	"	=	1 microgram

APPROXIMATE EQUIVALENTS

2.0 Gm.	=	grains	30
1.0 "	=	"	15
0.6 "	=	"	10
0.3 "	=	"	5
0.2 "	=	"	3
0.1 "	=	"	1½
65 mg.	=	grain	1
30 "	=	"	½
15 "	=	"	¼
7.5 "	=	"	⅛
4 "	=	"	1/16
3.2 "	=	"	1/20
2.7 "	=	"	1/25
2 "	=	"	1/30
0.6 "	=	"	1/100
0.4 "	=	"	1/150
0.3 "	=	"	1/200

APOTHECARIES' SYSTEM

TABLE OF WEIGHTS

		grains (gr.)	20	= 1 scruple	℈
3 scruples	or	"	60	= 1 dram	ℨ
8 drams	or	"	480	= 1 ounce	℥
12 ounces	or	"	5,760	= 1 pound	℔

APPROXIMATE EQUIVALENTS

1 grain = 0.065 Gm. (65 mg.)
1 dram = 4.0   "
1 ounce = 30.0   "

TABLE OF CAPACITY

60 minims = 1 fluid dram
8 drams = 1 ounce
16 ounces = 1 pint
2 pints   = 1 quart
4 quarts = 1 gallon

APPROXIMATE EQUIVALENTS

minim 1   =   0.065 ml.
minims 15   =   1.0   "
minims (3i) 60   =   4.0   "
1 ounce (480 m.)   =   30.0   "
1 pint (16 ounces)   =   500.0   "
1 quart (32 ounces)   =   1000.0   "

TABLE OF HOUSEHOLD EQUIVALENTS

3i or 4.0 Gm. = 1 level teaspoonful
3ii or 8.0 Gm. = 1   "   dessertspoonful
3iv or 16.0 Gm. = 1   "   tablespoonful

METRIC SYSTEM

The fundamental unit of measurement is the meter, which is about one ten-millionth part of the distance from the equator to the north pole. A meter is slightly longer than a yard, being equal to 39.37 inches, and is written 1 M. From fractional parts of the meter we derive the units of weight and capacity, e.g., a cubic centimeter measures 1 cm. on each side, and a gram is the weight of 1 cc. of pure water at 4° C.

Meter (M) .... Unit of length
Gram (Gm.) .... Unit of weight
Liter (L.) .... Unit of capacity

TABLE OF LENGTH

1,000	meters	= 1	Kilometer
100	"	= 1	Hectometer
10	"	= 1	Decameter
1.0	meter	=	Unit of length
0.1	"	= 1	Decimeter
0.01	"	= 1	Centimeter
0.001	"	= 1	Millimeter

APPROXIMATE EQUIVALENTS

1	meter	= 39.37	inches
1	centimeter	= ⅖	inch
5	centimeters	= 2	inches
30.5	centimeters	= 12	inches (1 foot)

SOLUTION TABLE WITH DOMESTIC MEASURES

1:1,000	 1	teaspoon	to 1 gallon
1:1,000 ⅒ of 1% }	 15	drops	to 1 quart
1:500	 2	teaspoons	to 1 gallon
1:500 ⅕ of 1% }	 30	drops	to 1 quart
1:200	 5	teaspoons	to 1 gallon
1:200 ½ of 1% }	. . . . 1¼	teaspoons	to 1 quart
1:100 or 1%.	2½	teaspoons	to 1 quart
1:50 or 2%.	5	teaspoons	to 1 quart
1:25 or 4%.	2½	tablespoons	to 1 quart
1:20 or 5%.	3	tablespoons	to 1 quart

TABLE OF CAPACITY

1	liter	=	Unit of capacity
0.1	"	= 1	deciliter
0.01	"	= 1	centiliter
0.001	"	= 1	milliliter
1	"	= 1,000	cc.
1	deciliter	= 100	cc.
1	centiliter	= 10	cc.
1	milliliter	= 1	cc.

APPROXIMATE EQUIVALENTS

1,000	ml. (1 liter)	=	1 quart
500	"	=	1 pint
30	"	=	1 ounce
4	"	=	1 dram
0.065	"	=	1 minim

THERMOMETER SCALES

To convert Centigrade to Fahrenheit multiply by 9/5 and add 32.

$$40° \text{ C.} \times 9/5 = 72 + 32 = 104° \text{ F.}$$

To convert Fahrenheit to Centigrade subtract 32 and multiply by 5/9.

$$104° \text{ F.} - 32 = 72 \times 5/9 = 40° \text{ C.}$$

OR

To convert Centigrade to Fahrenheit, add 40, multiply by 9/5 and subtract 40.

$$40° \text{ C.} + 40 = 80 \times 9/5 = 144 - 40 = 104° \text{ F.}$$

To convert Fahrenheit to Centigrade, add 40, multiply by 5/9 and subtract 40.

$$104° \text{ F.} + 40 = 144 \times 5/9 = 80 - 40 = 40° \text{ C.}$$

TABLE OF TEMPERATURE EQUIVALENTS

36° Centigrade	=	96.8°	Fahrenheit
37° "	=	98.6°	"
38° "	=	100.2°	"
39° "	=	102.2°	"
40° "	=	104.0°	"
41° "	=	105.8°	"
42° "	=	107.6°	"

POISONS: SYMPTOMS AND TREATMENT

Poison	Symptoms	Emergency Treatment	Supportive Treatment
Acids, corrosive	1. Severe burning in mouth, throat, stomach 2. Corrosion of mucous membranes of mouth, throat and esophagus 3. Epigastric pain, nausea and the vomiting of "coffee ground" material 4. Intense thirst 5. Circulatory collapse 6. Asphyxia due to glottic edema	1. Avoid lavage. Emetics should not be given. No carbonates or bicarbonates. 2. Give a neutralizer by mouth if possible (milk of magnesia or aluminum hydroxide gel, well diluted with water) 3. Large amount of water (if patient can swallow) 4. Demulcents: olive oil and egg whites *External Acid Burns* 1. Flood with water. 2. Cover with paste of sodium bicarbonate. 3. Eyes: (hold open the lids) flush for 10 to 15 minutes with water, then with 1% sodium bicarbonate, freshly prepared.	1. Keep patient warm. 2. Control of circulatory shock 3. I.V. sodium bicarbonate in the event of acidosis 4. Opiates for control of pain
Alcohols Ethyl (Ethanol)	1. Excitement 2. Inco-ordination and drowsiness; stupor, or coma 3. Flushing of face, rapid pulse, sweating 4. Peripheral vascular collapse, hypotension, hypothermia 5. Slow stertorous respirations 6. Respiratory failure, coma and death	1. Gastric lavage 2. Give an emetic if patient is conscious	1. Intramuscular caffeine sodium benzoate, or strong coffee by mouth 2. Oxygen if needed 3. Support circulation and respiration 4. Keep patient warm

Poison	Symptoms	Emergency Treatment	Supportive Treatment
Alcohols (Cont'd) Methyl (Methanol)	Often after a latency of 12 to 18 hours 1. Headache, anorexia, weakness, leg cramps, progressing to apathy and coma 2. Nausea and vomiting, violent abdominal pain 3. Visual disturbances often progressing to blindness 4. Respiratory or circulatory collapse	1. Gastric lavage with 3 to 5% sodium bicarbonate, leaving some solution in stomach 2. Whiskey (or 50% ethanol in water) 1 oz.	1. Continue with 1 ounce 50% ethanol every 3 to 4 hours until acidosis is corrected 2. 2 to 6 Gm. of sodium bicarbonate by mouth (if possible) every 2 hours until acidosis is corrected 3. Protects patient's eyes from light 4. Maintain body temperature
Alkalis (Corrosive lye, caustic soda, potash, sodium and potassium hydroxides, carbonates, oxides)	1. Mucous membranes of mouth appear soapy, swollen and white 2. Severe abdominal pain 3. Vomiting of blood and mucus	1. Large quantities of water or milk 2. Attempt to neutralize the caustic with a *weak* acid: diluted vinegar, lemon or orange juice 3. Wash contaminated skin and accessible areas of mucous membrane with running water	1. Treat for shock as necessary 2. Analgesics, liberally for pain
Arsenic	1. Sweetish metallic taste: garlic odor of breath and stools 2. Constriction in the throat; difficulty in swallowing 3. Burning and colicky pains in esophagus, stomach and bowel 4. Vomiting and profuse diarrhea. "Rice-water" stools 5. Dehydration with intense thirst 6. Cyanosis, feeble pulse, cold extremities 7. Coma and death	1. Gastric lavage: 2 to 3 liters of water, followed by 1% sodium thiosulfate solution 2. Dimercaprol (BAL) I.M.	1. Counteract dehydration 2. Morphine for pain if necessary 3. Treat shock 4. Oxygen if needed

[771]

POISONS: SYMPTOMS AND TREATMENT (Continued)

POISON	SYMPTOMS	EMERGENCY TREATMENT	SUPPORTIVE TREATMENT
Atropine (Belladonna)	1. Dryness of mucous membranes. Difficulty in swallowing; extreme thirst 2. Dilation of pupils. Become unreactive to light; photophobia 3. Skin becomes hot, dry, flushed 4. Tachycardia; palpitation; drop in blood pressure 5. Restlessness, excitement progressing to delirium 6. Occasionally coma, circulatory collapse	1. Activated charcoal 2. Lavage with 4% tannic acid	1. Short-acting barbiturates given with caution, to control excitement 2. Check for urinary retention, catheterize if necessary

Barbiturates and Other Hypnotics	1. Drowsiness
	2. Ataxia, vertigo, slurred speech
	3. Paresthesias, visual disturbances
	4. Stupor, progression to coma. Response to painful stimuli gradually ceases
	5. Respiration becomes irregular often progressing to Cheyne-Stokes
		1. Gastric lavage with water or potassium permanganate
		2. Aspiration precautions
		3. Leave 15 to 30 Gm. sodium sulfate in water in the stomach as cathartic
		4. Establish and maintain patent airway if gag reflex is absent
			Oxygen if necessary
			Picrotoxin, intravenously
			Observe closely:
			  vital signs
			  pupil size
			  light reflex
			  gag reflex
			  response to pain
			Good nursing care is essential

Carbolic Acid (cresol) (phenol)	*Ingested* 1. White corrosive burns of mucous membranes in mouth, esophagus and stomach. Abdominal pain; sometimes vomiting and bloody diarrhea 2. Watch for symptoms of shock 3. Scanty, dark-colored or "smoky" urine; moderate renal insufficiency may appear 4. Respiratory failure *External* Pain followed by numbness Skin becomes blanched	*Ingested* 1. Careful gastric lavage with olive oil or similar vegetable oil 2. Demulcents: egg white and milk 3. Avoid alcohol, internally or externally *External Burns* 1. Remove contaminated clothing immediately 2. Apply 50% alcohol 3. Wash with copious amounts of running water, until all odor of phenol is gone	1. Maintain body temperature for impending renal failure 2. Supportive measures for impending renal failure 3. Oxygen if needed 4. Hot tea or coffee (if possible)

Poison	Symptoms	Emergency Treatment	Supportive Treatment
Carbon Monoxide	1. Drowsiness 2. Flushed cherry-red face 3. Loss of consciousness 4. Deepening coma 5. Respiratory arrest	1. Fresh air immediately 2. Artificial respiration if necessary 3. Oxygen by most direct method available	Treatment to support the heart and combat shock
Cocaine shock	1. Short stage of excitement 2. Signs of severe shock 3. The blood pressure falls sharply. This state rapidly changes to deep coma often resulting in death	1. Administer adrenalin immediately 2. Clean the mucous membranes of cocaine which has been painted or instilled 3. Oxygen and a respiratory stimulant. Intubation for artificial respiration may be necessary 4. Calcium gluconate I.V. 5. Use of suction for saliva (anesthesia of swallow reflex)	Continued support of vital signs as necessary
Acute poisoning	Excitement and restlessness, tachycardia, redness of face. Sweating, hyperventilation	1. Activated charcoal 2. Gastric lavage (oral ingestion) potassium permanganate 0.1%	1. Sodium pentobarbital intravenously or by mouth for excitement 2. Stimulative drugs in depressive phase
Copper Compounds	1. Nausea and vomiting 2. Pain in mouth, esophagus and stomach 3. Diarrhea 4. Metallic taste in mouth 5. Severe headache, cold sweat, other symptoms of shock	1. Lavage stomach with 1% potassium ferrocyanide 2. Egg whites or milk	1. Control of pain 2. Maintain fluid balance 3. Control shock
Digitalis	1. Anorexia 2. Nausea, salivation and vomiting 3. Slow pulse (below 60) or sudden marked acceleration 4. Headache, fatigue, drowsiness	1. Stop drug 2. Activated charcoal 3. Lavage with warm water	1. Sedatives, with caution, for restlessness 2. Control of shock, support of respiration

POISONS: SYMPTOMS AND TREATMENT (Continued)

Poison	Symptoms	Emergency Treatment	Supportive Treatment
Food poisoning	1. Abdominal pain 2. Nausea or vomiting 3. Diarrhea	1. Try to ascertain source of poison 2. Control diarrhea, nausea and vomiting	1. Treat dehydration, nausea, persistent vomiting and diarrhea
Iodine	1. Nausea and vomiting (blue if starch is present in the stomach) 2. Abdominal pain and diarrhea 3. Watch for symptoms of shock	1. Flour or starch paste 2. Lavage with starch solution 3. Prepare for tracheotomy if necessary	Control 1. Dehydration 2. Shock 3. Treatment of acid-base imbalances
Lead Acute poisoning by ingestion	1. Metallic taste in the mouth, dry throat, thirst 2. Burning abdominal pain, nausea and vomiting 3. Circulatory collapse 4. Watch for symptoms of lead encephalopathy	1. Gastric lavage with 10% solution of sodium or magnesium sulfate 2. Demulcents	1. Control of abdominal pain 2. Control dehydration and shock 3. Treatment of electrolyte disturbances 4. Calcium disodium edetate (CaNa$_2$EDTA)
Mercury Salts	1. Burning pain, sense of constriction, ashen discoloration of the mucous membrane in mouth and pharynx 2. Intense epigastric pain. Almost continuous vomiting 3. Metallic taste, excessive salivation and thirst 4. Stomatitis	1. 2 to 6 egg whites, milk and activated charcoal 2. Induce vomiting if necessary 3. Lavage with egg white solution 4. Dimercarpol (BAL)	1. Treat for shock 2. Maintenance of nutritional status 3. Close observation of renal status
Opium and opium derivatives: (Morphine, Heroin, etc.)	1. Sleepiness, stupor or coma (depending upon dosage) 2. Marked slowing of respiratory rate 3. Pinpoint pupils 4. Slow pulse	1. Lavage with potassium permanganate 1:2000 2. Leave in the stomach 15 to 30 Gm. sodium sulfate in water 3. Establish and maintain patent airway; begin oxygen as necessary 4. Nalorphine 5 to 10 mg. intravenously	1. Precaution against aspiration 2. Maintain adequate rate and depth of respiration 3. Observe for urinary retention 4. Maintain body temperature 5. Good nursing is essential

POISON	SYMPTOMS	EMERGENCY TREATMENT	SUPPORTIVE TREATMENT
Phosphorus	*Ingested* 1. Warm or burning sensation in the throat and abdomen. Intense thirst 2. Nausea, vomiting, diarrhea, severe abdominal pain 3. Garlic odor from breath and excreta 4. Stools and vomitus phosphorescent (a symptom-free period of several days to several weeks is characteristic) 5. Nausea, vomiting often, massive hematemesis Liver tenderness, jaundice, pruritus Hemorrhages into skin Cardiovascular collapse, due to toxic action on the heart	1. Protect both patient and attendants from vomitus, gastric washings, and feces (phosphorus burns) 2. Gastric lavage with potassium permanganate solution 3. Do not give fats or oils	1. Supportive measures for hepatic insufficiency and renal failure 2. Control of pain 3. Combat shock
Silver Compounds (Silver Nitrate)	1. Burning sensation 2. Symptoms of severe gastro-enteritis	1. Lavage with sodium chloride solution 2. Give demulcents	As for other metallic poisons
Strychnine	1. Stiffness of muscles of face, neck, jaw. Twitching 2. Convulsions 3. Asphyxia 4. Trismus 5. Risus sardonicus	1. Tannic acid 2. Potassium permanganate solution, charcoal 3. Rapid acting barbiturate drugs for control of convulsions 4. Lavage before convulsions occur, or after control by sedation	1. Rest and quiet 2. Dark room 3. Protect from sensory stimuli 4. Support respiration as necessary 5. Observe for urinary retention. Catheterize if necessary

DIAGRAMS OF PRESSURE POINTS SHOWING RELATION TO ARTERIES AND BONES

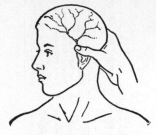

Pressure for scalp bleeding.

Pressure for face bleeding.

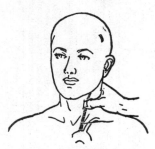

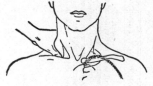

Pressure on subclavian artery for shoulder and high arm wounds.

Pressure for neck wounds.

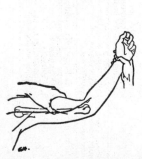

Pressure to stop bleeding in arm.

Pressure point for femoral artery.

Index

INDEX

INDEX

INDEX

Common Abbreviations Used in This Edition

(In the text, a descriptive phrase precedes any abbreviation. After the first use, the abbreviation is used alone.)

a = before
$\overline{aa}$ = of each
a.c. = before meals
ad = to; up to
ad lib. = freely
b.i.d. = twice a day
b.i.w. = twice a week
B.M.R. = basal metabolic rate
BSP = bromsulphalein
BUN = blood urea nitrogen
$\overline{c}$ = with
C. = centigrade
cc. = cubic centimeter
cm. = centimeter
C.N.S. = central nervous system
CO_2 = carbon dioxide
cu. mm. = cubic millimeter
EEG = electroencephalogram
EKG = electrocardiogram
ESR = erythrocyte sedimentation rate
F. = Fahrenheit
G.A.D. = glucose, acetone and diacetic acid urine test
G.I. = gastrointestinal
Gm. = gram
Gm./100 ml. = grams per 100 milliliters

gr. = grain
gtt. = drops
G.U. or g.u. = genitourinary
h.s. = at bedtime (hour of sleep)
I.M. = intramuscularly
I.Q. = intelligence quotient
I.V. = intravenously
Kg. = kilogram
L. = liter
lb. = pound
L./min. = liters per minute
m. = minim
mEq./L. = milliequivalents per liter
mg. = milligram
mg./L. = milligrams per liter
ml. = milliliter
N.F. = National Formulary
N.N.D. = New and Nonofficial Drugs
N.P.N. = nonprotein nitrogen
N.P.O. = nothing by mouth
O = a pint
o.d. = every day
o.m. = every morning
o.n. = every night